D0210004

Nursing Diagnoses in Psychiatric Nursing

CARE PLANS AND PSYCHOTROPIC MEDICATIONS

Sixth Edition

MARY C. TOWNSEND, RN, MN, CS

Clinical Nurse Specialist
Private Practice
Adult Psychiatric/Mental Health Nursing
McAlester, Oklahoma

Nurse Consultant
Counseling Center of S.E. Oklahoma
Antlers, Oklahoma

Former Assistant Professor and
Coordinator, Mental Health Nursing
Oklahoma City University
Oklahoma City, Oklahoma

F. A. Davis Company • Philadelphia

F. A. Davis Company
1915 Arch Street
Philadelphia, PA 19103
www.fadavis.com

Printed in United States of America

Last digit indicates print number: 10 9 8 7 6 5 4

Acquisitions Editor: Robert G. Martone
Production Manager: Robert C. Butler
Art & Design Manager: Louis J. Forgione

As new scientific information becomes available through basic and clinical research, recommended treatments and drug therapies undergo changes. The author(s) and publisher have done everything possible to make this book accurate, up to date, and in accord with accepted standards at the time of publication. The author(s), editors, and publisher are not responsible for errors or omissions or for consequences from application of the book, and make no warranty, expressed or implied, in regard to the contents of the book. Any practice described in this book should be applied by the reader in accordance with professional standards of care used in regard to the unique circumstances that may apply in each situation. The reader is advised always to check product information (package inserts) for changes and new information regarding dose and contraindications before administering any drug. Caution is especially urged when using new or infrequently ordered drugs.

Library of Congress Cataloging-in-Publication Data

Townsend, Mary C., 1941 -
Nursing diagnoses in psychiatric nursing : care plans and psychotropic medications /
Mary C. Townsend.— 6th ed.
p. cm.
Includes bibliographical references and index.
ISBN 10: 0-8036-1166-8 (hbk.) ISBN 13: 978-8036-1166-5
1. Psychiatric nursing—Diagnosis—Handbooks, manuals, etc. 2. Mental illness—Handbooks, manuals, etc. 3. Nursing diagnosis—Handbooks, manuals, etc. I.
Title.
RC440.T69 2004
616.89′0231—dc22

2003055455

This Book is Dedicated:

To my husband, Jim, who has encouraged and supported me throughout this project and whose love continues to nurture and sustain me, even after 42 years.

To my daughters, Kerry and Tina, who have brought joy that only a parent could understand, frustrations that only a parent could tolerate, happiness that only a parent could appreciate, and tears that only a parent could endure. You are truly loved.

To my faithful and beloved companions, Bucky, Chiro, and Angel, who make me laugh and bring pure pleasure into my life each and every day.

And finally, to my father and mother, Francis and Camalla Welsh, who reared my sister Francie and me without knowledge of psychology or developmental theories, but with the kind of unconditional love I have come to believe is so vital to the achievement and maintenance of emotional wellness.

MCT

Acknowledgments

My special thanks and appreciation:

To Bob Martone, who patiently provided assistance and guidance throughout the project.

To the editorial and production staffs of F.A. Davis, who are always willing to provide assistance when requested and whose consistent excellence in publishing makes me proud to be associated with them.

To the gracious individuals who read and critiqued the original manuscript, providing valuable input into the final product.

And finally, a special acknowledgment to the nurses who staff the psychiatric units of the clinical agencies where nursing students go to learn about psychiatric nursing; to those of you who willingly share your knowledge and expertise with, and act as role models for, these nursing students. If this book provides you with even a small amount of nursing assistance, please acknowledge it as my way of saying "thanks."

MCT

Consultants

Maude H. Alston, RN, PhD
Assistant Professor of Nursing
University of North Carolina at Greensboro
Greensboro, North Carolina

Betty J. Carmack, RN, EdD
Assistant Professor
University of San Francisco
School of Nursing
San Francisco, California

Doris K. DeVincenzo, PhD
Professor
Lienhard School of Nursing
Pace University
Pleasantville, New York

Mary Jo Gorney-Fadiman, RN, PhD
Assistant Professor
San Jose State University
School of Nursing
San Jose, California

Mary E. Martucci, RN, PhD
Associate Professor and Chairman
Saint Mary's College
Notre Dame, Indiana

Sheridan V. McCabe, BA, BSN, MSN, PhD
Assistant Professor of Nursing
University of Virginia
School of Nursing
Charlottesville, Virgina

Elizabeth Anne Rankin, PhD
Psychotherapist and Consultant
University of Maryland
School of Nursing
Baltimore, Maryland

Judith M. Saunders, DNS, FAAN
Postdoctoral Research Fellow
University of Washington
School of Nursing
Seattle, Washington

Gail Stuart, RN, CS, PhD
Associate Professor
Medical University of South Carolina
College of Nursing
Charleston, South Carolina

Contents

Index of DSM-IV-TR Psychiatric Diagnoses

Classification: Axes I and II Categories and Codes

How to Use This Book

In an attempt to standardize clinical nursing practice, the North American Nursing Diagnosis Association (NANDA) has published a list of nursing diagnoses that have been approved through the 2002 NANDA/NIC/NOC International Conference. Standardization of nursing actions and common terminology is important in the provision of consistent care over time, among nurses, across shifts, and even between different health-care agencies. This text incorporates the nomenclature of Taxonomy II that has been adopted by NANDA.

There are those individuals who believe that NANDA's list is incomplete. My intent is not to judge the completeness of this list but to suggest the need for clinical testing of what is available. NANDA encourages nurses to submit new diagnoses for consideration, after the nurses have conducted testing and research of the diagnoses in the clinical setting.

There are three essential components in a nursing diagnosis, which comprise the *PES format* (Gordon, 1987). The "P" identifies the health problem; the "E" represents the etiology (or cause) of the problem; and the "S" describes a cluster of signs and symptoms, or what has come to be known as "defining characteristics." These three parts are combined into one statement by the use of "connecting words." The diagnosis is then written as: Problem "related to" etiology "evidenced by" signs and symptoms (defining characteristics).

The problem can be identified as the human response to actual or potential health problems as assessed by the nurse. The etiology may be represented by past experiences of the individual, genetic influences, current environmental factors, or pathophysiological changes. The defining characteristics describe what the client says and what the nurse observes that indicate the existence of a particular problem.

Nursing diagnoses, then, become the basis for the care plan. This book may be used as a guide in the construction of care plans for various psychiatric clients. The concepts are presented in such a manner that they may be applied to various types of health-care settings: inpatient hospitalization, outpatient clinic, home health, partial hospitalization, and private practice, to name a few. Major divisions in the book are identified by psychiatric diagnostic categories, according to the order in which they appear in the *Diagnostic and Statistical Manual of Mental Disorders, 4th Edition, Text Revision (DSM-IV-TR,*

2000). The use of this format is not to imply that nursing diagnoses are based on, or flow from, medical diagnoses; it is meant only to enhance the usability of the book. In addition, I am not suggesting that the nursing diagnoses presented with each psychiatric category are all-inclusive.

It is valid, however, to state that certain nursing diagnoses are common to individuals with specific psychiatric disorders. The diagnoses presented in this book are meant to be used as guidelines for construction of care plans that must be individualized for each client, based on the nursing assessment. The interventions can also be used in areas in which interdisciplinary treatment plans take the place of a nursing care plan.

Each chapter in Unit II begins with an overview of information related to the medical diagnostic category, which may be useful to the nurse as background assessment data. Each chapter includes:

1. **The Disorder:** A definition and common types or categories that have been identified.
2. **Predisposing Factors:** Information regarding theories of etiology, which the nurse may use in formulating the "related to" portion of the nursing diagnosis as it applies to the client.
3. **Symptomatology:** Subjective and objective data identifying behaviors common to the disorder. These behaviors, as they apply to the individual client, may be pertinent to the "evidenced by" portion of the nursing diagnosis.

Information presented with each nursing diagnosis includes the following:

1. **Definition:** The approved NANDA definition is used for those nursing diagnoses for which a NANDA definition exists. I have suggested definitions for clarification of the other nursing diagnoses; these are identified by brackets [ ].
2. **Possible Etiologies ("related to"):** This section suggests possible causes for the problem identified. Those not approved by NANDA are identified by brackets [ ]. **Related/Risk Factors** are given for diagnoses for which the client is at risk. ***Note*: Defining characteristics do not exist in "Risk for" diagnoses.**
3. **Defining Characteristics ("evidenced by"):** This section includes signs and symptoms that may be evident to indicate that the problem exists. Again, as with definitions and etiologies, those not approved by NANDA are identified by brackets [ ].
4. **Goals:** These statements are made with client behavioral objective terminology. They are measurable short- and long-term goals to be used in evaluating the effectiveness of the nursing interventions in alleviating the identified problem. There may be more than one short-term goal, and each may be considered a "stepping stone" to fulfillment of the long-term goal. For the purposes of this book,

"long-term," in most instances, is designated as "by time of discharge," whether the client is in an inpatient or outpatient setting.

5. **Interventions with *Selected Rationales:*** Only those interventions that are appropriate to a particular nursing diagnosis within the context of the psychiatric setting are presented. Rationales for selected interventions are included to provide clarification beyond fundamental nursing knowledge and to assist in the selection of appropriate interventions for individual clients.
6. **Outcome Criteria:** These are behavioral changes that can be used as criteria to determine the extent to which the nursing diagnosis has been resolved.

To use this book in the preparation of psychiatric nursing care plans, find the section in the text applicable to the client's psychiatric diagnosis. Review background data pertinent to the diagnosis, if needed. Complete a biopsychosocial history and assessment of the client. Select and prioritize nursing diagnoses appropriate to the client. Using the list of NANDA-approved nursing diagnoses, be sure to include those that are client-specific and not just those that have been identified as "common" to a particular medical diagnosis. Select nursing interventions and outcome criteria appropriate to the client for each nursing diagnosis identified. Write all this information in the care plan, along with a date for evaluating the status of each problem. On the evaluation date, document success of the nursing interventions in achieving the goals of care, using the desired client outcomes as criteria. Modify the plan as required.

A new chapter on Loss and Bereavement has been added to Unit III. Unit IV, Psychotropic Medications, has been updated to include new medications that have been approved by the FDA since the last edition; for example, the antidepressant, escitalopram (Lexapro); the antipsychotic, aripiprazole (Abilify); and the agent for ADHD, atomoxetine (Strattera). Sections on drug interactions and route and dosage have been added. This new information should facilitate use of the book for nurses administering psychotropic medications and for nurse practitioners with prescriptive authority. The major categories of psychotropic medications are identified by chemical class. Information is presented related to indications, actions, contraindications and precautions, interactions, route and dosage, and adverse reactions and side effects. Examples of medications in each chemical class are presented by generic and trade name, along with information about half-life, controlled and pregnancy categories, and available forms of the medication. Therapeutic plasma level ranges are provided, where appropriate. Nursing diagnoses related to each category, along with nursing interventions, and client and family education guidelines are included in each chapter.

Another helpful feature is the table in Appendix I, which lists some client behaviors commonly observed in the psychiatric setting and the most appropriate nursing diagnosis for each. It is hoped that this information will broaden understanding of the need to use a variety of nursing diagnoses in preparing the client treatment plan.

This book helps to familiarize the nurse with the current NANDA-approved nursing diagnoses and provides suggestions for their use within the psychiatric setting. The book is designed to be used as a quick reference in the preparation of care plans, with the expectation that additional information will be required for each nursing diagnosis as the nurse individualizes care for psychiatric clients.

NANDA NURSING DIAGNOSES: Taxonomy II

Exchanging

- Imbalanced nutrition: More than body requirements
- Imbalanced nutrition: Less than body requirements
- Risk for imbalanced nutrition: More than body requirements
- Readiness for enhanced nutrition
- Risk for infection
- Risk for imbalanced body temperature
- Hypothermia
- Hyperthermia
- Ineffective thermoregulation
- Autonomic dysreflexia
- Risk for autonomic dysreflexia
- Constipation
- Perceived constipation
- Diarrhea
- Bowel incontinence
- Risk for constipation
- Impaired urinary elimination
- Readiness for enhanced urinary elimination
- Stress urinary incontinence
- Reflex urinary incontinence
- Urge urinary incontinence
- Functional urinary incontinence
- Total urinary incontinence
- Risk for urge urinary incontinence
- Urinary retention
- Ineffective tissue perfusion (specify type: renal, cerebral, cardiopulmonary, gastrointestinal, peripheral)
- Risk for imbalanced fluid volume
- Excess fluid volume
- Deficient fluid volume
- Risk for deficient fluid volume
- Readiness for enhanced fluid balance
- Decreased cardiac output

- Impaired gas exchange
- Ineffective airway clearance
- Ineffective breathing pattern
- Impaired spontaneous ventilation
- Dysfunctional ventilatory weaning response
- Risk for injury
- Risk for suffocation
- Risk for sudden infant death syndrome (SIDS)
- Risk for poisoning
- Risk for trauma
- Risk for aspiration
- Risk for disuse syndrome
- Latex allergy response
- Risk for latex allergy response
- Ineffective protection
- Impaired tissue integrity
- Impaired oral mucous membrane
- Impaired skin integrity
- Risk for impaired skin integrity
- Impaired dentition
- Decreased intracranial adaptive capacity
- Disturbed energy field

Communicating

- Impaired verbal communication
- Readiness for enhanced communication

Relating

- Impaired social interaction
- Social isolation
- Risk for loneliness
- Ineffective role performance
- Impaired parenting
- Risk for impaired parenting
- Readiness for enhanced parenting
- Risk for impaired parent/infant/child attachment
- Sexual dysfunction
- Interrupted family processes
- Readiness for enhanced family processes
- Caregiver role strain
- Risk for caregiver role strain
- Dysfunctional family processes: Alcoholism
- Parental role conflict
- Ineffective sexuality patterns

Valuing

- Spiritual distress
- Risk for spiritual distress
- Readiness for enhanced spiritual well-being
- Ineffective coping
- Readiness for enhanced coping
- Impaired adjustment
- Defensive coping
- Ineffective denial
- Disabled family coping
- Compromised family coping
- Readiness for enhanced family coping
- Readiness for enhanced community coping
- Ineffective community coping
- Ineffective therapeutic regimen management
- Readiness for enhanced therapeutic regimen management
- Noncompliance (specify)
- Ineffective family therapeutic regimen management
- Ineffective community therapeutic regimen management
- Effective therapeutic regimen management
- Decisional conflict (specify)
- Health-seeking behaviors (specify)

Moving

- Impaired physical mobility
- Risk for peripheral neurovascular dysfunction
- Risk for perioperative-positioning injury
- Impaired walking
- Risk for falls
- Wandering
- Impaired wheelchair mobility
- Impaired transfer ability
- Impaired bed mobility
- Activity intolerance
- Fatigue
- Risk for activity intolerance
- Disturbed sleep pattern
- Sleep deprivation
- Readiness for enhanced sleep
- Deficient diversional activity
- Impaired home maintenance
- Ineffective health maintenance
- Delayed surgical recovery
- Adult failure to thrive

- Feeding self-care deficit
- Impaired swallowing
- Ineffective breastfeeding
- Interrupted breastfeeding
- Effective breastfeeding
- Ineffective infant feeding pattern
- Bathing/hygiene self-care deficit
- Dressing/grooming self-care deficit
- Toileting self-care deficit
- Delayed growth and development
- Risk for delayed development
- Risk for disproportionate growth
- Relocation stress syndrome
- Risk for relocation stress syndrome
- Risk for disorganized infant behavior
- Disorganized infant behavior
- Readiness for enhanced organized infant behavior

Perceiving

- Disturbed body image
- Chronic low self-esteem
- Situational low self-esteem
- Risk for situational low self-esteem
- Readiness for enhanced self-concept
- Disturbed personal identity
- Disturbed sensory perception (specify: visual, auditory, kinesthetic, gustatory, tactile, olfactory)
- Unilateral neglect
- Hopelessness
- Powerlessness
- Risk for powerlessness

Knowing

- Deficient knowledge (specify)
- Readiness for enhanced knowledge of (specify)
- Impaired environmental interpretation syndrome
- Acute confusion
- Chronic confusion
- Disturbed thought processes
- Impaired memory

Feeling

- Acute pain
- Chronic pain
- Nausea
- Dysfunctional grieving

- Anticipatory grieving
- Chronic sorrow
- Risk for other-directed violence
- Self-mutilation
- Risk for self-mutilation
- Risk for self-directed violence
- Risk for suicide
- Post-trauma syndrome
- Rape-trauma syndrome
- Rape-trauma syndrome: Compound reaction
- Rape-trauma syndrome: Silent reaction
- Risk for post-trauma syndrome
- Anxiety
- Death anxiety
- Fear

SOURCE: *NANDA Nursing Diagnoses: Definitions & Classification 2003-2004.* Philadelphia: North American Nursing Diagnosis Association, 2003.

Internet References

- http://www.apna.org
- http://www.nanda.org
- http://www.nursecominc.com

UNIT ONE

THE FOUNDATION FOR PLANNING PSYCHIATRIC NURSING CARE

CHAPTER 1

Nursing Process: One Step to Professionalism

Nursing has struggled for many years to achieve recognition as a profession. Out of this struggle has emerged an awareness of the need to do the following:

1. Define the boundaries of nursing: what is nursing?
2. Identify a scientific method for delivering nursing care.

In its statement on social policy, the American Nurses Association (ANA) presented the following definition: "Nursing is the diagnosis and treatment of human responses to actual or potential health problems" (ANA, 1998). The nursing process has been identified as nursing's scientific method for delivering nursing care.

The curricula of most nursing schools include the nursing process as a component of their conceptual framework. The National Council of State Boards of Nursing (NCSBN) uses the nursing process as the basis for the Registered Nurse State Board Test Pool Examination (Schmitt, 1996). Questions about nursing behaviors in different client situations are presented according to the stages of the nursing process:

1. **Assessment:** Establishing a database about a client.
2. **Diagnosis:** Identifying the client's health-care needs and selecting care goals.
3. **Outcome Identification:** Establishing criteria for measuring achievement of desired outcomes.
4. **Planning:** Designing a strategy to achieve the care goals.
5. **Implementation:** Initiating and completing actions necessary to accomplish the goals.
6. **Evaluation:** Determining the extent to which care goals have been achieved.

By following these six steps, the nurse has a systematic framework for decision making and problem solving in the delivery of nursing care. The nursing process is dynamic, not static. It is an ongoing process that continues for as long as the nurse and client have interactions directed toward change in the client's physical or behavioral responses. Figure 1–1 is a schematic of the ongoing nursing process.

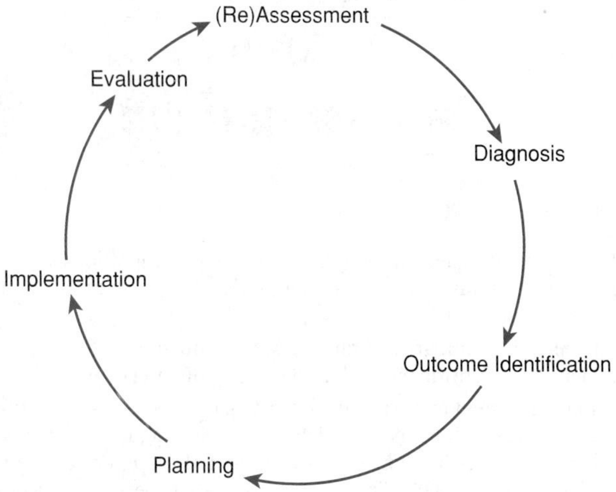

Figure 1–1 The ongoing nursing process.

Diagnosis is an integral part of the nursing process. In this step, the nurse identifies the "human responses to actual or potential health problems." In some states, diagnosing is identified within the Nurse Practice Acts as a legal responsibility of the professional nurse. Nursing diagnosis provides the basis for prescribing the specific interventions for which the nurse is accountable.

As an inherent part of the nursing process, nursing diagnosis is included in the ANA Standards of Practice. These standards provide one broad basis for evaluating practice and reflect a recognition of the rights of the person receiving nursing care (ANA, 1998).

The purpose of this book is to assist students and staff nurses as they endeavor to provide high-quality nursing care to their psychiatric clients. Following is an example of a nursing history and assessment tool that may be used to gather information about the client during the assessment phase.

INTERNET REFERENCES

- http://www.nursingworld.org
- http://www.sciencekomm.at/journals/medicine/nurse.html

I. NURSING HISTORY AND ASSESSMENT TOOL

General Information

Client name: ________________ Allergies: ________________
Room number: ________________ Diet: ________________
Doctor: ________________ Height/weight: ________________
Age: ________________ Vital signs: TPR/BP ________________
Sex: ________________ Name/number of significant other: ________________
Race: ________________
Dominant language: ________________ City of residence: ________________
Marital status: ________________ Diagnosis (admitting and current): ________________
Chief complaint: ________________

Conditions of admission:

Date: ________________ Time: ________________
Accompanied by: ________________
Route of admission (wheelchair; ambulatory; cart): ________________
Admitted from: ________________

II. Predisposing Factors

A. Genetic Influences

1. Family configuration (use genograms):
   Family of origin: Present family:

   Family dynamics (describe significant relationships between family members): ________________

2. Medical/Psychiatric History:
   a. Client: ________________
   b. Family members: ________________

3. Other genetic influences affecting present adaptation. This might include effects specific to gender, race, appearance [such as genetic physical defects], or any other factor related to genetics that is affecting the client's adaptation that has not been mentioned elsewhere in this assessment.
   ____

B. *Past Experiences*

1. CULTURAL AND SOCIAL HISTORY:
   a. Environmental factors (family living arrangements, type of neighborhood, special working conditions): ______
   ______
   ______
   b. Health beliefs and practices (personal responsibility for health; special self-care practices): ______
   ______
   ______
   c. Religious beliefs and practices: ______
   ______
   ______
   d. Educational background: ______
   ______
   ______
   e. Significant losses/changes (include dates): ______
   ______
   ______
   f. Peer/friendship relationships: ______
   ______
   ______
   g. Occupational history: ______
   ______
   ______
   h. Previous pattern of coping with stress: ______
   ______
   ______
   i. Other lifestyle factors contributing to present adaptation:
   ______
   ______

C. *Existing Conditions*

1. STAGE OF DEVELOPMENT (Erikson):
   a. Theoretically: ______
   b. Behaviorally: ______
   c. Rationale: ______
   ______
   ______
2. Support systems: ______
   ______
3. Economic security: ______
   ______
4. Avenues of productivity/contribution:
   a. Current job status: ______
   ______

b. Role contributions and responsibility for others: ________

____

III. Precipitating Event

Describe the situation or events that precipitated this illness/hospitalization: ________

____

____

IV. Client's Perception of the Stressor

Client's or family member's understanding or description of stressor/illness and expectations of hospitalization: ________

____

____

____

V. Adaptation Responses

A. Psychosocial

1. ANXIETY LEVEL (circle level, and check the behaviors that apply):

Mild Moderate Severe Panic

Calm ________ Friendly ________ Passive ________
Alert ________ Perceives environment correctly ________
Cooperative ________ Impaired attention ________
"Jittery" ________ Unable to concentrate ________
Hypervigilant ________ Tremors ________ Rapid speech ________
Withdrawn ________ Confused ________
Disoriented ________ Fearful ________ Hyperventilating ________
Misinterpreting the environment
(Hallucinations or delusions) ________
Depersonalization ________ Obsessions ________
Compulsions ________ Somatic complaints ________
Excessive hyperactivity ________ Other ________

2. MOOD/AFFECT (circle as many as apply):

Happiness Sadness Dejection Despair
Elation Euphoria Suspiciousness
Apathy (little emotional tone) Anger/Hostility

3. EGO DEFENSE MECHANISMS (describe how used by client):

Projection ________
Suppression ________
Undoing ________
Displacement ________
Intellectualization ________
Rationalization ________

Denial ______________________________
Repression ______________________________
Isolation ______________________________
Regression ______________________________
Reaction formation ______________________________
Splitting ______________________________
Religiosity ______________________________
Sublimation ______________________________
Compensation ______________________________

4. LEVEL OF SELF-ESTEEM (circle one):

Low Moderate High

Things client likes about self ______________________________

Things client would like to change about self ______________________________

Objective assessment of self-esteem:

Eye contact ______________________________

General appearance ______________________________

____

Personal hygiene ______________________________

Participation in group activities and interactions with others

____

5. STAGE AND MANIFESTATIONS OF GRIEF (circle one):

Denial Anger Bargaining Depression Acceptance

Describe client's behaviors that are associated with this stage of grieving in response to loss or change. ______________________________

____

____

6. THOUGHT PROCESSES (circle as many as apply):

Clear Logical Easy to follow Relevant Confused

Blocking Delusional Rapid flow of thoughts

Slowness In thought association

Suspicious

Recent Memory: Loss Intact

Remote Memory: Loss Intact

Other: ______________________________

____

7. COMMUNICATION PATTERNS (circle as many as apply):

Clear Coherent Slurred speech Incoherent

Neologisms Loose associations Flight of ideas

Aphasic Perseveration Rumination

Tangential speech Loquaciousness

Slow, impoverished speech

Speech impediment (describe) ______________________________

Other ______________________________

8. INTERACTION PATTERNS (describe client's pattern of interpersonal interactions with staff and peers in the unit, e.g., manipulative, withdrawn, isolated, verbally or physically hostile, argumentative, passive, assertive, aggressive, passive-aggressive, other): ____
____
____
____

9. REALITY ORIENTATION (check those that apply):
Oriented to: Time ______________ Person ______________
Place ______________ Situation ______________

10. IDEAS OF DESTRUCTION TO SELF/OTHERS? Yes No
If yes, consider plan; available means ______________________
____
____
____

B. *Physiological*

1. PSYCHOSOMATIC MANIFESTATIONS (describe any somatic complaints that may be stress-related): ______________________
____
____
____

2. DRUG HISTORY AND ASSESSMENT:
Use of prescribed drugs:

Name	*Dosage*	*Prescribed for*	*Results*
________	________	________	________
________	________	________	________
________	________	________	________
________	________	________	________

Use of over-the-counter drugs:

Name	*Dosage*	*Used for*	*Results*
________	________	________	________
________	________	________	________
________	________	________	________
________	________	________	________

Use of street drugs and/or alcohol:

Name	*Amount used*	*How often used*	*When last used*	*Effects produced*
________	________	________	________	________
________	________	________	________	________
________	________	________	________	________
________	________	________	________	________

3. PERTINENT PHYSICAL ASSESSMENTS:
   a. *Respirations*: Normal __________ Labored __________
   Rate ______________ Rhythm ______________

b. *Skin*: Warm ______ Dry ______ Moist ______
Cool ______ Clammy ______ Pink ______
Cyanotic ______ Poor turgor ______ Edematous ______
Evidence of: Rash ______ Bruising ______
Needle tracks ______ Hirsutism ______ Loss of hair ______
Other ______

c. *Musculoskeletal status*: Weakness Tremors
Degree of range of motion (describe limitations) ______
Pain (describe) ______
Skeletal deformities (describe) ______
Coordination (describe limitations) ______

d. *Neurological status*
History of (check all that apply): Seizures (describe method of control) ______
______
Headaches (describe location and frequency) ______
Fainting spells ______ Dizziness ______
Tingling/numbness (describe location) ______

e. *Cardiovascular*: B/P ______ Pulse ______
History of (check all that apply):
Hypertension ______ Palpitations ______
Heart murmur ______ Chest pain ______
Shortness of breath ______ Pain in legs ______
Phlebitis ______ Ankle/leg edema ______
Numbness/tingling in extremities ______
Varicose veins ______

f. *Gastrointestinal*
Usual diet pattern ______
Food allergies ______
Dentures? Upper ______ Lower ______
Any problems with chewing or swallowing? ______
Any recent change in weight? ______
Any problems with:
  Indigestion/heartburn? ______
    Relieved by ______
  Nausea/vomiting? ______
    Relieved by ______
  History of ulcers? ______
  Usual bowel pattern ______
    Constipation? ______ Diarrhea? ______
    Type of self-care assistance provided for either of the above problems ______

g. *Genitourinary/Reproductive*
Usual voiding pattern ______
Urinary hesitancy? ______ Frequency? ______
Nocturia? ______ Pain/burning? ______
Incontinence? ______
Any genital lesions? ______

Discharge? ______________ Odor? ____________
History of sexually transmitted disease? ____________________
If yes, please explain: ________________________________
____
Any concerns about sexuality/sexual activity? ______________
____
Method of birth control used ___________________________
Females:
Date of last menstrual cycle ___________________________
Length of cycle _______________________________________
Problems associated with menstruation? ___________________
____
Breasts: Pain/tenderness? ______________________________
Swelling? ________________ Discharge? ______________
Lumps? __________________ Dimpling? ______________
Practice breast self-examination? _________________________
Frequency? ____
Males:
Penile discharge? _____________________________________
Prostate problems? ____________________________________

h. *Eyes*

	YES	NO	EXPLAIN
Glasses?	____	____	____________
Contacts?	____	____	____________
Swelling?	____	____	____________
Discharge?	____	____	____________
Itching?	____	____	____________
Blurring?	____	____	____________
Double vision?	____	____	____________

i. *Ears*

	YES	NO	EXPLAIN
Pain?	____	____	____________
Drainage?	____	____	____________
Difficulty hearing?	____	____	____________
Hearing aid?	____	____	____________
Tinnitus?	____	____	____________

j. *Medication side effects*
What symptoms is the client experiencing that may be attributed to current medication usage? ____________________
____

k. *Altered laboratory values and possible significance* ____________
____
____

l. *Activity/rest patterns*
Exercise (amount, type, frequency) ______________________
____
Leisure time activities __________________________________
____

Patterns of sleep: Number of hours per night ______
Use of sleep aids? ______
Pattern of awakening during the night? ______
Feel rested upon awakening? ______

m. *Personal hygiene/activities of daily living*
Patterns of self-care: Independent ______
Requires assistance with: Mobility ______
Hygiene ______
Toileting ______
Feeding ______
Dressing ______
Other ______
Statement describing personal hygiene and general appearance
______
______

n. *Other pertinent physical assessments*
______
______

VI. SUMMARY OF INITIAL PSYCHOSOCIAL/ PHYSICAL ASSESSMENT

Knowledge Deficits Identified

Nursing Diagnoses Indicated

UNIT TWO

ALTERATIONS IN PSYCHOSOCIAL ADAPTATION

CHAPTER 2

Disorders Usually First Diagnosed In Infancy, Childhood, or Adolescence

BACKGROUND ASSESSMENT DATA

Several common psychiatric disorders may arise or become evident during infancy, childhood, or adolescence. Essential features of many disorders are identical, regardless of the age of the individual. Examples include the following:

Cognitive disorders	Personality disorders
Schizophrenia	Substance-related disorders
Schizophreniform disorder	Mood disorders
	Somatoform disorders
Adjustment disorder	Psychological factors affecting medical conditions
Sexual disorders	

There are, however, several disorders that appear during the early developmental years and are identified according to the child's ability or inability to perform age-appropriate tasks or intellectual functions. Selected disorders are presented here. It is essential that the nurse working with these clients understand normal behavior patterns characteristic of the infant, childhood, and adolescent years.

■ MENTAL RETARDATION

Defined

Mental retardation is defined by deficits in general intellectual functioning and adaptive functioning and is measured by an individual's performance on intelligence quotient (IQ) tests (APA, 2000). Mental retardation is coded on Axis II in the American Psychiatric Association (2000) *Diagnostic and Statistical Manual of Mental Disorders, Fourth Edition, Text Revision (DSM-IV-TR)* Classification. Codes include:

317: Mild Mental Retardation (IQ of 50 to 70)
318.0: Moderate Mental Retardation (IQ of 35 to 49)
318.1: Severe Mental Retardation (IQ of 20 to 34)
318.2: Profound Mental Retardation (IQ below 20)
319: Mental Retardation, Severity Unspecified

Predisposing Factors

1. **Physiological**
   a. About 5 percent of cases of mental retardation are caused by hereditary factors, such as Tay-Sachs disease, phenylketonuria, and hyperglycemia. Chromosomal disorders, such as Down's syndrome and Klinefelter's syndrome, have also been implicated.
   b. Events that occur during the prenatal period, such as maternal ingestion of alcohol or other drugs, maternal infections, toxemia, and uncontrolled diabetes, or during the perinatal period, such as birth trauma or premature separation of the placenta, can result in mental retardation.
   c. Mental retardation can occur as an outcome of childhood illnesses, such as encephalitis or meningitis, or be the result of poisoning or physical trauma in childhood.
2. **Psychosocial**
   a. Fifteen to 20 percent of cases of mental retardation are attributed to deprivation of nurturance and of social, linguistic, and other stimulation and to severe mental disorders, such as autistic disorder (APA, 2000).

Symptomatology (Subjective and Objective Data)

1. At the mild level (IQ of 50 to 70), the individual can live independently but requires some assistance. He or she is capable of sixth-grade-level work and can learn a vocational skill. Social skills are possible, but the individual functions best in a structured, sheltered setting. Coordination may be slightly affected.

2. At the moderate level (IQ of 35 to 49), the individual can perform some activities independently but requires supervision. Academic skill can be achieved to about the second-grade level. The individual may experience some limitation in speech communication and in interactions with others. Motor development may be limited to gross motor ability.
3. The severe level of mental retardation (IQ of 20 to 34) is characterized by the need for complete supervision. Systematic habit-training may be accomplished, but the individual does not have the ability for academic or vocational training. Verbal skills are minimal and psychomotor development is poor.
4. The profoundly mentally retarded individual (IQ of less than 20) has no capacity for independent living. Constant aid and supervision are required. No ability exists for academic or vocational training. There is a lack of ability for speech development, socialization skills, or fine or gross motor movements. The individual requires constant supervision and care.

Common Nursing Diagnoses and Interventions

(Interventions are applicable to various health-care settings, such as inpatient and partial hospitalization, community outpatient clinic, home health, and private practice.)

RISK FOR INJURY

Definition: ***At risk of injury as a result of environmental conditions interacting with the individual's adaptive and defensive resources.***

Related/Risk Factors ("related to")

Altered physical mobility
Aggressive behavior

Goals/Objectives

Short- /Long-Term Goal

Client will not experience injury.

Interventions with *Selected Rationales*

1. *To ensure client safety:*
   a. Create a safe environment for the client. Remove small items from the area where the client will be ambulating and move sharp items out of his or her reach.
   b. Store items that client uses frequently within easy reach.
   c. Pad side rails and headboard of client who has history of seizures.

d. Prevent physical aggression and acting-out behaviors by learning to recognize signs that client is becoming agitated.

Outcome Criteria

1. Client has experienced no physical harm.
2. Client responds to attempts to inhibit agitated behavior.

SELF-CARE DEFICIT

Definition: *Impaired ability to perform or complete [activities of daily living] independently.*

Possible Etiologies ("related to")

Altered physical mobility
Lack of maturity

Defining Characteristics ("evidenced by")

[Unwillingness or inability to keep self clean]
[Uncombed hair; offensive body and breath odor]
[Inability to obtain adequate nutrition without assistance]
[Inability to dress or groom self without assistance]
[Inability to toilet self without assistance]
[Incontinence]

Goals/Objectives

Short-Term Goal

Client will be able to participate in aspects of self-care.

Long-Term Goal

Client will have all self-care needs met.

Interventions with *Selected Rationales*

1. Identify aspects of self-care that may be within the client's capabilities. Work on one aspect of self-care at a time. Provide simple, concrete explanations. ***Because clients' capabilities vary so widely, it is important to know each client individually and to ensure that no client is set up to fail.***
2. Offer positive feedback for efforts at assisting with own self-care. ***Positive reinforcement enhances self-esteem and encourages repetition of desirable behaviors.***
3. When one aspect of self-care has been mastered to the best of the client's ability, move on to another. Encourage independence, but intervene when client is unable to perform. ***Client comfort and safety are nursing priorities.***

Outcome Criteria

1. Client assists with self-care activities to the best of his or her ability.
2. Client's self-care needs are being met.

IMPAIRED VERBAL COMMUNICATION

Definition: ***Decreased, delayed, or absent ability to receive, process, transmit, and use a system of symbols [to communicate].***

Possible Etiologies ("related to")

[Developmental alteration]

Defining Characteristics ("evidenced by")

Speaks or verbalizes with difficulty
Difficulty forming words or sentences
Difficulty expressing thought verbally
Inappropriate verbalizations
Does not or cannot speak

Goals/Objectives

Short-Term Goal

Client will establish trust with caregiver and a means of communication of needs.

Long-Term Goals

1. Client's needs are met through established means of communication.
2. If client cannot speak or communicate by other means, needs are met by caregiver's anticipation of client's needs.

Interventions with *Selected Rationales*

1. Maintain consistency of staff assignment over time. ***This facilitates trust and the ability to understand client's actions and communication.***
2. Anticipate and fulfill client's needs until satisfactory communication patterns are established. Learn (from family, if possible) special words client uses that are different from those of the norm.
3. Identify nonverbal gestures or signals that client may use to convey needs if verbal communication is absent. Practice these communication skills over and over. ***Some children with mental retardation, particularly at the severe level, can learn only by systematic habit-training.***

Outcome Criteria

1. Client is able to communicate with consistent caregiver.
2. (For client who is unable to communicate): Client's needs, as anticipated by caregiver, are being met.

IMPAIRED SOCIAL INTERACTION

Definition: ***Insufficient or excessive quantity or ineffective quality of social exchange.***

Possible Etiologies ("related to")

[Speech deficiencies]
[Difficulty adhering to conventional social behavior (because of delayed maturational development)]

Defining Characteristics ("evidenced by")

Observed use of unsuccessful social interaction behaviors
Dysfunctional interaction with peers, family, and/or others
Observed discomfort in social situations

Goals/Objectives

Short-Term Goal

Client will attempt to interact with others in the presence of trusted caregiver.

Long-Term Goal

Client will be able to interact with others using behaviors that are socially acceptable and appropriate to developmental level.

Interventions with *Selected Rationales*

1. Remain with client during initial interactions with others in the unit. ***The presence of a trusted individual provides a feeling of security.***
2. Explain to other clients the meaning of some of the client's nonverbal gestures and signals. ***Others may be more accepting of the client's differentness if they have a better understanding of his or her behavior.***
3. Use simple language to explain to client which behaviors are acceptable and which are not. Establish a procedure for behavior modification that offers rewards for appropriate behaviors and renders an aversive reinforcement in response to the use of inappropriate behaviors. ***Positive, negative, and aversive reinforcements can contribute to desired changes in behavior. The privileges and penalties are individually determined as staff learns the likes and dislikes of the client.***

Outcome Criterion

1. Client interacts with others in a socially appropriate manner.

■ 299.00 AUTISTIC DISORDER*

Defined

Autistic disorder is characterized by a withdrawal of the child into the self and into a fantasy world of his or her own creation. Activities and interests are restricted and may be considered somewhat bizarre. The disorder is rare but occurs four to five times more often in males than in females. Onset of symptoms is before age 3 years. The course is chronic and often persists into adulthood.

Predisposing Factors

1. **Physiological**
   a. ***Genetics.*** An increased risk of autistic disorder exists among siblings of individuals with the disorder (APA, 2000). Studies with both monozygotic and dizygotic twins have also provided evidence of a genetic involvement.
   b. ***Neurological Factors.*** Abnormalities in brain structures or functions have been correlated with autistic disorder (National Institute of Mental Health [NIMH], 2002). Certain developmental problems, such as postnatal neurological infections, congenital rubella, phenylketonuria, and fragile X syndrome, also have been implicated.

Symptomatology (Subjective and Objective Data)

1. Failure to form interpersonal relationships, characterized by unresponsiveness to people; lack of eye contact and facial responsiveness; indifference or aversion to affection and physical contact. In early childhood, there is a failure to develop cooperative play and friendships.
2. Impairment in communication (verbal and nonverbal) characterized by absence of language or, if language is developed, often an immature grammatical structure, incorrect use of words, echolalia, or inability to use abstract terms. Accompanying nonverbal expressions may be inappropriate or absent.
3. Bizarre responses to the environment, characterized by resistance or extreme behavioral reactions to minor occurrences; abnormal, obsessive attachment to peculiar objects; ritualistic behaviors.
4. Extreme fascination for objects that move (e.g., fans, trains). Special interest in music; playing with water, buttons, or parts of the body.

---

* Classification and criteria for this and all subsequent diagnoses in this chapter marked with an asterisk are from the *Diagnostic and Statistical Manual of Mental Disorders, Fourth Edition, Text Revision, 2000.* Used with permission from the American Psychiatric Association.

5. Unreasonable insistence on following routines in precise detail (e.g., insisting that exactly the same route always be followed when shopping).
6. Marked distress over changes in trivial aspects of environment (e.g., when a vase is moved from its usual position).
7. Stereotyped body movements (e.g., hand flicking or twisting, spinning, head banging, complex whole-body movements).

Common Nursing Diagnoses and Interventions

(Interventions are applicable to various health-care settings, such as inpatient and partial hospitalization, community outpatient clinic, home health, and private practice.)

RISK FOR SELF-MUTILATION

Definition: ***At risk for deliberate self-injurious behavior causing tissue damage with the intent of causing nonfatal injury to attain relief of tension.***

Related/Risk Factors ("related to")

[Neurological alterations]
[History of self-mutilative behaviors in response to increasing anxiety]
[Obvious indifference to environment or hysterical reactions to changes in the environment]

Goals/Objectives

Short-Term Goal

Client will demonstrate alternative behavior (e.g., initiating interaction between self and nurse) in response to anxiety within specified time. (Length of time required for this objective will depend on severity and chronicity of disorder.)

Long-Term Goal

Client will not inflict harm on self.

Interventions with *Selected Rationales*

1. Intervene to protect child when self-mutilative behaviors, such as head banging or other hysterical behaviors, become evident. ***The nurse is responsible for ensuring client safety.***
2. A helmet may be used to protect against head banging, hand mitts may be used to prevent hair pulling, and appropriate padding may be used to protect extremities from injury during hysterical movements.
3. Try to determine if self-mutilative behaviors occur in response to

increasing anxiety, and if so, to what the anxiety may be attributed. ***Mutilative behaviors may be averted if the cause can be determined.***
4. Work on one-to-one basis with child ***to establish trust.***
5. Offer self to child during times of increasing anxiety ***in order to decrease need for self-mutilative behaviors and provide feelings of security.***

Outcome Criteria

1. Anxiety is maintained at a level at which client feels no need for self-mutilation.
2. When feeling anxious, client initiates interaction between self and nurse.

IMPAIRED SOCIAL INTERACTION

Definition: *Insufficient or excessive quantity or ineffective quality of social exchange.*

Possible Etiologies ("related to")

Self-concept disturbance
Absence of available significant others
[Unfulfilled tasks of trust vs. mistrust]
[Neurological alterations]

Defining Characteristics ("evidenced by")

[Lack of responsiveness to, or interest in, people]
[Failure to cuddle]
[Lack of eye contact and facial responsiveness]
[Indifference or aversion to affection and physical contact]
[Failure to develop cooperative play and peer friendships]

Goals/Objectives

Short-Term Goal

Client will demonstrate trust in one caregiver (as evidenced by facial responsiveness and eye contact) within specified time (depending on severity and chronicity of disorder).

Long-Term Goal

Client will initiate social interactions (physical, verbal, nonverbal) with caregiver by time of discharge from treatment.

Interventions with *Selected Rationales*

1. Function in a one-to-one relationship with the child. ***Consistency of staff-client interaction enhances the establishment of trust.***

2. Provide child with familiar objects (favorite toys, blanket). ***These items will offer security during times when the child feels distressed.***
3. Convey a manner of warmth, acceptance, and availability as client attempts to fulfill basic needs. ***These characteristics enhance establishment and maintenance of a trusting relationship.***
4. Go slowly. Do not force interactions. Begin with positive reinforcement for eye contact. Gradually introduce touch, smiling, hugging. ***The autistic client may feel threatened by an onslaught of stimuli to which he or she is unaccustomed.***
5. Support client with your presence as he or she endeavors to relate to others in the environment. ***The presence of an individual with whom a trusting relationship has been established provides a feeling of security.***

Outcome Criteria

1. Client initiates interactions between self and others.
2. Client uses eye contact, facial responsiveness, and other nonverbal behaviors in interactions with others.
3. Client does not withdraw from physical contact.

IMPAIRED VERBAL COMMUNICATION

Definition: *Decreased, delayed, or absent ability to receive, process, transmit, and use a system of symbols [to communicate].*

Possible Etiologies ("related to")

[Inability to trust]
[Withdrawal into self]
[Neurological alterations]

Defining Characteristics ("evidenced by")

Does not or cannot speak
[Immature grammatical structure]
[Echolalia]
[Pronoun reversal]
[Inability to name objects]
[Inability to use abstract terms]
[Absence of nonverbal expression (e.g., eye contact, facial responsiveness, gestures)]

Goals/Objectives

Short-Term Goal

Client will establish trust with one caregiver (as evidenced by facial responsiveness and eye contact) by specified time (depending on severity and chronicity of disorder).

Long-Term Goal

Client will establish a means for communicating (verbally or nonverbally) needs and desires to staff by time of discharge from treatment.

Interventions with *Selected Rationales*

1. Maintain consistency of staff assignment over time. ***This facilitates trust and the ability to understand client's actions and communication.***
2. Anticipate and fulfill client's needs until satisfactory communication patterns are established.
3. Use the techniques of *consensual validation* and *seeking clarification* to decode communication patterns. (Examples: "I think you must have meant ..." or "Did you mean to say that ...?"). ***These techniques work to verify the accuracy of the message received or to clarify any hidden meanings within the message. Take caution not to "put words into the client's mouth."***
4. Use "en face" approach (face to face, eye to eye) to convey correct nonverbal expressions by example. ***Eye contact expresses genuine interest in and respect for the individual.***

Outcome Criteria

1. Client is able to communicate in a manner that is understood by others.
2. Client's nonverbal messages are congruent with verbalizations.
3. Client initiates verbal and nonverbal interaction with others.

DISTURBED PERSONAL IDENTITY

Definition: *Inability to distinguish between self and non-self.*

Possible Etiologies ("related to")

[Unfulfilled tasks of trust vs. mistrust]
[Neurological alterations]
[Inadequate sensory stimulation]

Defining Characteristics ("evidenced by")

[Inability to separate own physiological and emotional needs from those of others]
[Increased levels of anxiety resulting from contact with others]
[Inability to differentiate own body boundaries from those of others]
[Repeating words he or she hears others say or mimicking movements of others]

Goals/Objectives

Short-Term Goal

Client will name own body parts and body parts of caregiver within specified time (depending on severity and chronicity of disorder).

Long-Term Goal

Client will develop ego identity (evidenced by ability to recognize physical and emotional self as separate from others) by time of discharge from treatment.

Interventions with *Selected Rationales*

1. Function in a one-to-one relationship with the child. ***Consistency of staff-client interaction enhances the establishment of trust.***
2. Assist child to recognize separateness during self-care activities, such as dressing and feeding. ***These activities increase child's awareness of self as separate from others.***
3. Point out, and assist child in naming, own body parts. ***This activity may increase the child's awareness of self as separate from others.***
4. Gradually increase amount of physical contact, using touch to point out differences between client and nurse. Be cautious with touch until trust is established, ***because this gesture may be interpreted by the client as threatening.***
5. Use mirrors as well as drawings and pictures of the child to reinforce the child's learning of body parts and boundaries.

Outcome Criteria

1. Client is able to differentiate own body parts from those of others.
2. Client communicates ability to separate self from environment by discontinuing use of echolalia (repeating words heard) and echopraxia (imitating movements seen).

■ DISRUPTIVE BEHAVIOR DISORDERS

314.xx Attention-Deficit/Hyperactivity Disorder*

Defined

Attention-deficit/hyperactivity disorder (ADHD) is characterized by a persistent pattern of inattention and/or hyperactivity-impulsivity that is more frequent and severe than is typically observed in individuals at a comparable level of development (APA, 2000). The disorder is frequently not diagnosed until the child begins school because, before then, childhood behavior is much more variable than that of older children. ADHD is four to nine times more common in boys than in girls and may occur in as many as 3 to 7 percent of school-age children. The *DSM-IV-TR* further categorizes the disorder into the following subtypes:

314.01 Combined Type
314.00 Predominantly Inattentive Type
314.01 Predominantly Hyperactive-Impulsive Type

The course can be chronic, persisting into adulthood.

Predisposing Factors

1. **Physiological**
   a. ***Genetics.*** A number of studies indicate that hereditary factors may be implicated in the predisposition to ADHD. Siblings of hyperactive children are more likely than normal children to have the disorder.
   b. ***Biochemical.*** An elevation of the neurotransmitters dopamine and norepinephrine has been suggested as a causative factor (Dopheide, 2001).
   c. ***Prenatal and Perinatal Factors.*** Some studies link maternal smoking and substance use with ADHD in offspring. Premature birth, fetal distress, precipitated or prolonged labor, and perinatal asphyxia have also been implicated.
2. **Psychosocial**
   Environmental Influences: Disorganized or chaotic environments or a disruption in family equilibrium may predispose some individuals to ADHD. A high degree of psychosocial stress, maternal mental disorder, paternal criminality, low socioeconomic status, and foster care have been implicated (Dopheide and Theesen, 1999).

Symptomatology (Subjective and Objective Data)

The *DSM-IV-TR* identifies the following signs and symptoms of ADHD:

1. **Inattention**
   a. Often fails to give close attention to details or makes careless mistakes in schoolwork, work, or other activities.
   b. Often has difficulty sustaining attention in tasks or play activities.
   c. Often does not seem to listen when spoken to directly.
   d. Often does not follow through on instructions and fails to finish schoolwork, chores, or duties in the workplace (not because of oppositional behavior or failure to understand instructions).
   e. Often has difficulty organizing tasks and activities.
   f. Often avoids, dislikes, or is reluctant to engage in tasks that require sustained mental effort (such as schoolwork or homework).
   g. Often loses things necessary for tasks or activities (e.g., toys, school assignments, pencils, books, or tools).
   h. Often is easily distracted by extraneous stimuli.
   i. Often is forgetful in daily activities.

2. **Hyperactivity**
   a. Often fidgets with hands or feet or squirms in seat.
   b. Often leaves seat in classroom or in other situations in which remaining seated is expected.
   c. Often runs about or climbs excessively in situations in which it is inappropriate (in adolescents or adults, may be limited to subjective feelings of restlessness).
   d. Often has difficulty playing or engaging in leisure activities quietly.
   e. Often is "on the go" or often acts as if "driven by a motor."
   f. Often talks excessively.
3. **Impulsivity**
   a. Often blurts out answers before questions have been completed.
   b. Often has difficulty awaiting turn.
   c. Often interrupts or intrudes on others (e.g., butts into conversations or games).

312.xx Conduct Disorder*

Defined

The *DSM-IV-TR* describes the essential feature of this disorder as a repetitive and persistent pattern of conduct in which the basic rights of others or major age-appropriate societal norms or rules are violated. The conduct is more serious than the ordinary mischief and pranks of children and adolescents. The disorder is more common in boys than in girls, and the behaviors may continue into adulthood, often meeting the criteria for antisocial personality disorder. Conduct disorder is divided into the following subtypes:

312.81 Childhood-Onset Type. The onset of at least one characteristic of conduct disorder before age 10 years.

312.82 Adolescent-Onset Type. The absence of behaviors associated with conduct disorder before age 10 years.

312.89 Unspecified Onset. Age at onset is not known.

Predisposing Factors

1. **Physiological**
   a. ***Birth Temperament.*** The term "temperament" refers to personality traits that become evident very early in life and that may be present at birth. Evidence suggests a genetic component in temperament and an association between temperament and behavioral problems later in life (Bagley and Mallick, 2000).
2. **Psychosocial**
   a. ***Peer Relationships.*** Social groups have a significant impact on a child's development. Peers play an essential role in the socialization of interpersonal competence, and skills acquired in this manner affect the child's long-term adjustment. Studies

show that poor peer relations during childhood have consistently been implicated as a cause of later deviance (Ladd, 1999). Aggression has been found to be the principal cause of peer rejection, thus contributing to a cycle of maladaptive behavior.

b. ***Theory of Family Dynamics.*** The following factors related to family dynamics have been implicated as contributors in the predisposition to this disorder (Clunn, 1991; Popper and Steingard, 1994; Kaplan and Sadock, 1998):
   - Parental rejection
   - Inconsistent management and harsh discipline
   - Early institutional living
   - Frequent shifting of parental figures
   - Large family size
   - Absent father
   - Parents with antisocial personality disorder and/or alcohol dependence
   - Association with a delinquent subgroup
   - Marital conflict and divorce
   - Inadequate communication patterns
   - Parental permissiveness

Symptomatology (Subjective and Objective Data)

The *DSM-IV-TR* identifies the following signs and symptoms of conduct disorder:

1. Often bullies, threatens, or intimidates others
2. Often initiates physical fights
3. Has used a weapon that can cause serious physical harm to others (e.g., bat, brick, broken bottle, knife, gun)
4. Has been physically cruel to people
5. Has been physically cruel to animals
6. Has stolen while confronting a victim (e.g., mugging, purse snatching, extortion, armed robbery)
7. Has forced someone into sexual activity
8. Has deliberately engaged in setting fire with the intention of causing serious damage
9. Has deliberately destroyed others' property (other than by setting fire)
10. Has broken into someone's house, building, or car
11. Often lies to obtain goods or favors or to avoid obligations (i.e., "cons" others)
12. Has stolen items of nontrivial value without confronting a victim (e.g., shoplifting, but without breaking and entering; forgery)
13. Often stays out at night despite parental prohibitions, before age 13 years
14. Has run away from home overnight at least twice while living in

parental or parental surrogate home (or once without returning for a lengthy period)

15. Often is truant from school, before age 13 years

313.81 Oppositional Defiant Disorder*

Defined

The *DSM-IV-TR* defines this disorder as a pattern of negativistic, defiant, disobedient, and hostile behavior toward authority figures that occurs more frequently than is typically observed in individuals of comparable age and developmental level. The disorder typically begins by 8 years of age and usually not later than early adolescence. The disorder is more prevalent in boys than in girls and is often a developmental antecedent to conduct disorder.

Predisposing Factors

1. **Physiological**
   a. Refer to this section under Conduct Disorder (312.xx).
2. **Psychosocial**
   a. ***Theory of Family Dynamics.*** It is thought that some parents interpret average or increased levels of developmental oppositionalism as hostility and a deliberate effort on the part of the child to be in control. If power and control are issues for parents, or if they exercise authority for their own needs, a power struggle can be established between the parents and the child that sets the stage for the development of oppositional defiant disorder.

Symptomatology (Subjective and Objective Data)

The *DSM-IV-TR* identifies the following signs and symptoms of oppositional defiant disorder:

1. Often loses temper
2. Often argues with adults
3. Often actively defies or refuses to comply with adult requests or rules
4. Often deliberately annoys people
5. Often blames others for his or her mistakes or misbehavior
6. Is often touchy or easily annoyed by others
7. Is often angry and resentful
8. Is often spiteful or vindictive

Common Nursing Diagnoses and Interventions for Disruptive Behavior Disorders

(Interventions are applicable to various health-care settings, such as inpatient and partial hospitalization, community outpatient clinic, home health, and private practice.)

RISK FOR SELF-DIRECTED OR OTHER-DIRECTED VIOLENCE

Definition: ***At risk for behaviors in which an individual demonstrates that he/she can be physically, emotionally, and/or sexually harmful either to self or to others.***

Related/Risk Factors ("related to")

[Retarded ego development]
[Unsatisfactory parent-child relationship]
[Neurological alteration related to premature birth, fetal distress, precipitated or prolonged labor]
[Dysfunctional family system]
[Disorganized or chaotic environments]
[Child abuse or neglect]
[Birth temperament]
[Fears of abandonment]
Body language: rigid posture, clenching of fists and jaw, hyperactivity, pacing, breathlessness, and threatening stance.
[History or threats of violence toward self or others or of destruction to the property of others]
Impulsivity
History of cruelty to animals
Suicidal ideation, plan; available means

Goals/Objectives

Short-Term Goals

1. Client will seek out staff at any time if thoughts of harming self or others should occur.
2. Client will not harm self or others.

Long-Term Goal

Client will not harm self or others.

Interventions with *Selected Rationales*

1. Observe client's behavior frequently. Do this through routine activities and interactions to avoid appearing watchful and suspicious. ***Clients at high risk for violence require close observation to prevent harm to self or others.***
2. Observe for suicidal behaviors: verbal statements, such as "I'm going to kill myself" or "Very soon my mother won't have to worry herself about me any longer" or nonverbal behaviors, such as giving away cherished items or mood swings. ***Most clients who attempt suicide have communicated their intent, either verbally or nonverbally.***

3. Determine suicidal intent and available means. Ask, "Do you plan to kill yourself?" and "How do you plan to do it?" ***Direct, closed-ended questions are appropriate in this instance. The client who has a usable plan is at higher risk than one who does not.***
4. Obtain verbal or written contract from client agreeing not to harm self and agreeing to seek out staff in the event that such ideation occurs. ***Discussion of suicidal feelings with a trusted individual provides a degree of relief to the client. A contract gets the subject out in the open and places some of the responsibility for his or her safety with the client. An attitude of acceptance of the client as a worthwhile individual is conveyed.***
5. Help client to recognize when anger occurs and to accept those feelings as his or her own. Have client keep an "anger notebook" in which a record of anger experienced on a 24-hour basis is kept. Information regarding source of anger, behavioral response, and client's perception of the situation should also be noted. Discuss entries with client, suggesting alternative behavioral responses for those identified as maladaptive.
6. Act as a role model for appropriate expression of angry feelings, and give positive reinforcement to client for attempting to conform. ***It is vital that client express angry feelings, because suicide and other self-destructive behaviors are often viewed as a result of anger turned inward on the self.***
7. Remove all dangerous objects from client's environment. ***Client physical safety is a nursing priority.***
8. Try to redirect violent behavior with physical outlets for client's anxiety (e.g., punching bag, jogging, volleyball). ***Anxiety and tension can be relieved safely and with benefit to client in this manner.***
9. Be available to stay with client as anxiety level and tensions begin to rise. ***The presence of a trusted individual provides a feeling of security.***
10. Staff should maintain and convey a calm attitude to client. Anxiety is contagious and can be communicated from staff to client and vice versa. ***A calm attitude conveys a sense of control and a feeling of security to client.***
11. Have sufficient staff available to indicate a show of strength to client if it becomes necessary. ***This conveys to client evidence of control over the situation and provides some physical security for staff.***
12. Administer tranquilizing medications as ordered by physician, or obtain an order if necessary. Monitor medication for effectiveness and for adverse side effects. ***Short-term use of antianxiety medications (e.g., diazepam, chlordiazepoxide, alprazolam) provides relief from the immobilizing effects of anxiety and facilitates client's cooperation with therapy.***

13. Mechanical restraints or isolation room may be required if less restrictive interventions are unsuccessful. ***It is the client's right to expect use of techniques that ensure the safety of the client and others by the least restrictive means.***

Outcome Criteria

1. Anxiety is maintained at a level at which client feels no need for aggression.
2. Client seeks out staff to discuss true feelings.
3. Client recognizes, verbalizes, and accepts possible consequences of own maladaptive behaviors.
4. Client does not harm self or others.

DEFENSIVE COPING

Definition: ***Repeated projection of falsely positive self-evaluation based on a self-protective pattern that defends against underlying perceived threats to positive self-regard.***

Possible Etiologies ("related to")

[Low self-esteem]
[Retarded ego development]
[Negative role models]
[Lack of positive feedback]
[Repeated negative feedback, resulting in feelings of diminished self-worth]
[Unsatisfactory parent-child relationship]
[Disorganized or chaotic environments]
[Child abuse or neglect]
[Dysfunctional family system]
[Neurological alteration related to premature birth, fetal distress, precipitated or prolonged labor]

Defining Characteristics ("evidenced by")

Denial of obvious problems or weaknesses
Projection of blame or responsibility
Rationalization of failures
Hypersensitivity to criticism
Grandiosity
Superior attitude toward others
Difficulty establishing or maintaining relationships
Hostile laughter or ridicule of others
Difficulty in perception of reality
Lack of follow-through or participation in treatment or therapy

Goals/Objectives

Short-Term Goal

Client will verbalize personal responsibility for difficulties experienced in interpersonal relationships.

Long-Term Goal

Client will demonstrate ability to interact with others without becoming defensive, rationalizing behaviors, or expressing grandiose ideas.

Interventions with *Selected Rationales*

1. Recognize and support basic ego strengths. ***Focusing on positive aspects of the personality may help to improve self-concept.***
2. Encourage client to recognize and verbalize feelings of inadequacy and need for acceptance from others and to recognize how these feelings provoke defensive behaviors, such as blaming others for own behaviors. ***Recognition of the problem is the first step in the change process toward resolution.***
3. Provide immediate, matter-of-fact, nonthreatening feedback for unacceptable behaviors. ***Client may lack knowledge about how he or she is being perceived by others. Providing this information in a nonthreatening manner may help to eliminate these undesirable behaviors.***
4. Help client identify situations that provoke defensiveness and practice by role-playing more appropriate responses. ***Role-playing provides confidence to deal with difficult situations when they actually occur.***
5. Provide immediate positive feedback for acceptable behaviors. ***Positive feedback enhances self-esteem and encourages repetition of desirable behaviors.***
6. Help client set realistic, concrete goals and determine appropriate actions to meet those goals. ***Success increases self-esteem.***
7. With client, evaluate the effectiveness of the new behaviors and discuss any modifications for improvement. ***Because of limited problem-solving ability, assistance may be required to reassess and develop new strategies in the event that some new coping methods prove ineffective.***

Outcome Criteria

1. Client verbalizes and accepts responsibility for own behavior.
2. Client verbalizes correlation between feelings of inadequacy and need to defend the ego through rationalization and grandiosity.
3. Client does not ridicule or criticize others.
4. Client interacts with others in group situations without taking a defensive stance.

IMPAIRED SOCIAL INTERACTION

Definition: ***Insufficient or excessive quantity or ineffective quality of social exchange.***

Possible Etiologies ("related to")

[Self-concept disturbance]
[Retarded ego development]
[Neurological alterations related to premature birth, fetal distress, precipitated or prolonged labor]
[Dysfunctional family system]
[Disorganized or chaotic environments]
[Child abuse or neglect]
[Unsatisfactory parent-child relationship]
[Negative role models]

Defining Characteristics ("evidenced by")

Verbalized or observed discomfort in social situations
Verbalized or observed inability to receive or communicate a satisfying sense of belonging, caring, interest, or shared history
Observed use of unsuccessful social interaction behaviors
Dysfunctional interaction with peers, family, or others
[Behavior unaccepted for appropriate age by dominant cultural group]

Goals/Objectives

Short-Term Goal

Client will interact in age-appropriate manner with nurse in one-to-one relationship within 1 week.

Long-Term Goal

Client will be able to interact with staff and peers, by the time of discharge from treatment, with no indication of discomfort.

Interventions with *Selected Rationales*

1. Develop trusting relationship with client. Be honest; keep all promises; convey acceptance of client, separate from unacceptable behaviors ("It is not *you*, but *your behavior*, that is unacceptable"). ***Acceptance of client increases his or her feelings of self-worth.***
2. Offer to remain with client during initial interactions with others in the unit. ***Presence of a trusted individual provides client a feeling of security.***
3. Provide constructive criticism and positive reinforcement for client's efforts. ***Positive feedback enhances self-esteem and encourages repetition of desirable behaviors.***

4. Confront client and withdraw attention when client's interactions with others are manipulative or exploitative. ***Attention to unacceptable behavior may reinforce it.***
5. Act as role model for client through appropriate interactions with other clients and staff members.
6. Provide group situations for client. ***It is through these group interactions that client will learn socially acceptable behavior, with positive and negative feedback from his or her peers.***

Outcome Criteria

1. Client seeks out staff member for social as well as therapeutic interaction.
2. Client has formed and satisfactorily maintained one interpersonal relationship with another client.
3. Client willingly and appropriately participates in group activities.
4. Client verbalizes reasons for past inability to form close interpersonal relationships.

INEFFECTIVE COPING

Definition: *Inability to form a valid appraisal of the stressors, inadequate choices of practiced responses, and/or inability to use available resources.*

Possible Etiologies ("related to")

Situational crises
Maturational crises
[Inadequate support systems]
[Inadequate coping strategies]
[Negative role models]
[Neurological alteration related to premature birth, fetal distress, precipitated or prolonged labor]
[Retarded ego development]
[Low self-esteem]
[Dysfunctional family system]
[Disorganized or chaotic environments]
[Child abuse or neglect]

Defining Characteristics ("evidenced by")

[Inability to meet age-appropriate role expectations]
Inadequate problem-solving
Poor concentration
[Manipulation of others in the environment for purposes of fulfilling own desires]
[Verbal hostility toward staff and peers]

[Hyperactivity, evidenced by excessive motor activity, easy distraction, short attention span]
[Unable to delay gratification]
[Oppositional and defiant responses to adult requests or rules]

Goals/Objectives

Short-Term Goal

Within 7 days, client will demonstrate ability and willingness to follow unit rules.

Long-Term Goal

By time of discharge from treatment, client will develop and use age-appropriate, socially acceptable coping skills.

Interventions with *Selected Rationales*

1. If client is hyperactive, make environment safe for continuous large-muscle movement. Rearrange furniture and other objects to prevent injury. ***Client physical safety is a nursing priority.***
2. Provide large-motor activities in which client may participate. Nurse may join in some of these activities ***to facilitate relationship development. Tension is released safely and with benefit to client through physical activities.***
3. Provide frequent, nutritious snacks that client may "eat on the run" ***to ensure adequate calories to offset client's excessive use of energy.***
4. Set limits on manipulative behavior. ("I understand why you are saying these things [or doing these things], but I will not tolerate these behaviors from you.")
5. Identify for client the consequences of manipulative behavior. All staff must follow through and be consistent. ***Client may try to play one staff member against another, so consistency is vital if intervention is to be successful. Aversive reinforcement may work to decrease unacceptable behaviors.***
6. Do not debate, argue, rationalize, or bargain with client. ***Ignoring these attempts may work to decrease manipulative behaviors.***
7. Caution should be taken to avoid reinforcing manipulative behaviors by providing desired attention. ***Attention provides positive reinforcement and encourages repetition of the undesirable behavior.***
8. Confront client's use of manipulative behaviors, and explore their damaging effects on interpersonal relationships. ***Manipulative clients often deny responsibility for their behaviors.***
9. Encourage discussion of angry feelings. Help client identify the true object of the hostility. ***Dealing with feelings honestly and directly will discourage displacement of anger onto others.***
10. Explore with client alternative ways of handling frustration that would be most suited to his or her lifestyle. Provide support and

positive feedback to client as new coping strategies are tried. ***Positive feedback encourages use of acceptable behaviors.***

Outcome Criteria

1. Client is able to delay gratification without resorting to manipulation of others.
2. Client is able to express anger in a socially acceptable manner.
3. Client is able to verbalize alternative, socially acceptable, and lifestyle-appropriate coping skills he or she plans to use in response to frustration.

■ LOW SELF-ESTEEM

Definition: *Negative self-evaluation and feelings about self or self-capabilities.*

Possible Etiologies ("related to")

[Retarded ego development]
[Negative role models]
[Lack of positive feedback]
[Repeated negative feedback, resulting in diminished self-worth]
[Unsatisfactory parent-child relationship]
[Disorganized or chaotic environments]
[Child abuse or neglect]
[Dysfunctional family system]

Defining Characteristics ("evidenced by")

Self-negating verbalizations
Expressions of shame or guilt
Evaluates self as unable to deal with events
Rationalizes away or rejects positive feedback and exaggerates negative feedback about self
Hesitant to try new things or situations
[Denial of problems obvious to others]
[Projection of blame or responsibility for problems]
[Rationalization of personal failures]
[Hypersensitivity to criticism]
[Grandiosity]
Lack of eye contact

Goals/Objectives

Short-Term Goal

Client will independently direct own care and activities of daily living within 1 week.

Long-Term Goal

By time of discharge from treatment, client will exhibit increased feelings of self-worth as evidenced by verbal expression of positive aspects about self, past accomplishments, and future prospects.

Interventions with *Selected Rationales*

1. Ensure that goals are realistic. It is important for client to achieve something, so plan for activities in which the possibility for success is likely. ***Success enhances self-esteem.***
2. Convey unconditional positive regard for client. ***Communication of your acceptance of him or her as a worthwhile human being increases self-esteem.***
3. Spend time with client, both on a one-to-one basis and in group activities. ***This conveys to client that you feel he or she is worth your time.***
4. Assist client in identifying positive aspects of self and in developing plans for changing the characteristics he or she views as negative.
5. Help client decrease use of denial as a defense mechanism. Give positive reinforcement for problem identification and development of more adaptive coping behaviors. ***Positive reinforcement enhances self-esteem and increases client's use of acceptable behaviors.***
6. Encourage and support client in confronting the fear of failure by having client attend therapy activities and undertake new tasks. Offer recognition of successful endeavors and positive reinforcement for attempts made. ***Recognition and positive reinforcement enhance self-esteem.***

Outcome Criteria

1. Client verbalizes positive perception of self.
2. Client participates in new activities without exhibiting extreme fear of failure.

ANXIETY (MODERATE TO SEVERE)

Definition: *Vague, uneasy feeling of discomfort or dread accompanied by an autonomic response (the source is often nonspecific or unknown to the individual); a feeling of apprehension caused by anticipation of danger. It is an alerting signal that warns of impending danger and enables the individual to take measures to deal with threat.*

Possible Etiologies ("related to")

Situational and maturational crises
Threat to self-concept [perceived or real]
Threat of death

Unmet needs
[Fear of failure]
[Dysfunctional family system]
[Unsatisfactory parent-child relationship]
[Innately, easily agitated temperament since birth]

Defining Characteristics ("evidenced by")

Overexcited
Fearful
Feelings of inadequacy
Fear of unspecified consequences
Restlessness
Insomnia
Poor eye contact
Focus on self
[Continuous attention-seeking behaviors]
Difficulty concentrating
Impaired attention
Increased respiratory and heart rates

Goals/Objectives

Short-Term Goals

1. Within 7 days, client will be able to verbalize behaviors that become evident as anxiety starts to rise.
2. Within 7 days, client will be able to verbalize strategies to interrupt escalation of anxiety.

Long-Term Goal

By time of discharge from treatment, client will be able to maintain anxiety below the moderate level as evidenced by absence of disabling behaviors in response to stress.

Interventions with *Selected Rationales*

1. Establish a trusting relationship with client. Be honest, consistent in responses, and available. Show genuine positive regard. ***Honesty, availability, and acceptance promote trust in the nurse-client relationship.***
2. Provide activities geared toward reduction of tension and decreased anxiety (walking or jogging, volleyball, musical exercises, housekeeping chores, group games). ***Tension and anxiety are released safely and with benefit to the client through physical activities.***
3. Encourage client to identify true feelings and to acknowledge ownership of those feelings. ***Anxious clients often deny a relationship between emotional problems and their anxiety. Use of the defense mechanisms of projection and displacement is exaggerated.***

4. The nurse must maintain an atmosphere of calmness; ***anxiety is easily transmitted from one person to another.***
5. Offer support during times of elevated anxiety. Reassure client of physical and psychological safety. ***Client safety is a nursing priority.***
6. Use of touch is comforting to some clients. However, the nurse must be cautious with its use, ***because anxiety may foster suspicion in some individuals who might misinterpret touch as aggression.***
7. As anxiety diminishes, assist client to recognize specific events that preceded its onset. Work on alternative responses to future occurrences. ***A plan of action provides client with a feeling of security for handling a difficult situation more successfully, should it recur.***
8. Help client recognize signs of escalating anxiety, and explore ways client may intervene before behaviors become disabling.
9. Administer tranquilizing medication as ordered. Assess for effectiveness, and instruct client regarding possible adverse side effects. ***Short-term use of antianxiety medications (e.g., diazepam, chlordiazepoxide, alprazolam) provides relief from the immobilizing effects of anxiety and facilitates client's cooperation with therapy.***

Outcome Criteria

1. As anxiety starts to rise, client is able to verbalize behaviors that become evident and takes actions appropriate to interrupt progression of the condition.
2. Client is able to maintain anxiety at a manageable level.

NONCOMPLIANCE

Definition: *Behavior of person and/or caregiver that fails to coincide with a health-promoting or therapeutic plan agreed on by the person (and/or family and/or community) and health-care professional. In the presence of an agreed-on health-promoting or therapeutic plan, person's or caregiver's behavior is fully or partially nonadherent and may lead to clinically ineffective or partially ineffective outcomes.*

Possible Etiologies ("related to")

[Biochemical alteration]
[Neurological alteration related to premature birth, fetal distress, precipitated or prolonged labor]
[Negative temperament]
[Dysfunctional family system]
[Negative role models]
[Retarded ego development]
[Low frustration tolerance and short attention span]
[Denial of problems]

Defining Characteristics ("evidenced by")

Behavior indicative of failure to adhere [to treatment regimen]
[Inability to sit still long enough to complete a task]
[Expression of opposition to requests for participation]
[Refusal to follow directions or suggestions of treatment team]

Goals/Objectives

Short-Term Goal

Client will participate in and cooperate during therapeutic activities.

Long-Term Goal

Client will complete assigned tasks willingly and independently or with a minimum of assistance.

Interventions with *Selected Rationales*

(For the client with inattention and hyperactivity):

1. Provide an environment for task efforts that is as free of distractions as possible. ***Client is highly distractible and is unable to perform in the presence of even minimal stimulation.***
2. Provide assistance on a one-to-one basis, beginning with simple, concrete instructions. ***Client lacks the ability to assimilate information that is complicated or that has abstract meaning.***
3. Ask client to repeat instructions to you ***to determine client level of comprehension.***
4. Establish goals that allow client to complete a part of the task, rewarding completion of each step with a break for physical activity. ***Short-term goals are not so overwhelming to client with such a short attention span. The positive reinforcement (physical activity) increases self-esteem and provides incentive for client to pursue the task to completion.***
5. Gradually decrease the amount of assistance given to task performance while assuring the client that assistance will still be available if deemed necessary. ***This encourages the client to perform independently while providing a feeling of security with the presence of a trusted individual.***

   (For the client with oppositional tendencies):
6. Set forth a structured plan of therapeutic activities. Start with minimum expectations and increase as client begins to manifest evidence of compliance. ***Structure provides security, and one or two activities may not seem as overwhelming as the whole schedule of activities presented at one time.***
7. Establish a system of rewards for compliance with therapy and consequences for noncompliance. Ensure that the rewards and consequences are concepts of value to the client. ***Positive and negative reinforcements can contribute to desired changes in behavior.***
8. Convey acceptance of client separate from the undesirable behav-

iors being exhibited. ("It is not *you*, but *your behavior*, that is unacceptable.") ***Unconditional acceptance enhances client's self-worth and may contribute to a decrease in the need for passive-aggressive behavior toward others.***

Outcome Criteria

1. Client cooperates with staff in an effort to complete assigned tasks.
2. Client complies with treatment by participating in therapies without negativism.
3. Client takes direction from staff without becoming defensive.

■ 307.23 TOURETTE'S DISORDER*

Defined

Tourette's disorder is characterized by the presence of multiple motor tics and one or more vocal tics that may appear simultaneously or at different periods during the illness (APA, 2000). Onset of the disorder can be as early as age 2 years, but it occurs most commonly during childhood (around age 6 to 7 years). Tourette's disorder is more common in boys than in girls. The duration of the disorder may be lifelong, although there may be periods of remission that last from weeks to years (APA, 2000). The symptoms usually diminish during adolescence and adulthood and, in some cases, disappear altogether by early adulthood.

Predisposing Factors

1. **Physiological**
   a. ***Genetics.*** Family studies show that Tourette's disorder is more common in relatives of individuals with the disorder than in the general population. Autosomal-dominant transmission may be involved (Kaplan and Sadock, 1998).
   b. ***Brain Alterations.*** Altered levels of neurotransmitters and dysfunction in the area of the basal ganglia have been implicated as a cause of Tourette's disorder.
   c. ***Biochemical Factors.*** Abnormalities in levels of dopamine, serotonin, dynorphin, gamma-aminobutyric acid, acetylcholine, and norepinephrine have been associated with Tourette's disorder (Popper and Steingard, 1994).
2. **Psychosocial**
   a. The genetic predisposition to Tourette's disorder may be reinforced by certain factors in the environment, such as increased prenatal complications, low birth weight, and emotional stress during pregnancy.

Symptomatology (Subjective and Objective Data)

The *DSM-IV-TR* identifies the following signs and symptoms of Tourette's disorder:

1. The disorder may begin with a single motor tic, such as eye

blinking, neck jerking, shoulder shrugging, facial grimacing, or coughing.

2. Complex motor tics may follow, which include touching, squatting, hopping, skipping, deep knee bending, retracing steps, and twirling when walking.
3. Vocal tics include various sounds such as clicks, grunts, yelps, barks, sniffs, snorts, or coughs; in about 10 percent of cases, a complex vocal tic involves uttering obscenities.
4. Vocal tics may include repeating certain words or phrases out of context, repeating one's own sounds or words (palilalia), or repeating what others say (echolalia).
5. The movements and vocalizations are experienced as compulsive and irresistible, but they can be suppressed for varying amounts of time.
6. Tics are exacerbated by stress and attenuated during periods in which the individual becomes totally absorbed by an activity.
7. Tics are markedly diminished during sleep.

Common Nursing Diagnoses and Interventions

(Interventions are applicable to various health-care settings, such as inpatient and partial hospitalization, community outpatient clinic, home health, and private practice.)

■ RISK FOR SELF-DIRECTED OR OTHER-DIRECTED VIOLENCE

Definition: ***At risk for behaviors in which an individual demonstrates that he/she can be physically, emotionally, and/or sexually harmful either to self or to others.***

Related/Risk Factors ("related to")

[Low tolerance for frustration]
[Abnormalities in brain neurotransmitters]
Body language: rigid posture, clenching of fists and jaw, hyperactivity, pacing, breathlessness, and threatening stances
[History or threats of violence toward self or others or of destruction to the property of others]
Impulsivity
Suicidal ideation, plan, available means

Goals/Objectives

Short-Term Goals

1. Client will seek out staff or support person at any time if thoughts of harming self or others should occur.
2. Client will not harm self or others.

Long-Term Goal

Client will not harm self or others.

Interventions with *Selected Rationales*

1. Observe client's behavior frequently through routine activities and interactions. Become aware of behaviors that indicate a rise in agitation. ***Stress commonly increases tic behaviors. Recognition of behaviors that precede the onset of aggression may provide the opportunity to intervene before violence occurs.***
2. Monitor for self-destructive behavior and impulses. A staff member may need to stay with the client to prevent self-mutilation. ***Client physical safety is a nursing priority.***
3. Provide hand coverings and other restraints that prevent the client from self-mutilative behaviors. ***Provide immediate external controls against self-aggressive behaviors.***
4. Redirect violent behavior to provide physical outlets for frustration. ***Excess energy is released through physical activities, and a feeling of relaxation is induced.***
5. Administer medication as ordered by the physician. Several medications have been used to treat Tourette's disorder. The most common include the following:
   a. **Haloperidol** (**Haldol**). Haloperidol has been the drug of choice for Tourette's disorder. Children on this medication must be monitored for adverse effects associated with most antipsychotic medications (see Chapter 27). Because of the potential for adverse effects, haloperidol should be reserved for children with severe symptoms or with symptoms that interfere with their ability to function. Usual dosage for children 3 to 12 years of age is 0.05 to 0.075 mg/kg/d.
   b. **Pimozide** (**Orap**). The response rate and side-effect profile of pimozide are similar to those of haloperidol. Pimozide is used to manage severe motor or vocal tics that have failed to respond to more conventional treatment. It is not recommended for children younger than age 12 years. Recommended dosage is 0.05 to 0.2 mg/kg, not to exceed 10 mg/d.
   c. **Clonidine** (**Catapres**). Clonidine is an antihypertensive medication, the efficacy of which in the treatment of Tourette's disorder has been mixed. Some physicians like it and use it as a drug of first choice because of its relative safety and few side effects. Recommended dosage is 150 to 200 μg/d.
   d. **Ziprasidone (Geodon).** The antipsychotic ziprasidone has been found to reduce the severity and frequency of tic symptoms safely in adolescents and children as young as 7 years of age. The benefits of the drug appear to be somewhat less than those achieved with the traditional neuroleptics, but it has a more positive side-effect profile, with an absence of extrapyramidal symptoms or weight gain. However, ziprasidone has a

greater capacity to prolong the QT interval compared with several other antipsychotics. Dosage is initiated at 5 mg/d and titrated up to a maximum of 40 mg/d.

Outcome Criteria

1. Anxiety is maintained at a level at which client feels no need for aggression.
2. Client seeks out staff or support person for expression of true feelings.
3. Client has not harmed self or others.

IMPAIRED SOCIAL INTERACTION

Definition: *Insufficient or excessive quantity or ineffective quality of social exchange.*

Possible Etiologies ("related to")

Self-concept disturbance
[Low tolerance for frustration]
[Impulsiveness]
[Oppositional behavior]
[Aggressive behavior]

Defining Characteristics ("evidenced by")

Verbalized or observed discomfort in social situations
Verbalized or observed inability to receive or communicate a satisfying sense of belonging, caring, interest, or shared history
Observed use of unsuccessful social interaction behaviors
Dysfunctional interaction with peers, family, or others

Goals/Objectives

Short-Term Goal

Client will develop a one-to-one relationship with a nurse or support person within 1 week.

Long-Term Goal

Client will be able to interact with staff and peers using age-appropriate, acceptable behaviors.

Interventions with *Selected Rationales*

1. Develop a trusting relationship with client. Convey acceptance of the person separate from the unacceptable behavior. ***Unconditional acceptance increases client's feelings of self-worth.***
2. Discuss with client which behaviors are and are not acceptable. Describe in matter-of-fact manner the consequences of unaccept-

able behavior. Follow through. ***Aversive reinforcement can alter undesirable behaviors.***
3. Provide group situations for client. ***Appropriate social behavior is often learned from positive and negative feedback of peers.***
4. Act as a role model for client through appropriate interactions with others. ***Role-modeling of a respected individual is one of the strongest forms of learning.***

Outcome Criteria

1. Client seeks out staff or support person for social as well as for therapeutic interaction.
2. Client verbalizes reasons for past inability to form close interpersonal relationships.
3. Client interacts with others, using age-appropriate, acceptable behaviors.

LOW SELF-ESTEEM

Definition: *Negative self-evaluation and feelings about self or self-capabilities.*

Possible Etiologies ("related to")

[Shame associated with tic behaviors]

Defining Characteristics ("evidenced by")

Lack of eye contact
Self-negating verbalizations
Expressions of shame or guilt
Hesitant to try new things or situations
[Manipulation of others]

Goals/Objectives

Short-Term Goal

Client will verbalize positive aspects about self not associated with tic behaviors.

Long-Term Goal

Client will exhibit increased feeling of self-worth as evidenced by positive verbal expression about aspects of self, past accomplishments, and future prospects.

Interventions with *Selected Rationales*

1. Convey unconditional acceptance and positive regard. ***Communication of client as worthwhile human being may increase self-esteem.***

2. Set limits on manipulative behavior. Take caution not to reinforce manipulative behaviors by providing desired attention. Identify the consequences of manipulation. Administer consequences matter-of-factly when manipulation occurs. ***Aversive reinforcement may work to decrease unacceptable behaviors.***
3. Help client understand that he or she uses this behavior in order to try to increase own self-esteem. Interventions should reflect other actions to accomplish this goal. ***When client feels better about self, need to manipulate others will diminish.***
4. If client chooses to suppress tics in the presence of others, provide a specified "tic time" during which client "vents" tics, feelings, and behaviors (alone or with staff). ***Allows for release of tics and assists in sense of control and management of symptoms (Rosner and Pollice, 1991).***
5. Ensure that client has regular one-to-one time with staff or support person. ***Provides opportunity for educating about illness and teaching management tactics. Assists in exploring feelings around illness and incorporating illness into a healthy sense of self (Rosner and Pollice, 1991).***

Outcome Criteria

1. Client verbalizes positive perception of self.
2. Client willingly participates in new activities and situations.

■ 309.21 SEPARATION ANXIETY DISORDER*

Defined

The APA (2000) defines separation anxiety disorder as excessive anxiety concerning separation from the home or from those to whom the person is attached. Onset may occur as early as preschool age, rarely as late as adolescence, but always before age 18 years and is more common in girls than in boys.

Predisposing Factors

1. **Physiological**
   a. ***Genetics.*** Studies indicate that a greater number of children with relatives who manifest anxiety problems develop anxiety disorders themselves than do children with no such family patterns.
   b. ***Temperament.*** Studies show that differences in temperamental characteristics at birth may be correlated to the acquisition of fear and anxiety disorders in childhood. This may denote an inherited vulnerability or predisposition toward developing these disorders.
2. **Psychosocial**
   a. ***Stressful Life Events.*** Studies indicate that children who are

predisposed to anxiety disorders may be affected significantly by stressful life events.

b. ***Family Influences.*** Several theories relate the development of separation anxiety to the following dynamics within the family:
   - An overattachment to the mother (primary caregiver)
   - Separation conflicts between parent and child
   - Enmeshment of members within a family
   - Overprotection of the child by the parents
   - Transfer of parents' fears and anxieties to the children through role-modeling

Symptomatology (Subjective and Objective Data)

The *DSM-IV-TR* identifies the following signs and symptoms of separation anxiety disorder:

1. Recurrent, excessive distress when separation from home or major attachment figures occurs or is anticipated
2. Persistent and excessive worry about losing, or about possible harm befalling, major attachment figures
3. Persistent and excessive worry that an untoward event will lead to separation from a major attachment figure
4. Persistent reluctance or refusal to go to school or elsewhere because of fear of separation
5. Persistent and excessive fear or reluctance to be alone or without major attachment figures at home or without significant adults in other settings
6. Persistent reluctance or refusal to go to sleep without being near a major attachment figure or to sleep away from home
7. Repeated nightmares involving the theme of separation
8. Repeated complaints of physical symptoms, such as headaches, stomachaches, nausea, or vomiting, when separation from major attachment figures occurs or is anticipated

Common Nursing Diagnoses and Interventions

(Interventions are applicable to various health-care settings, such as inpatient and partial hospitalization, community outpatient clinic, home health, and private practice.)

ANXIETY (SEVERE)

Definition: *Vague, uneasy feeling of discomfort or dread accompanied by an autonomic response (the source is often nonspecific or unknown to the individual); a feeling of apprehension caused by anticipation of danger. It is an alerting signal that warns of impending danger and enables the individual to take measures to deal with threat.*

Possible Etiologies ("related to")

Family history
[Birth temperament]
[Overattachment to parent]
[Negative role-modeling]

Defining Characteristics ("evidenced by")

[Excessive distress when separated from attachment figure]
[Fear of anticipation of separation from attachment figure]
[Fear of being alone or without attachment figure]
[Reluctance or refusal to go to school or anywhere else without attachment figure]
[Nightmares about being separated from attachment figure]
[Somatic symptoms occurring as a result of fear of separation]

Goals/Objectives

Short-Term Goal

Client will discuss fears of separation with trusted individual.

Long-Term Goal

Client will maintain anxiety at no higher than moderate level in the face of events that formerly precipitated panic.

Interventions with *Selected Rationales*

1. Establish an atmosphere of calmness, trust, and genuine positive regard. ***Trust and unconditional acceptance are necessary for satisfactory nurse-client relationship. Calmness is important because anxiety is easily transmitted from one person to another.***
2. Assure client of his or her safety and security. ***Symptoms of panic anxiety are very frightening.***
3. Explore the child's or adolescent's fears of separating from the parents. Explore with the parents possible fears they may have of separation from the child. ***Some parents may have an underlying fear of separation from the child of which they are unaware and which they are unconsciously transferring to the child.***
4. Help parents and child initiate realistic goals (e.g., child to stay with sitter for 2 hours with minimal anxiety; child to stay at friend's house without parents until 9:00 PM without experiencing panic anxiety). ***Parents may be so frustrated with the child's clinging and demanding behaviors that assistance with problem-solving may be required.***
5. Give, and encourage parents to give, positive reinforcement for desired behaviors. ***Positive reinforcement encourages repetition of desirable behaviors.***

Outcome Criteria

1. Client and parents are able to discuss their fears regarding separation.
2. Client experiences no somatic symptoms from fear of separation.
3. Client maintains anxiety at moderate level when separation occurs or is anticipated.

INEFFECTIVE COPING

Definition: ***Inability to form a valid appraisal of the stressors, inadequate choices of practiced responses, and/or inability to use available resources.***

Possible Etiologies ("related to")

[Unresolved separation conflicts]
[Inadequate coping skills]

Defining Characteristics ("evidenced by")

[Somatic complaints in response to occurrence or anticipation of separation from attachment figure]

Goals/Objectives

Short-Term Goal

Client will verbalize correlation of somatic symptoms to fear of separation.

Long-Term Goal

Client will demonstrate use of more adaptive coping strategies (than physical symptoms) in response to stressful situations.

Interventions with *Selected Rationales*

1. Encourage child or adolescent to discuss specific situations in life that produce the most distress and to describe his or her response to these situations. Include parents in the discussion. ***Client and family may be unaware of the correlation between stressful situations and the exacerbation of physical symptoms.***
2. Help child or adolescent who is perfectionistic to recognize that self-expectations may be unrealistic. Connect times of unmet self-expectations to the exacerbation of physical symptoms. ***Recognition of maladaptive patterns is the first step in the change process.***
3. Encourage parents and child to identify more adaptive coping strategies that the child could use in the face of anxiety that feels overwhelming. Practice through role-play. ***Practice facilitates use***

of desired behavior when the individual is actually faced with the stressful situation.

Outcome Criteria

1. Client and family verbalize the correlation between separation anxiety and somatic symptoms.
2. Client verbalizes the correlation between unmet self-expectations and somatic symptoms.
3. Client responds to stressful situations without exhibiting physical symptoms.

IMPAIRED SOCIAL INTERACTION

Definition: *Insufficient or excessive quantity or ineffective quality of social exchange.*

Possible Etiologies ("related to")

[Reluctance to be away from attachment figure]

Defining Characteristics ("evidenced by")

[Symptoms of severe anxiety]
Verbalized or observed discomfort in social situations
Verbalized or observed inability to receive or communicate a satisfying sense of belonging, caring, interest, or shared history
Observed use of unsuccessful social interaction behaviors
Dysfunctional interaction with others

Goals/Objectives

Short-Term Goal

Client will spend time with staff or other support person, without presence of attachment figure, without excessive anxiety.

Long-Term Goal

Client will be able to spend time with others (without presence of attachment figure) without excessive anxiety.

Interventions with *Selected Rationales*

1. Develop a trusting relationship with client. ***This is the first step in helping client learn to interact with others.***
2. Attend groups with the child, and support efforts to interact with others. Give positive feedback. ***Presence of a trusted individual provides security during times of distress. Positive feedback encourages repetition.***
3. Convey to the child the acceptability of his or her not participat-

ing in group in the beginning. Gradually encourage small contributions until client is able to participate more fully. ***Small successes will gradually increase self-confidence and decrease self-consciousness so that client will feel less anxious in the group situation.***

4. Help client set small personal goals (e.g., "Today I will speak to one person I don't know"). ***Simple, realistic goals provide opportunities for success that increase self-confidence and may encourage client to attempt more difficult objectives in the future.***

Outcome Criteria

1. Client spends time with others using acceptable, age-appropriate behaviors.
2. Client is able to interact with others away from the attachment figure without excessive anxiety.

■ INTERNET REFERENCES

Additional information about ADHD is located at the following websites:

- http://www.chadd.org
- http://www.laurus.com/Library/HealthGuide/IllnessConditions/topic.asp?hwid=hw166083
- http://www.nimh.nih.gov/publicat/adhdmenu.cfm

Additional information about medications to treat ADHD is located at the following websites:

- http://www.fadavis.com/townsend
- http://www.laurus.com/library/healthguide/DrugGuide
- http://www.nimh.nih.gov/publicat/childmedmenu.cfm

Additional information about autism is located at the following websites:

- http://www.autism-society.org
- http://www.nimh.nih.gov/publicat/autismmenu.cfm

CHAPTER 3

*Delirium, Dementia, and Amnestic Disorders**

BACKGROUND ASSESSMENT DATA

293.0 Delirium

Defined

The American Psychiatric Association (2000) *Diagnostic and Statistical Manual of Mental Disorders, Fourth Edition, Text Revision (DSM-IV-TR)* defines delirium as a disturbance of consciousness and a change in cognition that develop rapidly over a short period (APA, 2000). The symptoms of delirium usually begin quite abruptly, and the duration is usually brief (e.g., 1 week; rarely more than 1 month). The disorder subsides completely on recovery from the underlying determinant. If the underlying condition persists, the delirium may gradually shift to the syndrome of dementia or progress to coma. The individual then recovers, becomes chronically vegetative, or dies.

Predisposing Factors

The *DSM-IV-TR* differentiates among the disorders of delirium by their etiology, although they share a common symptom presentation. Categories of delirium include the following:

1. **Delirium due to a General Medical Condition.** Certain medical conditions, such as systemic infections, metabolic disorders, fluid and electrolyte imbalances, liver or kidney disease, thiamine deficiency, postoperative states, hypertensive encephalopathy, postictal states, and sequelae of head trauma, can cause the symptoms of delirium.
2. **Substance-Induced Delirium.** The symptoms of delirium can be induced by the exposure to a toxin or the ingestion of a medication, such as anticonvulsants, neuroleptics, anxiolytics, antidepressants, cardiovascular medications, antineoplastics, analgesics, antiasthmatic agents, antihistamines, antiparkinsonian drugs, corticosteroids, and gastrointestinal medications.

---

* Classification and criteria from the *Diagnostic and Statistical Manual of Mental Disorders, Fourth Edition, Text Revision, 2000.* Used with permission from the American Psychiatric Association.

3. **Substance-Intoxication Delirium.** Delirium symptoms can occur in response to taking high doses of cannabis, cocaine, hallucinogens, alcohol, anxiolytics, or narcotics.
4. **Substance-Withdrawal Delirium.** Reduction or termination of long-term, high-dose use of certain substances, such as alcohol, sedatives, hypnotics, or anxiolytics, can result in withdrawal delirium symptoms.
5. **Delirium due to Multiple Etiologies.** Symptoms of delirium may be related to more than one general medical condition or to the combined effects of a general medical condition and substance use.

Symptomatology (Subjective and Objective Data)

The following symptoms have been identified with the syndrome of delirium:

1. Altered consciousness ranging from hypervigilance to stupor or semicoma.
2. Extreme distractibility with difficulty focusing attention.
3. Disorientation to time and place.
4. Impaired reasoning ability and goal-directed behavior.
5. Disturbance in the sleep-wake cycle.
6. Emotional instability as manifested by fear, anxiety, depression, irritability, anger, euphoria, or apathy.
7. Misperceptions of the environment, including illusions and hallucinations.
8. Autonomic manifestations, such as tachycardia, sweating, flushed face, dilated pupils, or elevated blood pressure.
9. Incoherent speech.
10. Impairment of recent memory.

294.xx Dementia

Defined

Dementia is defined as a syndrome of acquired, persistent intellectual impairment with compromised function in multiple spheres of mental activity, such as memory, language, visuospatial skills, emotion or personality, and cognition (Wise and Gray, 1994). The disease usually has a slow, insidious onset and is chronic, progressive, and irreversible.

Predisposing Factors

The *DSM-IV-TR* identifies the following etiological categories for the syndrome of dementia:

1. **Dementia of the Alzheimer's Type.** The exact cause of Alzheimer's disease is unknown, but several theories have been proposed, such as reduction in brain acetylcholine, accumulation of aluminum in the brain, immune system alterations, head trauma, and genetic factors. Pathological changes in the brain include atrophy, enlarged ventricles, and the presence of numerous neurofibrillary plaques and tangles. Definitive diagnosis is by

biopsy or autopsy examination of brain tissue, although refinement of diagnostic criteria and new diagnostic tools enable clinicians to use specific clinical features to identify the disease at an accuracy rate of 85 to 90 percent.

2. **Vascular Dementia.** This type of dementia is caused by significant cerebrovascular disease. The client suffers the equivalent of small strokes caused by arterial hypertension or cerebral emboli or thrombi, which destroy many areas of the brain. The onset of symptoms is more abrupt than in Alzheimer's disease and runs a highly variable course, progressing in steps rather than as a gradual deterioration.
3. **Dementia due to HIV Disease.** The immune dysfunction associated with HIV can lead to brain infections by other organisms. HIV also appears to cause dementia directly.
4. **Dementia due to Head Trauma.** The syndrome of symptoms associated with dementia can be brought on by a traumatic brain injury.
5. **Dementia due to Parkinson's Disease.** Parkinson's disease is caused by a loss of nerve cells in the substantia nigra of the basal ganglia. The symptoms of dementia associated with Parkinson's disease closely resemble those of Alzheimer's disease.
6. **Dementia due to Huntington's Disease.** This disease is transmitted as a mendelian dominant gene, and damage occurs in the areas of the basal ganglia and the cerebral cortex. The average course of the disease to complete incapacitation and death is about 15 years (Nowak and Handford, 1994).
7. **Dementia due to Pick's Disease.** Pathological effects occur from atrophy in the frontal and temporal lobes of the brain. Symptoms are strikingly similar to those of Alzheimer's disease, and Pick's disease is often misdiagnosed as Alzheimer's.
8. **Dementia due to Creutzfeldt-Jakob Disease.** This form of dementia is caused by a transmissible virus. The clinical presentation is typical of the syndrome of dementia, and the course is extremely rapid, with progressive deterioration and death within 1 year.
9. **Dementia due to Other General Medical Conditions.** These include endocrine, hepatic, renal, cardiopulmonary, and neurological conditions, brain lesions, and systemic infections.
10. **Substance-Induced Persisting Dementia.** This type of dementia is related to the persisting effects of substances such as alcohol, inhalants, sedatives, hypnotics, anxiolytics, other medications, and environmental toxins. The term "persisting" indicates that the dementia persists long after the effects of substance intoxication or substance withdrawal have subsided.

Symptomatology (Subjective and Objective Data)

The following symptoms have been identified with the syndrome of dementia:

1. Memory impairment (impaired ability to learn new information or to recall previously learned information).
2. Impairment in abstract thinking, judgment, and impulse control.
3. Impairment in language ability, such as difficulty naming objects. In some instances, the individual may not speak at all (aphasia).
4. Personality changes.
5. Impaired ability to execute motor activities despite intact motor abilities (apraxia).
6. Disorientation.
7. Wandering.
8. Delusions (particularly delusions of persecution).

294.0 Amnestic Disorders

Defined

Amnestic disorders are characterized by an inability to learn new information (short-term memory deficit) despite normal attention and an inability to recall previously learned information (long-term memory deficit). No other cognitive deficits exist.

Predisposing Factors

The *DSM-IV-TR* identifies the following etiological categories for the syndrome of amnestic disorders:

1. **Amnestic Disorder due to a General Medical Condition**. The symptoms may be associated with head trauma, cerebrovascular disease, cerebral neoplastic disease, cerebral anoxia, herpes simplex encephalitis, poorly controlled insulin-dependent diabetes, or surgical intervention to the brain (APA, 2000; Wise and Gray, 1994). Transient amnestic syndromes can also occur from epileptic seizures, electroconvulsive therapy, severe migraine, and drug overdose (Wise and Gray, 1994).
2. **Substance-Induced Persisting Amnestic Disorder**. This type of amnestic disorder is related to the persisting effects of substances such as alcohol, sedatives, hypnotics, anxiolytics, other medications, and environmental toxins. The term "persisting" indicates that the symptoms persist long after the effects of substance intoxication or substance withdrawal have subsided.

Symptomatology (Subjective and Objective Data)

The following symptoms have been identified with amnestic disorders:

1. Disorientation to place and time may occur with profound amnesia.
2. There is an inability to recall events from the recent past and from the remote past. (Events from the very remote past are often more easily recalled than recently occurring ones.)
3. The individual is prone to confabulation, the creation of imaginary events to fill in memory gaps.
4. Apathy, lack of initiative, and emotional blandness are common.

Common Nursing Diagnoses and Interventions for Delirium, Dementia, and Amnestic Disorders

(Interventions are applicable to various health-care settings, such as inpatient and partial hospitalization, community outpatient clinic, home health, and private practice.)

RISK FOR TRAUMA

Definition: ***[The client has] accentuated risk of accidental tissue injury (e.g., wound, burn, fracture).***

Related/Risk Factors ("related to")

[Chronic alteration in structure or function of brain tissue, secondary to the aging process, multiple infarcts, HIV disease, head trauma, chronic substance abuse, or progressively dysfunctional physical condition, resulting in the following symptoms:
Disorientation; confusion
Weakness
Muscular incoordination
Seizures
Memory impairment
Poor vision
Extreme psychomotor agitation observed in the late stages of delirium]
[Frequent shuffling of feet and stumbling]
[Falls caused by muscular incoordination or seizures]
[Bumping into furniture]
[Exposing self to frigid conditions with insufficient protective clothing]
[Cutting self when using sharp instruments]
[History of attempting to light burner or oven and leaving gas on in house]
[Smoking and leaving burning cigarettes in various places; smoking in bed; falling asleep sitting on couch or chair with lighted cigarette in hand]
[Purposeless, thrashing movements; hyperactivity that is out of touch with the environment]

Goals/Objectives

Short-Term Goal

Client will call for assistance when ambulating or carrying out other activities.

Long-Term Goal

Client will not experience physical injury.

Interventions with Selected Rationales

1. Assess client's level of disorientation and confusion to determine specific requirements for safety. ***Knowledge of client's level of functioning is necessary to formulate appropriate plan of care.***
2. Institute appropriate safety measures, such as the following:
   a. Place furniture in room in an arrangement that best accommodates client's disabilities.
   b. Observe client behaviors frequently; assign staff on one-to-one basis if condition warrants; accompany and assist client when ambulating; use wheelchair for transporting long distances.
   c. Store items that client uses frequently within easy access.
   d. Remove potentially harmful articles from client's room: cigarettes, matches, lighters, sharp objects.
   e. Remain with client while he or she smokes.
   f. Pad side rails and headboard of client with seizure disorder. Institute seizure precautions as described in procedure manual of individual institution. ***Client safety is a nursing priority.***
3. Frequently orient client to reality and surroundings. ***Disorientation may endanger client safety if he or she unknowingly wanders away from safe environment.***
4. Use tranquilizing medications and soft restraints, as prescribed by physician, for client's protection during periods of excessive hyperactivity. ***Use restraints judiciously, because they can increase agitation. They may be required, however, to provide for client safety.***
5. Teach prospective caregivers methods that have been successful in preventing client injury. ***These caregivers will be responsible for client's safety after discharge from the hospital. Sharing successful interventions may be helpful.***

Outcome Criteria

1. Client is able to accomplish daily activities within the environment without experiencing injury.
2. Prospective caregivers are able to verbalize means of providing safe environment for client.

RISK FOR SELF-DIRECTED OR OTHER-DIRECTED VIOLENCE

Definition: *At risk for behaviors in which an individual demonstrates that he/she can be physically, emotionally, and/or sexually harmful either to self or to others.*

Related/Risk Factors ("related to")

[Chronic alteration in structure or function of brain tissue, secondary to the aging process, multiple infarcts, HIV disease, head trauma,

chronic substance abuse, or progressively dysfunctional physical condition, resulting in the following symptoms:
Delusional thinking
Suspiciousness of others
Hallucinations
Illusions
Disorientation or confusion
Impairment of impulse control]
[Inaccurate perception of the environment]
Body language—rigid posture, clenching of fists and jaw, hyperactivity, pacing, breathlessness, and threatening stances.
Suicidal ideation, plan, available means
Cognitive impairment
[Depressed mood]

Goals/Objectives

Short-Term Goals

1. Client will maintain agitation at manageable level so as not to become violent.
2. Client will not harm self or others.

Long-Term Goal

Client will not harm self or others.

Interventions with *Selected Rationales*

1. Assess client's level of anxiety and behaviors that indicate that anxiety is increasing. ***Recognizing these behaviors, the nurse may be able to intervene before violence occurs.***
2. Maintain low level of stimuli in client's environment (low lighting, few people, simple decor, low noise level). ***Anxiety increases in a highly stimulating environment.***
3. Remove all potentially dangerous objects from client's environment. ***In a disoriented, confused state, the client may use these objects to harm self or others.***
4. Have sufficient staff available to execute a physical confrontation, if necessary. ***Assistance may be required from others to provide for physical safety of client or primary nurse or both.***
5. Maintain a calm manner with client. Attempt to prevent frightening the client unnecessarily. Provide continual reassurance and support. ***Anxiety is contagious and can be transferred to the client.***
6. Interrupt periods of unreality and reorient. ***Client safety is jeopardized during periods of disorientation. Correcting misinterpretations of reality enhances client's feelings of self-worth and personal dignity.***
7. Use tranquilizing medications and soft restraints, as prescribed by physician, ***for protection of client and others during periods***

of elevated anxiety. Use restraints judiciously, ***because agitation sometimes increases; however, they may be required to ensure client safety.***

8. Sit with client and provide one-to-one observation if client assessed to be actively suicidal. ***Client safety is a nursing priority.***
9. Teach relaxation exercises ***to intervene in times of increasing anxiety.***
10. Teach prospective caregivers to recognize client behaviors that indicate anxiety is increasing and ways to intervene before violence occurs.

Outcome Criteria

1. Prospective caregivers are able to verbalize behaviors that indicate an increasing anxiety level and ways they may assist client to manage the anxiety before violence occurs.
2. Client is able to control impulse to perform acts of violence against self or others, with assistance from caregivers.

DISTURBED THOUGHT PROCESSES

Definition: *Disruption in cognitive operations and activities.*

Possible Etiologies ("related to")

[Alteration in structure/function of brain tissue, secondary to the following conditions:
Advanced age
Vascular disease
Hypertension
Cerebral hypoxia
Long-term abuse of mood- or behavior-altering substances
Exposure to environmental toxins
Other physical disorders that predispose to cerebral abnormalities (see Predisposing Factors)] AU2

Defining Characteristics ("evidenced by")

[Delusional thinking]
Inaccurate interpretation of environment
Memory deficit or problems [and confabulation]
[Altered attention span]
Distractibility
[Disorientation to time, place, person, circumstances, and events]
[Impaired ability to make decisions, problem-solve, reason, abstract or conceptualize, calculate]
Inappropriate or nonreality-based thinking

Goals/Objectives

Short-Term Goal

Client will accept explanations of inaccurate interpretations of the environment within 5 days.

Long-Term Goal

With assistance from caregiver, client will be able to interrupt nonreality-based thinking.

Interventions with *Selected Rationales*

1. Frequently orient client to reality and surroundings. Allow client to have familiar objects around him or her. Use other items, such as clock, calendar, and daily schedules, to assist client in maintaining reality orientation. ***Client safety is jeopardized during periods of disorientation. Maintaining reality orientation enhances client's sense of self-worth and personal dignity.***
2. Teach prospective caregivers how to orient client to time, person, place, and circumstances, as required. ***These caregivers will be responsible for client safety after discharge from the hospital. Sharing successful interventions may be helpful.***
3. Give positive feedback when client thinking and behavior are appropriate or when client verbalizes that certain ideas expressed are not based in reality. ***Positive feedback increases self-esteem and enhances desire to repeat appropriate behaviors.***
4. Use simple explanations and face-to-face interaction when communicating with client. Do not shout message into client's ear. ***Speaking slowly and in a face-to-face position is most effective when communicating with an elderly individual experiencing a hearing loss. Visual cues facilitate understanding. Shouting causes distortion of high-pitched sounds and in some instances creates a feeling of discomfort for the client.***
5. Express reasonable doubt if client relays suspicious beliefs in response to delusional thinking. Discuss with client the potential personal negative effects of continued suspiciousness of others. Reinforce accurate perception of people and situations. ***Expressions of doubt by a trusted individual may foster in client similar uncertainties about delusions.***
6. Do not permit rumination on false ideas. When this begins, talk to client about real people and real events. ***Reality orientation increases client's sense of self-worth and personal dignity.***
7. Close observation of client's behavior is indicated if delusional thinking reveals an intention for violence. ***Client safety is a nursing priority.***

Outcome Criteria

1. With assistance from caregiver, client is able to distinguish between reality-based and nonreality-based thinking.

2. Prospective caregivers are able to verbalize ways of orienting client to reality, as needed.

SELF-CARE DEFICIT

Definition: *Impaired ability to perform or complete [activities of daily living (ADLs)] independently.*

Possible Etiologies ("related to")

[Disorientation]
[Confusion]
[Memory deficits]

Defining Characteristics ("evidenced by")

[Inability to fulfill ADLs]

Goals/Objectives

Short-Term Goal

Client will participate in ADLs with assistance from caregiver.

Long-Term Goal

Client will accomplish ADLs to the best of his or her ability. Unfulfilled needs will be met by caregiver.

Interventions with *Selected Rationales*

1. Provide a simple, structured environment ***to minimize confusion:***
   a. Identify self-care deficits, and provide assistance as required.
   b. Allow plenty of time for client to perform tasks.
   c. Provide guidance and support for independent actions by talking the client through a task one step at a time.
   d. Provide a structured schedule of activities that does not change from day to day.
   e. Ensure ADLs follow home routine as closely as possible.
   f. Provide for consistency in assignment of daily caregivers.
2. In planning for discharge:
   a. Perform ongoing assessment of client's ability to fulfill nutritional needs, ensure personal safety, follow medication regimen, and communicate need for assistance with those activities that he or she cannot accomplish independently. ***Client safety and security are nursing priorities.***
   b. Assess prospective caregivers' ability to anticipate and fulfill client's unmet needs. Provide information to assist caregivers with this responsibility. Ensure that caregivers are aware of available community support systems from which they can seek

assistance when required. ***This will facilitate transition to discharge from treatment center.***

c. National support organizations can provide information:
National Parkinson Foundation Inc.
1501 NW 9th Ave.
Miami, FL 33136
1-800-327-4545

Alzheimer's Association
919 N. Michigan Ave., Suite 1000
Chicago, IL 60611
1-800-272-3900

The Centers for Disease Control and Prevention (CDC)
AIDS Hotline
1-800-342-AIDS
(24 hours/day, 7 days/week)

Outcome Criteria

1. Client willingly participates in ADLs.
2. Client accomplishes ADLs to the best of his or her ability.
3. Client's unfulfilled needs are met by caregivers.

DISTURBED SENSORY PERCEPTION (Specify)

Definition: *Change in the amount or patterning of incoming stimuli [either internally or externally initiated] accompanied by a diminished, exaggerated, distorted, or impaired response to such stimuli.*

Possible Etiologies ("related to")

[Alteration in structure/function of brain tissue, secondary to the following conditions:
Advanced age
Vascular disease
Hypertension
Cerebral hypoxia
Abuse of mood- or behavior-altering substances
Exposure to environmental toxins
Various other physical disorders that predispose to cerebral abnormalities (see Predisposing Factors)]
AU3

Defining Characteristics ("evidenced by")

[Disorientation to time, place, person, or circumstances]
[Inability to concentrate]
[Visual and auditory distortions]
[Inappropriate responses]
[Talking and laughing to self]

[Suspiciousness]
Hallucinations

Goals/Objectives

Short-Term Goal

With assistance from caregiver, client will maintain orientation to time, place, person, and circumstances for specified period.

Long-Term Goal

Client will demonstrate accurate perception of the environment by responding appropriately to stimuli indigenous to the surroundings.

Interventions with *Selected Rationales*

1. Decrease the amount of stimuli in client's environment (e.g., low noise level, few people, simple decor). ***This decreases the possibility of client's forming inaccurate sensory perceptions.***
2. Do not reinforce the hallucination. Let client know that you do not share the perception. Maintain reality through reorientation and focus on real situations and people. ***Reality orientation decreases false sensory perceptions and enhances client's sense of self-worth and personal dignity.***
3. Provide reassurance of safety if client responds with fear to inaccurate sensory perception. ***Client safety and security are nursing priorities.***
4. Correct client's description of inaccurate perception, and describe the situation as it exists in reality. ***Explanation of and participation in real situations and real activities interfere with client's ability to respond to hallucinations.***
5. Teach prospective caregivers how to recognize signs and symptoms of client's inaccurate sensory perceptions. Explain techniques they may use to restore reality to the situation.
6. Allow for care to be given by same personnel on a regular basis, if possible, ***to provide client a feeling of security and stability in the environment.***

Outcome Criteria

1. With assistance from caregiver, client is able to recognize when perceptions of the environment are inaccurate.
2. Prospective caregivers are able to verbalize ways in which to correct inaccurate perceptions and restore reality to the situation.

LOW SELF-ESTEEM

Definition: *Negative self-evaluation or feelings about self or self capabilities.*

Possible Etiologies ("related to")

[Loss of independent functioning]
[Loss of capacity for remembering]
[Loss of capability for effective verbal communication]

Defining Characteristics ("evidenced by")

[Withdraws into social isolation]
[Lack of eye contact]
[Excessive crying alternating with expressions of anger]
[Refusal to participate in therapies]
[Refusal to participate in own self-care activities]
[Becomes increasingly dependent on others to perform ADLs]
Expressions of shame or guilt

Goals/Objectives

Short-Term Goal

Client will voluntarily spend time with staff and peers in dayroom activities within 1 week.

Long-Term Goal

By time of discharge, client will exhibit increased feelings of self-worth as evidenced by voluntary participation in own self-care and interaction with others.

Interventions with *Selected Rationales*

1. Encourage client to express honest feelings in relation to loss of prior level of functioning. Acknowledge pain of loss. Support client through process of grieving. ***Client may be fixed in anger stage of grieving process, which is turned inward on the self, resulting in diminished self-esteem.***
2. Devise methods for assisting client with memory deficit. Examples follow:
   a. Name sign on door identifying client's room.
   b. Identifying sign on outside of dining-room door.
   c. Identifying sign on outside of restroom door.
   d. Large clock, with oversized numbers and hands, placed appropriately.
   e. Large calendar, indicating one day at a time, with month, day, and year identified in bold print.
   f. Printed, structured daily schedule, with one copy for client and one posted on unit wall.
   g. "News board" on unit wall where current national and local events may be posted. ***These aids may assist client to function more independently, thereby increasing self-esteem.***
3. Encourage client's attempts to communicate. If verbalizations are not understandable, express to client what you think he or she

intended to say. It may be necessary to reorient client frequently. ***The ability to communicate effectively with others may enhance self-esteem.***

4. Encourage reminiscence and discussion of life review. Also discuss present-day events. Sharing picture albums, if possible, is especially good. ***Reminiscence and life review help the client resume progression through the grief process associated with disappointing life events and increase self-esteem as successes are reviewed.***
5. Encourage participation in group activities. Caregiver may need to accompany client at first until client feels secure that the group members will be accepting, regardless of limitations in verbal communication. ***Positive feedback from group members will increase self-esteem.***
6. Offer support and empathy when client expresses embarrassment at inability to remember people, events, and places. Focus on accomplishments ***to lift self-esteem.***
7. Encourage client to be as independent as possible in self-care activities. Provide written schedule of tasks to be performed. Intervene in areas where client requires assistance. ***The ability to perform independently preserves self-esteem.***

Outcome Criteria

1. Client initiates own self-care according to written schedule and willingly accepts assistance as needed.
2. Client interacts with others in group activities, maintaining anxiety at minimal level in response to difficulties with verbal communication.

CAREGIVER ROLE STRAIN

Definition: *Difficulty in performing family caregiver role.*

Possible Etiologies ("related to")

[Severity of the care receiver's illness]
[Duration of the care receiver's illness]
[Lack of respite and recreation for the caregiver]
Caregiver's competing role commitments
Inadequate physical environment for providing care
Family or caregiver isolation
Complexity and amount of caregiving tasks

Defining Characteristics ("evidenced by")

Apprehension about possible institutionalization of care receiver
Apprehension about future regarding care receiver's health and caregiver's ability to provide care

Difficulty performing required activities
[Inability to complete caregiving tasks]
Apprehension about care receiver's care when caregiver becomes ill or dies

Goals/Objectives

Short-Term Goal

Caregiver will verbalize understanding of ways to facilitate the caregiver role.

Long-Term Goal

Caregiver will demonstrate effective problem-solving skills and develop adaptive coping mechanisms to regain equilibrium.

Interventions with *Selected Rationales*

1. Assess caregivers' ability to anticipate and fulfill client's unmet needs. Provide information to assist caregivers with this responsibility. ***Caregivers may be unaware of what client will realistically be able to accomplish. They may be unaware of the progressive nature of the illness.***
2. Ensure that caregivers are aware of available community support systems from which they can seek assistance when required. Examples include adult day-care centers, housekeeping and homemaker services, respite-care services, and a local chapter of the Alzheimer's Disease and Related Disorders Association. This organization sponsors a nationwide 24-hour hot line to provide information and link families who need assistance with nearby chapters and affiliates. The hot line number is 1-800-272-3900. ***Caregivers require relief from the pressures and strain of providing 24-hour care for their loved ones. Studies show that elder abuse arises out of caregiving situations that place overwhelming stress on the caregivers.***
3. Encourage caregivers to express feelings, particularly anger. ***Release of these emotions can serve to prevent psychopathology, such as depression or psychophysiological disorders, from occurring.***
4. Encourage participation in support groups composed of members with similar life situations. ***Hearing others who are experiencing the same problems discuss ways in which they have coped may help caregiver adopt more adaptive strategies. Individuals who are experiencing similar life situations provide empathy and support for each other.***

Outcome Criteria

1. Caregivers are able to problem-solve effectively regarding care of elderly client.
2. Caregivers demonstrate adaptive coping strategies for dealing with stress of caregiver role.

3. Caregivers express feelings openly.
4. Caregivers express desire to join support group of other caregivers.

■ INTERNET REFERENCES

Additional information about Alzheimer's Disease is located at the following websites:

- http://www.alz.org
- http://www.alzheimers.org/adear
- http://www.brain.nwu.edu/
- http://www.ninds.nih.gov/health_and_medical/disorders/alzheimersdisease_doc.htm
- http://www.ahcpr.gov/clinic/alzcons.htm

Additional information on caregiving is located at the following website:

- http://www.aarp.org

Additional information about medications to treat Alzheimer's disease is located at the following websites:

- http://www.fadavis.com/townsend
- http://www.aafp.org/afp/981001ap/delagarz.html

CHAPTER 4

Substance-Related Disorders

■ BACKGROUND ASSESSMENT DATA

The substance-related disorders are composed of two groups: the substance-use disorders (dependence and abuse) and the substance-induced disorders (intoxication and withdrawal). Other substance-induced disorders (delirium, dementia, amnesia, psychosis, mood disorder, anxiety disorder, sexual dysfunction, and sleep disorders) are included in the chapters with which they share symptomatology (e.g., substance-induced mood disorders are included in Chapter 6; substance-induced sexual dysfunction is included in Chapter 10, etc.).

■ SUBSTANCE-USE DISORDERS

Substance Abuse*

Defined

The *DSM-IV-TR* defines substance abuse as a maladaptive pattern of substance use manifested by recurrent and significant adverse consequences related to repeated use of the substance. Criteria include the following:

1. Recurrent substance use resulting in a failure to fulfill major role obligations at work, school, or home.
2. Recurrent substance use in situations in which it is physically hazardous.
3. Recurrent substance-related legal problems.
4. Continued substance use despite having persistent or recurrent social or interpersonal problems caused or exacerbated by the effects of the substance.

---

* Classification and criteria for this and all subsequent diagnoses in this chapter marked with an asterisk are from the *Diagnostic and Statistical Manual of Mental Disorders, Fourth Edition, Text Revision, 2000.* Used with permission from the American Psychiatric Association.

Substance Dependence*

Defined

The *DSM-IV-TR* defines substance dependence by the following criteria:

1. Evidence of tolerance, as identified by either of the following:
   a. A need for increased amounts of the substance to achieve intoxication or the desired effect.
   b. Markedly diminished effect with continued use of the same amount of the substance.
2. Evidence of withdrawal symptoms, as manifested by either of the following:
   a. The characteristic withdrawal syndrome for the substance.
   b. The same (or closely related) substance is taken to relieve or avoid withdrawal symptoms.
3. The substance is often taken in larger amounts or over a longer period than was intended.
4. There is a persistent desire or unsuccessful effort to decrease or control substance use.
5. A great deal of time is spent in activities necessary to obtain or use the substance or to recover from the effects of the substance.
6. Important social, occupational, or recreational activities are given up or reduced because of substance use.
7. The substance use is continued despite knowledge of having a persistent or recurrent physical or psychological problem that is likely to have been caused or exacerbated by the substance.

■ SUBSTANCE-INDUCED DISORDERS

Substance Intoxication*

Defined

The *DSM-IV-TR* defines substance intoxication by the following criteria:

1. The development of a reversible substance-specific syndrome caused by recent ingestion of or exposure to a substance.
2. Clinically significant maladaptive behavior or psychological changes that are caused by the effect of the substance on the central nervous system (CNS) and that develop during or shortly after use of the substance.
3. The symptoms are not caused by a general medical condition and are not better accounted for by another mental disorder.

Substance Withdrawal*

Defined

The *DSM-IV-TR* defines substance withdrawal by the following criteria:

1. The development of a substance-specific syndrome caused by the cessation of or reduction in heavy and prolonged substance use.

2. The substance-specific syndrome causes clinically significant distress or impairment in social, occupational, or other important areas of functioning.
3. The symptoms are not caused by a general medical condition and are not better accounted for by another mental disorder.

CLASSIFICATION OF SUBSTANCES

Alcohol

303.90 Alcohol Dependence
305.00 Alcohol Abuse
303.00 Alcohol Intoxication
291.81 Alcohol Withdrawal

Even though alcohol is a depressant, it is discussed here instead of two sections later because of the complex effects and widespread nature of its use. Low to moderate consumption produces a feeling of well-being and reduced inhibitions. At higher concentrations, motor and intellectual functioning are impaired, mood becomes very labile, and behaviors characteristic of depression, euphoria, and aggression are exhibited. The only medical use for alcohol (with the exception of its inclusion in a number of pharmacological concentrates) is as an antidote for methanol consumption.

Examples: Beer, wine, bourbon, scotch, gin, vodka, rum, tequila, liqueurs.

Common substances containing alcohol and used by some dependent individuals to satisfy their need include liquid cough medications, liquid cold preparations, mouthwashes, isopropyl rubbing alcohol, nail polish removers, colognes, and aftershave and preshave preparations.

Opioids

304.00 Opioid Dependence
305.50 Opioid Abuse
292.89 Opioid Intoxication
292.0 Opioid Withdrawal

Opioids have a medical use as analgesics, antitussives, and antidiarrheals. They produce the effects of analgesia and euphoria by stimulating the opiate receptors in the brain, thereby mimicking the naturally occurring endorphins.

Examples: Opium, morphine, codeine, heroin, hydromorphone, meperidine, methadone.

Common street names: Horse, junk, H (heroin); black stuff, poppy, big O (opium); M, morph (morphine); dollies (methadone); terp (terpin hydrate or cough syrup with codeine).

CNS Depressants

304.10 Sedative, Hypnotic, or Anxiolytic Dependence
305.40 Sedative, Hypnotic, or Anxiolytic Abuse

292.89 Sedative, Hypnotic, or Anxiolytic Intoxication
292.0 Sedative, Hypnotic, or Anxiolytic Withdrawal

CNS depressants have a medical use as antianxiety agents, sedatives, hypnotics, anticonvulsants, and anesthetics. They depress the action of the CNS, resulting in an overall calming, relaxing effect on the individual. At higher dosages they can induce sleep.

Examples: Benzodiazepines, barbiturates, chloral hydrate, meprobamate.

Common street names: Peter, Mickey (chloral hydrate); green and whites, roaches (Librium); blues (Valium, 10 mg); yellows (Valium, 5 mg); red birds, red devils (secobarbital); blue birds (Amytal capsules); yellow birds (Nembutal); downers (barbiturates, tranquilizers).

CNS Stimulants

304.40 Amphetamine Dependence
305.70 Amphetamine Abuse
292.89 Amphetamine Intoxication
292.0 Amphetamine Withdrawal
305.90 Caffeine Intoxication
304.20 Cocaine Dependence
305.60 Cocaine Abuse
292.89 Cocaine Intoxication
292.0 Cocaine Withdrawal
305.1 Nicotine Dependence
292.0 Nicotine Withdrawal

CNS stimulants have a medical use in the management of hyperkinesia, narcolepsy, and weight control. They stimulate the action of the CNS, resulting in increased alertness, excitation, euphoria, increased pulse rate and blood pressure, insomnia, and loss of appetite.

Examples: Amphetamines, methylphenidate (Ritalin), phendimetrazine (Prelu-2), cocaine, hydrochloride cocaine, caffeine, tobacco.

Common street names: Bennies, wake-ups, uppers, speed (amphetamines); coke, snow, gold dust, girl (cocaine); crack, rock (hydrochloride cocaine); speedball (mixture of heroin and cocaine).

Hallucinogens

304.50 Hallucinogen Dependence
305.30 Hallucinogen Abuse
292.89 Hallucinogen Intoxication
304.60 Phencyclidine Dependence
305.90 Phencyclidine Abuse
292.89 Phencyclidine Intoxication

Hallucinogens act as sympathomimetic agents, producing effects resembling those resulting from stimulation of the sympathetic nervous system (e.g., excitation, increased energy, distortion of the senses). Therapeutic medical uses for lysergic acid diethylamide (LSD) have been proposed in the treatment of chronic alcoholism and in the reduction of intractable pain, such as terminal malignant disease and phantom limb sensations. At this time there is no real evidence of the safety and efficacy of the drug in humans.

Examples: LSD, mescaline, phencyclidine (PCP).

Common street names: Acid, cube, big D, California sunshine (LSD); angel dust, hog, peace pill, crystal (PCP); cactus, mescal, mesc (mescaline).

Cannabinols

304.30 Cannabis Dependence
305.20 Cannabis Abuse
292.89 Cannabis Intoxication

Cannabinols depress higher centers in the brain and consequently release lower centers from inhibitory influence. They produce an anxiety-free state of relaxation characterized by a feeling of extreme well-being. Large doses of the drug can produce hallucinations. Marijuana has been used therapeutically in the relief of nausea and vomiting associated with antineoplastic chemotherapy.

Examples: Marijuana, hashish.

Common street names: Joints, reefers, pot, grass, Mary Jane (marijuana); hash (hashish).

A profile summary of these psychoactive substances is presented in Table 4–1.

Predisposing Factors

1. **Physiological**
   a. ***Genetics.*** A genetic link may be involved in the development of substance-related disorders. This is especially evident in alcoholism, less so with other substances. Children of alcoholics are four times more likely than other children to become alcoholics (American Academy of Child & Adolescent Psychiatry, 1999). Studies with monozygotic and dizygotic twins support the genetic hypothesis.
   b. ***Biochemical.*** A second physiological hypothesis is the possibility that alcohol may produce morphine-like substances in the brain responsible for alcohol addiction. This occurs when the products of alcohol metabolism react with biologically active amines.
2. **Psychosocial**
   a. ***Psychodynamic Theory.*** The psychodynamic approach to the cause of substance abuse focuses on a punitive superego and fixation at the oral stage of psychosexual development (Kaplan and Sadock, 1998). Individuals with punitive superegos turn to alcohol to diminish unconscious anxiety. Kaplan and Sadock stated, "Anxiety in people fixated at the oral stage may be reduced by taking substances, such as alcohol, by mouth."

Table 4–1 Psychoactive Substances: A Profile Summary

Class of Drugs	Symptoms of Use	Therapeutic Uses	Symptoms of Overdose	Trade Names	Common Names
CNS Depressants Alcohol	Relaxation, loss of inhibitions, lack of concentration, drowsiness, slurred speech, sleep	Antidote for methanol consumption; ingredient in many pharmacological concentrates	Nausea, vomiting; shallow respirations; cold, clammy skin; weak, rapid pulse; coma; possible death	Ethyl alcohol, beer, gin, rum, vodka, bourbon, whiskey, liqueurs, wine, brandy, sherry, champagne	Booze, alcohol, liquor, drinks, cocktails, highballs, nightcaps, moonshine, white lightning, firewater
Other (barbiturates and nonbarbiturates)	Same as alcohol	Relief from anxiety and insomnia; as anticonvulsants and anesthetics	Anxiety, fever, agitation, hallucinations, disorientation, tremors, delirium, convulsions, possible death	Seconal, Nembutal, Amytal Valium Librium Noctec Miltown	Red birds, yellow birds Blues/yellows Green & whites Mickies Downers
CNS Stimulants Amphetamines and related drugs	Hyperactivity, agitation, euphoria, insomnia, loss of appetite	Management of narcolepsy, hyperkinesia, and weight control	Cardiac arrhythmias, headache, convulsions, hypertension, rapid heart rate, coma, possible death	Dexedrine, Didrex, Tenuate, Prelu-2, Ritalin, Fastin, Cylert, Meridia, Plegine	Uppers, pep pills, wake-ups, bennies, eye-openers, speed, black beauties, sweet A's

TABLE 4–1 Psychoactive Substances: A Profile Summary *(Continued)*

Class of Drugs	Symptoms of Use	Therapeutic Uses	Symptoms of Overdose	Trade Names	Common Names
Cocaine	Euphoria, hyperactivity, restlessness, talkativeness, increased pulse, dilated pupils, rhinitis	Topical anesthetic	Hallucinations, convulsions, pulmonary edema, respiratory failure, coma, cardiac arrest, possible death	Cocaine hydrochloride	Coke, flake, snow, dust, happy dust, gold dust, girl, cecil, C, toot, blow, crack
Opioids	Euphoria, lethargy, drowsiness, lack of motivation, constricted pupils	As analgesics; methadone in substitution therapy; heroin has no therapeutic use	Shallow breathing, slowed pulse, clammy skin, pulmonary edema, respiratory arrest, convulsions, coma, possible death	Heroin	Snow, stuff, H, harry, horse,
				Morphine	M, morph, Miss Emma
				Codeine	Schoolboy
				Dilaudid	Lords
				Demerol	Doctors
				Dolophine	Dollies
				Percodan	Perkies
				Talwin	T's
				Opium	Big O, black stuff

(Continued on the following page)

TABLE 4–1 Psychoactive Substances: A Profile Summary *(Continued)*

Class of Drugs	Symptoms of Use	Therapeutic Uses	Symptoms of Overdose	Trade Names	Common Names
Hallucinogens	Visual hallucinations, disorientation, confusion, paranoid delusions, euphoria, anxiety, panic, increased pulse	LSD has been proposed in the treatment of chronic alcoholism and in the reduction of intractable pain. No therapeutic use at this time.	Agitation, extreme hyperactivity, violence, hallucinations, psychosis, convulsions, possible death	LSD	Acid, cube, big D
				PCP	Angel dust, hog, peace pill
				Mescaline	Mesc
				DMT	Businessman's trip
				STP	Serenity and peace
Cannabinols	Relaxation, talkativeness, lowered inhibitions, euphoria, mood swings	Marijuana has been used for relief of nausea and vomiting associated with antineoplastic chemotherapy and to reduce eye pressure in glaucoma	Fatigue, paranoia, delusions, hallucinations, possible psychosis	Cannabis	Marijuana, pot, grass, joint, Mary Jane, MJ,
				Hashish	Hash, rope, sweet Lucy

Alcohol may also serve to increase feelings of power and self-worth in these individuals.

b. ***Social Learning Theory.*** The effects of modeling, imitation, and identification on behavior can be observed from early childhood onward. In relation to drug consumption, the family appears to be an important influence. Various studies show that children and adolescents are more likely to use substances if they have parents who provide a model for substance use (Hermes, 1993). Peers often exert a great deal of influence on a child or adolescent to encourage use of substances for the first time. Modeling may continue to be a factor in the use of substances once the individual enters the work force. This is particularly true in the work setting that provides plenty of leisure time with coworkers and where drinking is valued and is used to express group cohesiveness.

■ COMMON PATTERNS OF USE IN SUBSTANCE-RELATED DISORDERS

Symptomatology (Subjective and Objective Data)

Alcohol Abuse/Dependence

1. Begins with social drinking that provides feeling of relaxation and well-being. Soon requires more and more drinking to produce the same effects.
2. Drinks in secret; hides bottles of alcohol; drinks first thing in the morning (to "steady my nerves") and at any other opportunity that arises during the day.
3. As the disease progresses, may drink in binges. During a binge, drinking continues until the individual is too intoxicated or too sick to consume any more. Behavior borders on the psychotic, with the individual wavering in and out of reality.
4. Begins to have blackouts. Periods of amnesia occur (in the absence of intoxication or loss of consciousness) during which the individual is unable to remember periods of time or events that have occurred.
5. Experiences multisystem physiological impairments from chronic use that include (but are not limited to) the following:
   a. ***Peripheral Neuropathy:*** Numbness, tingling, pain in the extremities (caused by thiamine deficiency).
   b. ***Wernicke-Korsakoff Syndrome:*** Mental confusion, agitation, diplopia (caused by thiamine deficiency). Rapid deterioration to coma and death will occur without immediate thiamine replacement.
   c. ***Alcoholic Cardiomyopathy:*** Enlargement of the heart caused by an accumulation of excess lipids in myocardial cells. Symptoms of tachycardia, dyspnea, and arrhythmias may be evident.
   d. ***Esophagitis:*** Inflammation of and pain in the esophagus

e. ***Esophageal Varices:*** Distended veins in the esophagus, with risk of rupture and subsequent hemorrhage.
f. ***Gastritis:*** Inflammation of lining of the stomach caused by irritation from the alcohol, resulting in pain, nausea, vomiting, and possibility of bleeding because of erosion of blood vessels.
g. ***Pancreatitis:*** Inflammation of the pancreas, resulting in pain, nausea and vomiting, and abdominal distention. With progressive destruction to the gland, symptoms of diabetes mellitus could occur.
h. ***Alcoholic Hepatitis:*** Inflammation of the liver, resulting in enlargement, jaundice, right upper quadrant pain, and fever.
i. ***Cirrhosis of the Liver:*** Fibrous and degenerative changes occurring in response to chronic accumulation of large amounts of fatty acids in the liver. In cirrhosis, symptoms of alcoholic hepatitis progress to include the following:
   - **Portal Hypertension:** Elevation of blood pressure through the portal circulation resulting from defective blood flow through the cirrhotic liver.
   - **Ascites:** An accumulation of serous fluid in the peritoneal cavity.
   - **Hepatic Encephalopathy:** Liver disorder caused by inability of the liver to convert ammonia to urea (the body's natural method of discarding excess ammonia); as serum ammonia levels rise, confusion occurs, accompanied by restlessness, slurred speech, and fever. Without intervention, there is an eventual progression to coma and death.

Alcohol Intoxication

1. Symptoms of alcohol intoxication include disinhibition of sexual or aggressive impulses, mood lability, impaired judgment, impaired social or occupational functioning, slurred speech, incoordination, unsteady gait, nystagmus, and flushed face.
2. Intoxication usually occurs at blood alcohol levels between 100 and 200 mg/dL.

Alcohol Withdrawal

1. Occurs within 4 to 12 hours of cessation of or reduction in heavy and prolonged (several days or longer) alcohol use.
2. Symptoms include coarse tremor of hands, tongue, or eyelids; nausea or vomiting; malaise or weakness; tachycardia; sweating, elevated blood pressure; anxiety; depressed mood or irritability; transient hallucinations or illusions; headache; and insomnia.
3. Without aggressive intervention, the individual may progress to *alcohol withdrawal delirium* about the second or third day following cessation of or reduction in prolonged, heavy alcohol use. Symptoms include those described under the syndrome of delirium (see Chapter 3).

Amphetamine (or Amphetamine-like) Dependence/Abuse

1. The use of amphetamines is often initiated for their appetite-suppressant effect in an attempt to lose or control weight.
2. Amphetamines are also taken for the initial feeling of well-being and confidence.
3. They are typically taken orally, intravenously, or by nasal inhalation.
4. Chronic daily (or almost daily) use usually results in an increase in dosage over time to produce the desired effect.
5. Episodic use often occurs as binges, followed by an intense and unpleasant "crash" in which the individual experiences anxiety, irritability, and feelings of fatigue and depression.
6. Continued use appears to be related to a "craving" for the substance rather than to prevention or alleviation of withdrawal symptoms.

Amphetamine (or Amphetamine-like) Intoxication

1. Amphetamine intoxication usually begins with a "high" feeling, followed by the development of symptoms such as euphoria with enhanced vigor, gregariousness, hyperactivity, restlessness, hypervigilance, interpersonal sensitivity, talkativeness, anxiety, tension, alertness, grandiosity, stereotypical and repetitive behavior, anger, fighting, and impaired judgment (APA, 2000).
2. Physical signs and symptoms that occur include tachycardia or bradycardia, pupillary dilation, elevated or lowered blood pressure, perspiration or chills, nausea or vomiting, psychomotor retardation or agitation, muscular weakness, respiratory depression, chest pain or cardiac arrhythmias, confusion, seizures, dyskinesias, dystonias, or coma (APA, 2000).

Amphetamine (or Amphetamine-like) Withdrawal

1. Amphetamine withdrawal symptoms occur after cessation of or reduction in amphetamine (or a related substance) use that has been heavy and prolonged.
2. Symptoms of withdrawal develop within a few hours to several days and include fatigue; vivid, unpleasant dreams; insomnia or hypersomnia; increased appetite; and psychomotor retardation or agitation.

Cannabis Dependence/Abuse

1. Cannabis preparations are almost always smoked but may also be taken orally.
2. It is commonly regarded incorrectly to be a substance without potential for dependence.
3. Tolerance to the substance may result in increased frequency of its use.
4. Abuse is evidenced by participation in hazardous activities while motor coordination is impaired from cannabis use.

Cannabis Intoxication

1. Cannabis intoxication is characterized by impaired motor coordination, euphoria, anxiety, sensation of slowed time, impaired judgment, and social withdrawal that develops during or shortly after cannabis use (APA, 2000).
2. Physical symptoms include conjunctival injection, increased appetite, dry mouth, and tachycardia.
3. The impairment of motor skills lasts for 8 to 12 hours.

Cocaine Dependence/Abuse

1. Various forms are smoked, inhaled, injected, or taken orally.
2. Chronic daily (or almost daily) use usually results in an increase in dosage over time to produce the desired effect.
3. Episodic use often occurs as binges, followed by an intense and unpleasant "crash" in which the individual experiences anxiety, irritability, and feelings of fatigue and depression.
4. The drug user often abuses or is dependent on a CNS depressant to relieve the residual effects of cocaine.
5. Cocaine abuse and dependence lead to tolerance of the substance and subsequent use of increasing doses.
6. Continued use appears to be related to a "craving" for the substance rather than to prevention or alleviation of withdrawal symptoms.

Cocaine Intoxication

1. Symptoms develop during or shortly after use of cocaine.
2. Symptoms include euphoria or affective blunting, changes in sociability, hypervigilance, interpersonal sensitivity, anxiety, tension, anger, stereotyped behaviors, impaired judgment, and impaired social or occupational functioning.
3. Physical symptoms include tachycardia or bradycardia, pupillary dilation, elevated or lowered blood pressure, perspiration or chills, nausea or vomiting, psychomotor agitation or retardation, muscular weakness, respiratory depression, chest pain or cardiac arrhythmias, confusion, seizures, dyskinesias, dystonias, and coma.

Cocaine Withdrawal

1. Symptoms of withdrawal occur after cessation of or reduction in cocaine use that has been heavy and prolonged.
2. Symptoms of cocaine withdrawal include dysphoric mood; fatigue; vivid, unpleasant dreams; insomnia or hypersomnia; increased appetite; and psychomotor retardation or agitation.

Hallucinogen Dependence/Abuse

1. Hallucinogenic substances are taken orally.
2. Because the cognitive and perceptual impairment may last for up to 12 hours, use is generally episodic, because the individual must organize time during the daily schedule for its use.

3. Frequent use results in tolerance to the effects of the substance.
4. Dependence is rare, and most people are able to resume their previous lifestyle, following a period of hallucinogen use, without much difficulty.
5. Flashbacks may occur following cessation of hallucinogen use. These episodes consist of visual or auditory misperceptions usually lasting only a few seconds but sometimes lasting up to several hours.
6. Hallucinogens are highly unpredictable in the effects they may induce each time they are used.

Hallucinogen Intoxication

1. Symptoms of intoxication develop during or shortly after hallucinogen use.
2. Symptoms include marked anxiety or depression, ideas of reference, fear of losing one's mind, paranoid ideation, impaired judgment, and impaired social or occupational functioning.
3. Other symptoms include subjective intensification of perceptions, depersonalization, derealization, illusions, hallucinations, and synesthesias.

Inhalant Dependence/Abuse

1. Effects are induced by inhaling the vapors of volatile substances through the nose or mouth.
2. Examples of substances include glue, gasoline, paint, paint thinners, various cleaning chemicals, and typewriter correction fluid.
3. Use of inhalants often begins in childhood, and considerable family dysfunction is characteristic.
4. Use may be daily or episodic, and chronic use may continue into adulthood.
5. Tolerance has been reported among individuals with heavy use, but a withdrawal syndrome from these substances has not been well documented.

Inhalant Intoxication

1. Symptoms of intoxication develop during or shortly after use of or exposure to volatile inhalants.
2. Symptoms include belligerence, assaultiveness, apathy, impaired judgment, and impaired social or occupational functioning.
3. Physical symptoms include dizziness, nystagmus, incoordination, slurred speech, unsteady gait, lethargy, depressed reflexes, psychomotor retardation, tremor, generalized muscle weakness, blurred vision or diplopia, stupor or coma, and euphoria.

Nicotine Dependence

1. The effects of nicotine are induced through inhaling the smoke of cigarettes, cigars, or pipe tobacco or orally through the use of snuff or chewing tobacco.

2. Continued use results in a "craving" for the substance.
3. Nicotine is commonly used to relieve or to avoid withdrawal symptoms that occur when the individual has been in a situation where use is restricted.
4. Continued use despite knowledge of medical problems related to smoking is a particularly important health problem.

Nicotine Withdrawal

1. Symptoms of withdrawal develop within 24 hours after abrupt cessation of or reduction in nicotine use.
2. Symptoms include dysphoric or depressed mood, insomnia, irritability, frustration, anger, anxiety, difficulty concentrating, restlessness, decreased heart rate, and increased appetite.

Opioid Dependence/Abuse

1. Various forms are taken orally, intravenously, by nasal inhalation, and by smoking.
2. Dependence occurs after recreational use of the substance "on the street" or after prescribed use of the substance for relief of pain or cough.
3. Chronic use leads to remarkably high levels of tolerance.
4. Once abuse or dependence is established, substance procurement often comes to dominate the person's life.
5. Cessation or decreased consumption results in a "craving" for the substance and produces a specific syndrome of withdrawal.

Opioid Intoxication

1. Symptoms of intoxication develop during or shortly after opioid use.
2. Symptoms include euphoria (initially) followed by apathy, dysphoria, psychomotor agitation or retardation, impaired judgment, and impaired social or occupational functioning.
3. Physical symptoms include pupillary constriction, drowsiness or coma, slurred speech, and impairment in attention or memory.

Opioid Withdrawal

1. Symptoms occur after cessation of or reduction in heavy and prolonged opioid use. Symptoms can also occur after administration of an opioid antagonist after a period of opioid use.
2. Symptoms can occur within minutes to several days following use (or antagonist) and include dysphoric mood, nausea or vomiting, muscle aches, lacrimation or rhinorrhea, pupillary dilation, piloerection, sweating, abdominal cramping, diarrhea, yawning, fever, and insomnia.

Phencyclidine Dependence/Abuse

1. Phencyclidine (PCP) is taken orally, intravenously, or by smoking or inhaling.
2. Use can be on a chronic daily basis but is more often episodic in binges that can last several days.

3. Abuse or dependence can occur after only a short period of occasional use.
4. Unclear if tolerance or withdrawal symptoms develop with use of PCP.

PCP Intoxication

1. Symptoms develop during or shortly after PCP use.
2. Symptoms include belligerence, assaultiveness, impulsiveness, unpredictability, psychomotor agitation, impaired judgment, and impaired social or occupational functioning.
3. Physical symptoms occur within an hour or less of PCP use and include vertical or horizontal nystagmus, hypertension or tachycardia, numbness or diminished responsiveness to pain, ataxia, dysarthria, muscle rigidity, seizures or coma, and hyperacusis.

Sedative, Hypnotic, or Anxiolytic Dependence/Abuse

1. Effects are produced from oral intake of these substances.
2. Dependence can occur following recreational use of the substance "on the street" or after prescribed use of the substance for relief of anxiety or insomnia.
3. Chronic use leads to remarkably high levels of tolerance.
4. Once dependence develops, there is evidence of strong substance-seeking behaviors (obtaining prescriptions from several physicians or resorting to illegal sources to maintain adequate supplies of the substance).
5. Abrupt cessation of these substances can result in life-threatening withdrawal symptoms.

Sedative, Hypnotic, or Anxiolytic Intoxication

1. Symptoms of intoxication develop during or shortly after intake of sedatives, hypnotics, or anxiolytics.
2. Symptoms include inappropriate sexual or aggressive behavior, mood lability, impaired judgment, and impaired social or occupational functioning.
3. Physical symptoms of sedative, hypnotic, or anxiolytic intoxication include slurred speech, incoordination, unsteady gait, nystagmus, impairment in attention or memory, and stupor or coma.

Sedative, Hypnotic, or Anxiolytic Withdrawal

1. Withdrawal symptoms occur after cessation of or reduction in heavy and prolonged use of sedatives, hypnotics, or anxiolytics.
2. Symptoms occur within several hours to a few days after abrupt cessation or reduction in use of the drug.
3. Symptoms include autonomic hyperactivity (e.g., sweating or pulse rate higher than 100); increased hand tremors; insomnia; nausea or vomiting; transient visual, tactile, or auditory hallucinations or illusions; psychomotor agitation; anxiety; and grand mal seizures.

A summary of symptoms associated with the syndromes of intoxication and withdrawal is presented in Table 4–2.

TABLE 4–2 Summary of Symptoms Associated with the Syndromes of Intoxication and Withdrawal

Class of Drugs	Intoxication	Withdrawal	Comments
Alcohol	Aggressiveness, impaired judgment, impaired attention, irritability, euphoria, depression, emotional lability, slurred speech, incoordination, unsteady gait, nystagmus, flushed face	Tremors, nausea/vomiting, malaise, weakness, tachycardia, sweating, elevated blood pressure, anxiety, depressed mood, irritability, hallucinations, headache, insomnia, seizures	Alcohol withdrawal begins within 4–6 hours after last drink. May progress to delirium tremens on second or third day. Use of Librium or Serax is common for substitution therapy.
Amphetamines and related substances	Fighting, grandiosity, hypervigilance, psychomotor agitation, impaired judgment, tachycardia, pupillary dilation, elevated blood pressure, perspiration or chills, nausea and vomiting.	Anxiety, depressed mood, irritability, craving for the substance, fatigue, insomnia or hypersomnia, psychomotor agitation, paranoid and suicidal ideation.	Withdrawal symptoms usually peak within 2–4 days, although depression and irritability may persist for months. Antidepressants may be used.
Caffeine	Restlessness, nervousness, excitement, insomnia, flushed face, diuresis, gastrointestinal complaints, muscle twitching, rambling flow of thought and speech, cardiac arrhythmia, periods of inexhaustibility, psychomotor agitation	Headache, fatigue, anxiety, irritability, depression, nausea, vomiting, muscle pain and stiffness.	Caffeine is contained in coffee, tea, colas, cocoa, chocolate, some over-the-counter analgesics, "cold" preparations, and stimulants.
Cannabis	Euphoria, anxiety, suspiciousness, sensation of slowed time, impaired judgment, social withdrawal, tachycardia, conjunctival redness, increased appetite, hallucinations	Restlessness, irritability, insomnia, loss of appetite	Intoxication occurs immediately and lasts about 3 hours. Oral ingestion is more slowly absorbed and has longer-lasting effects.

TABLE 4–2 Summary of Symptoms Associated with the Syndromes of Intoxication and Withdrawal *(Continued)*

Class of Drugs	Intoxication	Withdrawal	Comments
Cocaine	Euphoria, fighting, grandiosity, hypervigilance, psychomotor agitation, impaired judgment, tachycardia, elevated blood pressure, pupillary dilation, perspiration or chills, nausea/vomiting, hallucinations, delirium	Depression, anxiety, irritability, fatigue, insomnia or hypersomnia, psychomotor agitation, paranoid or suicidal ideation, apathy, social withdrawal	Large doses of the drug can result in convulsions or death from cardiac arrhythmias or respiratory paralysis.
Inhalants	Belligerence, assaultiveness, apathy, impaired judgment, dizziness, nystagmus, slurred speech, unsteady gait, lethargy, depressed reflexes, tremor, blurred vision, stupor or coma, euphoria, irritation around eyes, throat, and nose		Intoxication occurs within 5 minutes of inhalation. Symptoms last 60–90 minutes. Large doses can result in death from CNS depression or cardiac arrhythmia.
Nicotine		Craving for the drug, irritability, anger, frustration, anxiety, difficulty concentrating, restlessness, decreased heart rate, increased appetite, weight gain, tremor, headaches, insomnia	Symptoms of withdrawal begin within 24 hours of last drug use and decrease in intensity over days, weeks, or sometimes longer.

(Continued on the following page)

TABLE 4–2 Summary of Symptoms Associated with the Syndromes of Intoxication and Withdrawal *(Continued)*

Class of Drugs	Intoxication	Withdrawal	Comments
Opioids	Euphoria, lethargy, somnolence, apathy, dysphoria, impaired judgment, pupillary constriction, drowsiness, slurred speech, constipation, nausea, decreased respiratory rate and blood pressure	Craving for the drug, nausea or vomiting, muscle aches, lacrimation or rhinorrhea, pupillary dilation, piloerection or sweating, diarrhea, yawning, fever, insomnia	Withdrawal symptoms appear within 6–8 hours after last dose, reach a peak in the second or third day, and disappear in 7–10 days.
Phencyclidine and related substances	Belligerence, assaultiveness, impulsiveness, psychomotor agitation, impaired judgment, nystagmus, increased heart rate and blood pressure, diminished pain response, ataxia, dysarthria, muscle rigidity, seizures, hyperacusis, delirium		Delirium can occur within 24 hours after use of phencyclidine or may occur up to a week following recovery from an overdose.
Sedatives, hypnotics, and anxiolytics	Disinhibition of sexual or aggressive impulses, mood lability, impaired judgment, slurred speech, incoordination, unsteady gait, impairment in attention or memory disorientation, confusion	Nausea or vomiting, malaise, weakness, tachycardia, sweating, anxiety, irritability, orthostatic hypotension, tremor, insomnia, seizures	Withdrawal may progress to delirium, usually within 1 week of last use. Long-acting barbiturates or benzodiazepines may be used in withdrawal substitution therapy.

Common Nursing Diagnoses and Interventions

(Interventions are applicable to various health-care settings, such as inpatient and partial hospitalization, community outpatient clinic, home health, and private practice.)

RISK FOR INJURY

Definition: ***At risk for injury as a result of [internal or external] environmental conditions interacting with the individual's adaptive and defensive resources.***

Related/Risk Factors ("related to")

[Substance intoxication]
[Substance withdrawal]
[Disorientation]
[Seizures]
[Hallucinations]
[Psychomotor agitation]
[Unstable vital signs]
[Delirium]
[Flashbacks]
[Panic level of anxiety]

Goals/Objectives

Short-Term Goal

Client's condition will stabilize within 72 hours.

Long-Term Goal

Client will not experience physical injury.

Interventions with *Selected Rationales*

1. Assess client's level of disorientation to determine specific requirements for safety. ***Knowledge of client's level of functioning is necessary to formulate appropriate plan of care.***
2. Obtain a drug history, if possible, to determine the following:
   a. Type of substance(s) used.
   b. Time of last ingestion and amount consumed.
   c. Length and frequency of consumption.
   d. Amount consumed on a daily basis.
3. Obtain a urine sample for laboratory analysis of substance content. ***Subjective history is often not accurate. Knowledge of substance ingestion is important for accurate assessment of client condition.***
4. Place client in quiet, private room. ***Excessive stimuli increase client agitation.***

5. Institute necessary safety precautions as follows:
   a. Observe client behaviors frequently; assign staff on one-to-one basis if condition is warranted; accompany and assist client when ambulating; use wheelchair for transporting client long distances.
   b. Be sure that side rails are up when client is in bed.
   c. Pad headboard and side rails of bed with thick towels to protect client in case of seizure.
   d. Use mechanical restraints as necessary to protect client if excessive hyperactivity accompanies disorientation. ***Client safety is a nursing priority.***
6. Ensure that smoking materials and other potentially harmful objects are stored away from client's access. ***Client may harm self or others in disoriented, confused state.***
7. Frequently orient client to reality and surroundings. ***Disorientation may endanger client safety if he or she unknowingly wanders away from safe environment.***
8. Monitor client's vital signs every 15 minutes initially and less frequently as acute symptoms subside. ***Vital signs provide the most reliable information about client condition and need for medication during acute detoxification period.***
9. Follow medication regimen, as ordered by physician. Common medical intervention for detoxification from the following substances includes:
   a. **Alcohol.** Chlordiazepoxide (Librium) is given orally every 4 to 8 hours in decreasing doses until withdrawal is complete. For clients with liver disease, accumulation of the longer-acting agents, such as chlordiazepoxide, may be problematic, and the use of the shorter-acting benzodiazepine, oxazepam (Serax), is more appropriate. Some physicians may order anticonvulsant medication to be used prophylactically; however, this is not a universal intervention. Multivitamin therapy, in combination with daily thiamine (either orally or by injection), is common protocol.
   b. **Narcotics.** Narcotic antagonists, such as naloxone (Narcan), naltrexone (ReVia), or nalmefene (Revex), are administered intravenously for narcotic overdose. Withdrawal is managed with rest and nutritional therapy. Substitution therapy to decrease withdrawal symptoms may include propoxyphene (Darvon) for weaker effects or methadone (Dolophine) for longer effects.
   c. **Depressants.** Substitution therapy to decrease withdrawal symptoms may include a long-acting barbiturate, such as phenobarbital (Luminal). The dosage required to suppress withdrawal symptoms is given. When stabilization has been achieved, the dose is gradually decreased by 30 mg/d until with-

drawal is complete. Long-acting benzodiazepines are commonly used for substitution therapy when the abused substance is a nonbarbiturate CNS depressant.

d. **Stimulants.** Treatment of overdose is geared toward stabilization of vital signs. Intravenous antihypertensives may be used, along with IV diazepam (Valium) to control seizures. Treatment is usually aimed at reducing drug craving and managing severe depression. The client is placed in a quiet atmosphere and allowed to sleep and eat as much as is needed or desired. Suicide precautions may need to be instituted. Therapy with tricyclic antidepressants (e.g., desipramine [Norpramin]) has been successful in treating the symptoms of cocaine withdrawal (Julien, 2001).
e. **Hallucinogens and Cannabinols.** Medications are normally not prescribed for withdrawal from these substances. However, in the event of overdose, diazepam (Valium) or chlordiazepoxide (Librium) may be given as needed to decrease agitation. Should psychotic reactions occur, they may be treated with antipsychotics, such as phenothiazines, haloperidol, or one of the newer atypical antipsychotic medications.

Outcome Criteria

1. Client is no longer exhibiting any signs or symptoms of substance intoxication or withdrawal.
2. Client shows no evidence of physical injury obtained during substance intoxication or withdrawal.

INEFFECTIVE DENIAL

Definition: *Conscious or unconscious attempt to disavow knowledge or meaning of an event in order to reduce anxiety or fear, but leading to the detriment of health.*

Possible Etiologies ("related to")

[Weak, underdeveloped ego]
[Underlying fears and anxieties]
[Low self-esteem]
[Fixation in early level of development]

Defining Characteristics ("evidenced by")

[Denies substance abuse or dependence]
[Denies that substance use creates problems in his or her life]
[Continues to use substance, knowing it contributes to impairment in functioning or exacerbation of physical symptoms]

[Uses substance(s) in physically hazardous situations]
[Use of rationalization and projection to explain maladaptive behaviors]
Unable to admit impact of disease on life pattern

Goals/Objectives

Short-Term Goal

Client will divert attention away from external issues and focus on behavioral outcomes associated with substance use.

Long-Term Goal

Client will verbalize acceptance of responsibility for own behavior and acknowledge association between substance use and personal problems.

Interventions with *Selected Rationales*

1. Begin by working to develop a trusting nurse-client relationship. Be honest. Keep all promises. ***Trust is the basis of a therapeutic relationship.***
2. Convey an attitude of acceptance to the client. Ensure that he or she understands "It is not *you* but your *behavior* that is unacceptable." ***An attitude of acceptance promotes feelings of dignity and self-worth.***
3. Provide information to correct misconceptions about substance abuse. Client may rationalize his or her behavior with statements such as, "I'm not an alcoholic. I can stop drinking any time I want. Besides, I only drink beer." or "I only smoke pot to relax before class. So what? I know lots of people who do. Besides, you can't get hooked on pot." ***Many myths abound regarding use of specific substances. Factual information presented in a matter-of-fact, nonjudgmental way explaining what behaviors constitute substance-related disorders may help the client focus on his or her own behaviors as an illness that requires help.***
4. Identify recent maladaptive behaviors or situations that have occurred in the client's life, and discuss how use of substances may have been a contributing factor. ***The first step in decreasing use of denial is for client to see the relationship between substance use and personal problems.***
5. Use confrontation with caring. Do not allow client to fantasize about his or her lifestyle (for example: "It is my understanding that the last time you drank alcohol, you . . ." or "The lab report shows that you were under the influence of alcohol when you had the accident that injured three people"). ***Confrontation interferes with client's ability to use denial; a caring attitude preserves self-esteem and avoids putting the client on the defensive.***
6. Do not accept rationalization or projection as client attempts to make excuses for or blame his or her behavior on other people or

situations. ***Rationalization and projection prolong denial that problems exist in the client's life because of substance use.***
7. Encourage participation in group activities. ***Peer feedback is often more accepted than feedback from authority figures. Peer pressure can be a strong factor as well as association with individuals who are experiencing or who have experienced similar problems.***
8. Offer immediate positive recognition of client's expressions of insight gained regarding illness and acceptance of responsibility for own behavior. ***Positive reinforcement enhances self-esteem and encourages repetition of desirable behaviors.***

Outcome Criteria

1. Client verbalizes understanding of the relationship between personal problems and use of substances.
2. Client verbalizes acceptance of responsibility for own behavior.
3. Client verbalizes understanding of substance dependence and abuse as an illness requiring ongoing support and treatment.

INEFFECTIVE COPING

Definition: *Inability to form a valid appraisal of the stressors, inadequate choices of practiced responses, and/or inability to use available resources.*

Possible Etiologies ("related to")

[Inadequate support systems]
[Inadequate coping skills]
[Underdeveloped ego]
[Possible hereditary factor]
[Dysfunctional family system]
[Negative role-modeling]
[Personal vulnerability]

Defining Characteristics ("evidenced by")

[Low self-esteem]
[Chronic anxiety]
[Chronic depression]
Inability to meet role expectations
[Alteration in societal participation]
Inability to meet basic needs
[Inappropriate use of defense mechanisms]
Abuse of chemical agents
[Low frustration tolerance]
[Need for immediate gratification]
[Manipulative behavior]

Goals/Objectives

Short-Term Goal

Client will express true feelings about using substances as a method of coping with stress.

Long-Term Goal

Client will be able to verbalize use of adaptive coping mechanisms, instead of substance abuse, in response to stress.

Interventions with *Selected Rationales*

1. Establish trusting relationship with client (be honest; keep appointments; be available to spend time). ***The therapeutic nurse-client relationship is built on trust.***
2. Set limits on manipulative behavior. Be sure that the client knows what is acceptable, what is unacceptable, and the consequences for violating the limits set. Ensure that all staff maintain consistency with this intervention. ***Client is unable to establish own limits, so limits must be set for him or her. Unless administration of consequences for violation of limits is consistent, manipulative behavior will not be eliminated.***
3. Encourage client to verbalize feelings, fears, anxieties. Answer any questions he or she may have regarding the disorder. ***Verbalization of feelings in a nonthreatening environment may help client come to terms with long-unresolved issues.***
4. Explain the effects of substance abuse on the body. Emphasize that prognosis is closely related to abstinence. ***Many clients lack knowledge regarding the deleterious effects of substance abuse on the body.***
5. Explore with client the options available to assist with stressful situations rather than resorting to substance abuse (e.g., contacting various members of Alcoholics Anonymous or Narcotics Anonymous, physical exercise, relaxation techniques, meditation). ***Client may have persistently resorted to chemical abuse and thus may possess little or no knowledge of adaptive responses to stress.***
6. Provide positive reinforcement for evidence of gratification delayed appropriately. ***Positive reinforcement enhances self-esteem and encourages client to repeat acceptable behaviors.***
7. Encourage client to be as independent as possible in own self-care. Provide positive feedback for independent decision making and effective use of problem-solving skills.

Outcome Criteria

1. Client is able to verbalize adaptive coping strategies as alternatives to substance use in response to stress.
2. Client is able to verbalize the names of support people from whom he or she may seek help when the desire for substance use is intense.

IMBALANCED NUTRITION: LESS THAN BODY REQUIREMENTS

Definition: *Intake of nutrients insufficient to meet metabolic needs.*

Possible Etiologies ("related to")

[Drinking alcohol instead of eating nourishing food]
[Eating only "junk food"]
[Eating nothing (or very little) while on a "binge"]
[No money for food (having spent what is available on substances)]
[Problems with malabsorption caused by chronic alcohol abuse]

Defining Characteristics ("evidenced by")

Loss of weight
Pale conjunctiva and mucous membranes
Poor muscle tone
[Poor skin turgor]
[Edema of extremities]
[Electrolyte imbalances]
[Cheilosis (cracks at corners of mouth)]
[Scaly dermatitis]
[Weakness]
[Neuropathies]
[Anemias]
[Ascites]

Goals/Objectives

Short-Term Goals

Client will gain 2 lb during next 7 days.
Client's electrolytes will be restored to normal within 1 week.

Long-Term Goal

Client will exhibit no signs or symptoms of malnutrition by discharge. (This is not a realistic goal for a chronic alcoholic client in the end stages of the disease. For such a client, it is more appropriate to establish short-term goals, as realistic step objectives, to use in the evaluation of care given.)

Interventions with *Selected Rationales*

1. In collaboration with dietitian, determine number of calories required to provide adequate nutrition and realistic (according to body structure and height) weight gain.
2. Maintain strict documentation of intake, output, and calorie count. ***This information is necessary to make an accurate nutritional assessment and maintain client safety.***

3. Weigh daily. ***Weight loss or gain is important assessment information.***
4. Determine client's likes and dislikes, and collaborate with dietitian to provide favorite foods. ***Client is more likely to eat foods that he or she particularly enjoys.***
5. Ensure that client receives small, frequent feedings, including a bedtime snack, rather than three larger meals. ***Large amounts of food may be objectionable, or even intolerable, to the client.***
6. Administer vitamin and mineral supplements, as ordered by physician, ***to improve nutritional state.***
7. If appropriate, ask family members or significant others to bring in special foods that client particularly enjoys.
8. Monitor laboratory results, and report significant changes to physician.
9. Explain the importance of adequate nutrition. ***Client may have inadequate or inaccurate knowledge about the contribution of good nutrition to overall wellness.***

Outcome Criteria

1. Client has achieved and maintained at least 90 percent of normal body weight.
2. Client's vital signs, blood pressure, and laboratory serum studies are within normal limits.
3. Client is able to verbalize importance of adequate nutrition.

CHRONIC LOW SELF-ESTEEM

Definition: *Long-standing negative self-evaluation and feelings about self or self-capabilities.*

Possible Etiologies ("related to")

[Retarded ego development]
[Dysfunctional family system]
[Lack of positive feedback]
[Perceived failures]

Defining Characteristics ("evidenced by")

[Difficulty accepting positive reinforcement]
[Failure to take responsibility for self-care]
[Self-destructive behavior (substance abuse)]
Lack of eye contact
[Withdraws into social isolation]
[Highly critical and judgmental of self and others]
[Sense of worthlessness]
[Fear of failure]

[Unable to recognize own accomplishments]
[Setting self for failure by establishing unrealistic goals]
[Unsatisfactory interpersonal relationships]
[Negative or pessimistic outlook]
[Denial of problems obvious to others]
[Projection of blame or responsibility for problems]
[Rationalizing personal failures]
[Hypersensitivity to slight criticism]
[Grandiosity]

Goals/Objectives

Short-Term Goal

Client will accept responsibility for personal failures and verbalize the role substances played in those failures.

Long-Term Goal

By time of discharge, client will exhibit increased feelings of self-worth as evidenced by verbal expression of positive aspects about self, past accomplishments, and future prospects.

Interventions with *Selected Rationales*

1. Be accepting of client and his or her negativism. ***An attitude of acceptance enhances feelings of self-worth.***
2. Spend time with client ***to convey acceptance and contribute toward feelings of self-worth.***
3. Help client recognize and focus on strengths and accomplishments. Discuss past (real or perceived) failures, but minimize amount of attention devoted to them beyond client's need to accept responsibility for them. ***Client must accept responsibility for own behavior before change in behavior can occur. Minimizing attention to past failures may help to eliminate negative ruminations and increase client's sense of self-worth.***
4. Encourage participation in group activities ***from which client may receive positive feedback and support from peers.***
5. Help client identify areas he or she would like to change about self and assist with problem-solving toward this effort. ***Low self-worth may interfere with client's perception of own problem-solving ability. Assistance may be required.***
6. Ensure that client is not becoming increasingly dependent and that he or she is accepting responsibility for own behaviors. ***Client must be able to function independently if he or she is to be successful within the less structured community environment.***
7. Ensure that therapy groups offer client simple methods of achievement. Offer recognition and positive feedback for actual accomplishments. ***Successes and recognition increase self-esteem.***
8. Provide instruction in assertiveness techniques: the ability to recognize the difference among passive, assertive, and aggressive

behaviors and the importance of respecting the human rights of others while protecting one's own human rights. ***Self-esteem is enhanced by the ability to interact with others in an assertive manner.***

9. Teach effective communication techniques, such as the use of "I" messages and placing emphasis on ways to avoid making judgmental statements.

Outcome Criteria

1. Client is able to verbalize positive aspects of self.
2. Client is able to communicate assertively with others.
3. Client is able to express an optimistic outlook for the future.

DEFICIENT KNOWLEDGE (EFFECTS OF SUBSTANCE ABUSE ON THE BODY)

Definition: *Absence or deficiency of cognitive information related to [the effects of substance abuse on the body and its interference with achievement and maintenance of optimal wellness].*

Possible Etiologies ("related to")

Lack of interest in learning
[Low self-esteem]
[Denial of need for information]
[Denial of risks involved with substance abuse]
Unfamiliarity with information resources

Defining Characteristics ("evidenced by")

[Abuse of substances]
[Statement of lack of knowledge]
[Statement of misconception]
[Request for information]
Verbalization of the problem

Goals/Objectives

Short-Term Goal

Client will be able to verbalize effects of [substance used] on the body following implementation of teaching plan.

Long-Term Goal

Client will verbalize the importance of abstaining from use of [substance] to maintain optimal wellness.

Interventions with *Selected Rationales*

1. Assess client's level of knowledge regarding effects of [substance]

on body. ***Baseline assessment of knowledge is required to develop appropriate teaching plan for client.***

2. Assess client's level of anxiety and readiness to learn. ***Learning does not take place beyond moderate level of anxiety.***
3. Determine method of learning most appropriate for client (e.g., discussion, question and answer, use of audio or visual aids, oral or written method). ***Level of education and development are important considerations as to methodology selected.***
4. Develop teaching plan, including measurable objectives for the learner. ***Measurable objectives provide criteria on which to base evaluation of the teaching experience.***
5. Include significant others, if possible. ***Lifestyle changes often affect all family members.***
6. Implement teaching plan at a time that facilitates and in a place that is conducive to optimal learning (e.g., in the evening when family members visit, in an empty, quiet classroom or group therapy room). ***Learning is enhanced by an environment with few distractions.***
7. Begin with simple concepts and progress to the more complex. ***Retention is increased if introductory material presented is easy to understand.***
8. Include information on physical effects of [substance]: substance's capacity for creating physiological and psychological dependence, its effects on family functioning, its effects on a fetus (and the importance of contraceptive use until abstinence has been achieved), and the importance of regular participation in an appropriate treatment program.
9. Provide activities for client and significant others in which to participate actively during the learning exercise. ***Active participation increases retention.***
10. Ask client and significant others to demonstrate knowledge gained by verbalizing information presented. ***Verbalization of knowledge gained is measurable in evaluating the teaching experience.***
11. Provide positive feedback for participation as well as for accurate demonstration of knowledge gained. ***Positive feedback enhances self-esteem and encourages repetition of acceptable behaviors.***
12. Evaluate teaching plan. Identify strengths and weaknesses as well as any changes that may enhance the effectiveness of the plan.

Outcome Criteria

1. Client is able to verbalize effects of [substance] on the body.
2. Client verbalizes understanding of risks involved in use of [substance].
3. Client is able to verbalize community resources for obtaining knowledge of and support with substance-related problems.

DYSFUNCTIONAL FAMILY PROCESSES: ALCOHOLISM

Definition: ***Psychosocial, spiritual, and physiological functions of the family unit are chronically disorganized, which leads to conflict, denial of problems, resistance to change, ineffective problem solving, and a series of self-perpetuating crises***

Possible Etiologies ("related to")

Abuse of alcohol
Genetic predisposition
Lack of problem-solving skills
Inadequate coping skills
Family history of alcoholism, resistance to treatment
Biochemical influences
Addictive personality

Defining Characteristics ("evidenced by")

Anxiety, anger/suppressed rage; shame and embarrassment
Emotional isolation/loneliness; vulnerability; repressed emotions
Disturbed family dynamics; closed communication systems, ineffective spousal communication and marital problems
Altered role function/disruption of family roles
Manipulation; dependency; criticizing; rationalization/denial of problems
Enabling to maintain drinking; refusal to get help/inability to accept and receive help appropriately

Goals/Objectives

Short-Term Goals

Family members will participate in individual family programs and support groups.
Family members will identify ineffective coping behaviors and consequences.
Family will initiate and plan for necessary lifestyle changes.

Long-Term Goal

Family members will take action to change self-destructive behaviors and alter behaviors that contribute to client's addiction.

Interventions with *Selected Rationales**

1. Review family history; explore roles of family members, circum-

* From Doenges, ME, Townsend, MC, and Moorhouse, MF: *Psychiatric Care Plans: Guidelines for Individualizing Care,* ed 3. Philadelphia, F.A. Davis, 1998.

stances involving alcohol use, strengths, areas of growth. ***This information determines areas for focus and potential for change.***

2. Explore how family members have coped with the client's addiction (e.g., denial, repression, rationalization, hurt, loneliness, projection). ***Persons who enable also suffer from the same feelings as the client and use ineffective methods for dealing with the situation, necessitating help in learning new and effective coping skills.***
3. Determine understanding of current situation and previous methods of coping with life's problems. ***Provides information on which to base present plan of care.***
4. Assess current level of functioning of family members. ***Affects individual's ability to cope with the situation.***
5. Determine extent of enabling behaviors being evidenced by family members; explore with each individual and client. ***Enabling is doing for the client what he or she needs to do for self (rescuing). People want to be helpful and do not want to feel powerless to help their loved one to stop substance use and change the behavior that is so destructive. However, the substance abuser often relies on others to cover up own inability to cope with daily responsibilities.***
6. Provide information about enabling behavior and addictive disease characteristics for both the user and nonuser. ***Awareness and knowledge of behaviors (e.g., avoiding and shielding, taking over responsibilities, rationalizing, and subserving) provide opportunity for individuals to begin the process of change.***
7. Identify and discuss sabotage behaviors of family members. ***Even though family members may verbalize a desire for the individual to become substance-free, the reality of interactive dynamics is that they may unconsciously not want the individual to recover, as this would affect the family members' own roles in the relationship. Additionally, they may receive sympathy or attention from others (secondary gain).***
8. Encourage participation in therapeutic writing, e.g., journaling (narrative), guided or focused. ***Serves as a release for feelings (e.g., anger, grief, stress); helps move client forward in treatment process.***
9. Provide factual information to client and family about the effects of addictive behaviors on the family and what to expect after discharge. ***Many people are unaware of the nature of addiction. If client is using legally obtained drugs, he or she may believe this does not constitute abuse.***
10. Encourage family members to be aware of their own feelings, to look at the situation with perspective and objectivity. They can ask themselves: "Am I being conned? Am I acting out of fear, shame, guilt, or anger? Do I have a need to control?" ***When the enabling family members become aware of their own actions***

that perpetuate the client's problems, they need to decide to change themselves. If they change, the client can then face the consequences of own actions and may choose to get well.

11. Provide support for enabling family members. ***For change to occur, families need support as much as the person who has the problem with alcohol.***
12. Assist the client's partner to become aware that client's abstinence and drug use are not the partner's responsibility. ***Partners need to learn that the client's use of substances may or may not change despite partner's involvement in treatment.***
13. Help a recovering (former user) partner who is enabling to distinguish between destructive aspects of own behavior and genuine motivation to aid the client. ***Enabling behavior can be a recovering individual's attempts at personal survival.***
14. Note how the partner relates to the treatment team and staff. ***Determines enabling style. A parallel exists between how partner relates to client and to staff, based on the partner's feelings about self and situation.***
15. Explore conflicting feelings the enabling partner may have about treatment (e.g., feelings similar to those of the substance abuser [blend of anger, guilt, fear, exhaustion, embarrassment, loneliness, distrust, grief, and possibly relief]). ***This is useful in establishing the need for therapy for the partner. This individual's own identity may have been lost—he or she may fear self-disclosure to staff and may have difficulty giving up the dependent relationship.***
16. Involve family in discharge referral plans. ***Alcohol abuse is a family illness. Because the family has been so involved in dealing with the substance abuse behavior, family members need help adjusting to the new behavior of sobriety/abstinence. Incidence of recovery is almost doubled when the family is treated along with the client.***
17. Be aware of staff's enabling behaviors and feelings about client and enabling family members. ***Lack of understanding of enabling and codependence can result in nontherapeutic approaches to clients and their families.***
18. Encourage involvement with self-help associations, such as Alcoholics Anonymous, Al-Anon, Alateen, and professional family therapy. ***Puts client and family in direct contact with support systems necessary for continued sobriety and assists with problem resolution.***

Outcome Criteria

1. Family verbalizes understanding of dynamics of enabling behaviors.
2. Family members demonstrate patterns of effective communication.

3. Family members regularly participate in self-help support programs.
4. Family members demonstrate behaviors required to change destructive patterns of behavior that contribute to and enable dysfunctional family process.

INTERNET REFERENCES

Additional information on addictions is located at the following websites:

- http://www.addictions.org/recoveryworks/
- http://www.ncbi.nlm.nih.gov
- http://www.liebertpub.com
- http://www.drugs.indiana.edu

Additional information on self-help organizations is located at the following websites:

- http://www.ca.org (Cocaine Anonymous)
- http://www.aa.org (Alcoholics Anonymous)
- http://www.na.org (Narcotics Anonymous)

Additional information about medications for treatment of alcohol and drug dependence is located at the following websites:

- http://www.fadavis.com/townsend
- http://www.nlm.nih.gov/medlineplus

CHAPTER 5

Schizophrenia and Other Psychotic Disorders

BACKGROUND ASSESSMENT DATA

The syndrome of symptoms associated with schizophrenia and other psychotic disorders reveals alterations in content and organization of thoughts, perception of sensory input, affect or emotional tone, sense of identity, volition, psychomotor behavior, and ability to establish satisfactory interpersonal relationships.

Categories*

295.30 Paranoid Schizophrenia

This type is characterized by extreme suspiciousness of others and by delusions and hallucinations of a persecutory or grandiose nature. The individual is often tense and guarded and may be argumentative, hostile, and aggressive.

295.10 Disorganized Schizophrenia

Behavior is typically regressive and primitive. Affect is inappropriate, with common characteristics being silliness, incongruous giggling, facial grimaces, and extreme social withdrawal. Communication is consistently incoherent.

295.20 Catatonic Schizophrenia

This type manifests itself in the form of *stupor* (marked psychomotor retardation, mutism, waxy flexibility [posturing], negativism, and rigidity) or *excitement* (extreme psychomotor agitation, leading to exhaustion or the possibility of hurting self or others if not curtailed).

---

* Classification and criteria for this and all subsequent diagnoses in this chapter marked with an asterisk are from the *Diagnostic and Statistical Manual of Mental Disorders, Fourth Edition, Text Revision, 2000.* Used with permission from the American Psychiatric Association.

295.90 Undifferentiated Schizophrenia

This is characterized by disorganized behaviors and psychotic symptoms (e.g., delusions, hallucinations, incoherence, and grossly disorganized behavior), which may appear in more than one category.

295.60 Residual Schizophrenia

Behavior is eccentric, but psychotic symptoms, if present at all, are not prominent. Social withdrawal and inappropriate affect are characteristic. The patient has a history of at least one episode of schizophrenia in which psychotic symptoms were prominent.

295.70 Schizoaffective Disorder

The behaviors are characteristic of schizophrenia, in addition to those indicative of disorders of mood, such as depression or mania.

298.8 Brief Psychotic Disorder

The essential features include a sudden onset of psychotic symptoms in response to a severe psychosocial stressor. The symptoms last at least 1 day but less than 1 month, with a virtual return to the premorbid level of functioning. The diagnosis is further specified by whether it follows a severe identifiable stressor or whether the onset occurs within 4 weeks postpartum.

295.40 Schizophreniform Disorder

The essential features are identical to the characteristic symptoms of schizophrenia (i.e.: delusions, hallucinations, disorganized speech and behaviors), with the exception that the duration is at least 1 month but less than 6 months. The diagnosis is termed "provisional" if a diagnosis must be made prior to recovery.

297.1 Delusional Disorder

Delusional disorder is characterized by the presence of one or more nonbizarre delusions that persist for at least 1 month. Hallucinatory activity is not prominent. Apart from the delusions, behavior is not bizarre. The following types are based on the predominant delusional theme (APA, 2000):

1. **Persecutory Type.** Delusions that one is being malevolently treated in some way.
2. **Jealous Type.** Delusions that one's sexual partner is unfaithful.
3. **Erotomanic Type.** Delusions that another person of higher status is in love with him or her.
4. **Somatic Type.** Delusions that the person has some physical defect, disorder, or disease.
5. **Grandiose Type.** Delusions of inflated worth, power, knowledge, or special identity or special relationship to a deity or famous person.

297.3 Shared Psychotic Disorder (Folie à Deux)

A delusional system develops in the context of a close relationship with another person who already has a psychotic disorder with prominent delusions.

293.xx Psychotic Disorder due to a General Medical Condition

The *DSM-IV-TR* identifies the essential features of this disorder as prominent hallucinations and delusions that can be directly attributed to a general medical condition. Examples of general medical conditions that may cause psychotic symptoms include neurological conditions (e.g., neoplasms, Huntington's disease, central nervous system [CNS] infections), endocrine conditions (e.g., hyperthyroidism, hypothyroidism, hypoadrenocorticism), metabolic conditions (e.g., hypoxia, hypercarbia, hypoglycemia), autoimmune disorders (e.g., systemic lupus erythematosus), and others (e.g., fluid or electrolyte imbalances, hepatic or renal diseases).

Substance-Induced Psychotic Disorder (See Chapter 4 for substance-specific codes)

The essential features are the presence of prominent hallucinations and delusions that are judged to be directly attributable to the physiological effects of a substance (i.e., a drug of abuse, a medication, or toxin exposure) (APA, 2000).

Predisposing Factors

1. **Physiological**
   a. ***Genetics.*** Studies (Black and Andreasen, 1994; Kaplan and Sadock, 1998) indicate that certain genetic factors may be involved in the development of a psychotic disorder. Results show that individuals are at higher risk for the disorder if there is a familial pattern of involvement (parents, siblings, other relatives).
   b. ***Histological Changes.*** Scheibel (1991) suggested that schizophrenic disorders may in fact be a birth defect, occurring in the hippocampus region of the brain, and related to an influenza virus encountered by the mother during the second trimester of pregnancy. The studies show a "disordering" of the pyramidal cells in the brains of schizophrenics, but the cells in the brains of nonschizophrenic individuals appeared to be arranged in an orderly fashion. Further research is required to determine the possible link between this birth defect and the development of schizophrenia.
   c. ***The Dopamine Hypothesis.*** A biochemical theory suggests the involvement of elevated levels of the neurotransmitter dopamine, which is thought to produce the symptoms of overactivity and fragmentation of associations that are commonly observed in psychoses (Hollandsworth, 1990).

d. ***Anatomical Abnormalities.*** Computed tomographic scan abnormalities occur in up to 40 percent of schizophrenic patients (Black and Andreasen, 1999). Ventricular enlargement is the most consistent finding; however sulci enlargement and cerebellar atrophy are also reported.

2. **Environmental**

a. ***Sociocultural Factors.*** Many studies have attempted to link schizophrenia to social class. Indeed, epidemiological statistics show that greater numbers of individuals from the lower socioeconomic classes experience symptoms associated with schizophrenia than do those from the higher socioeconomic groups (Black and Andreasen, 1994). This may occur as a result of the conditions associated with living in poverty, such as congested housing accommodations, inadequate nutrition, absence of prenatal care, few resources for dealing with stressful situations, and feelings of hopelessness for changing one's lifestyle of poverty.

An alternative view is that of the *downward drift hypothesis* (Kaplan and Sadock, 1998). This hypothesis relates the schizophrenic's move into or failure to move out of the low socioeconomic group to the tendency for social isolation and the segregation of self from others—characteristics of the disease process itself. Proponents of this notion view poor social conditions as a consequence rather than as a cause of schizophrenia.

b. ***Stressful Life Events.*** Some studies have tried to determine whether psychotic episodes may be precipitated by stressful life events. There is no scientific evidence to indicate that stress causes schizophrenia. However, it is very probable that stress may contribute to the severity and course of the illness. It is known that extreme stress can precipitate psychotic episodes (Sackeim and Mukherjee, 1992). Stress may precipitate symptoms in an individual who possesses a genetic vulnerability to schizophrenia. Kaplan and Sadock (1998) state: "The stress can be biological, environmental, or both. The environmental component can be either biological (e.g., an infection) or psychological (e.g., a stressful family situation)." (p. 459)

Stressful life events may be associated with exacerbation of schizophrenic symptoms and increased rates of relapse.

Symptomatology (Subjective/Objective Data)

1. **Autism.** There is a focus inward. The psychotic individual may create his or her own world. Words and events may take on special meaning of a highly symbolic nature that only the individual can understand.
2. **Emotional Ambivalence.** Powerful emotions of love, hate, and fear produce much conflict within the psychotic individual. Each

emotion tends to balance the other until an emotional neutralization occurs and the individual experiences apathy or indifference.

3. **Inappropriate Affect.** The affect is blunted or flat and often inappropriate (e.g., person who laughs when told of the death of a parent).
4. **Associative Looseness.** This term describes the very disorganized thoughts and verbalizations of the psychotic person. Ideas shift from one unrelated subject to another. When the condition is severe, speech may be incoherent.
5. **Echolalia.** The psychotic person often repeats words he or she hears.
6. **Echopraxia.** The psychotic person often repeats movements he or she sees in others. (Echolalia and echopraxia are products of the person's very weak ego boundaries.)
7. **Neologisms.** Words that are invented by the psychotic person are meaningless to others but have symbolic meaning to the individual.
8. **Concrete Thinking.** The psychotic person has difficulty thinking on the abstract level and may use literal translations concerning aspects of the environment.
9. **Clang Associations.** The psychotic individual uses rhyming words in a nonsensical pattern.
10. **Word Salad.** The psychotic person may put together a random jumble of words.
11. **Mutism.** Psychotic individuals may refuse or be unable to speak.
12. **Circumstantiality.** This is a psychotic person's delay in reaching the point of a communication because of unnecessary and tedious details.
13. **Tangentiality.** Tangentiality differs from circumstantiality in that the psychotic person never gets to the point of the communication. Unrelated topics are introduced, and the original discussion is lost.
14. **Perseveration.** The psychotic individual may persistently repeat the same word or idea in response to different questions.
15. **Delusions.** These are false ideas or beliefs. Types of delusions include the following:
    a. ***Grandeur.*** The psychotic person has an exaggerated feeling of importance or power.
    b. ***Persecution.*** The psychotic person feels threatened and believes others intend harm or persecution toward him or her in some way.
    c. ***Reference.*** All events within the environment are referred by the psychotic person to himself or herself.
    d. ***Control or Influence.*** The psychotic individual believes certain objects or people have control over his or her behavior.
16. **Hallucinations.** Hallucinations are false sensory perceptions that may involve any of the five senses. Auditory and visual hallucina-

tions are most common, although olfactory, tactile, and gustatory hallucinations can occur.

17. **Regression.** This is a primary ego defense mechanism used in psychoses. Childlike mannerisms and comfort techniques are employed. Socially inappropriate behavior may be evident.
18. **Religiosity.** The psychotic person becomes preoccupied with religious ideas, a defense mechanism thought to be used in an attempt to provide stability and structure to disorganized thoughts and behaviors.

Common Nursing Diagnoses and Interventions

(Interventions are applicable to various health-care settings, such as inpatient and partial hospitalization, community outpatient clinic, home health, and private practice.)

■ RISK FOR SELF-DIRECTED OR OTHER-DIRECTED VIOLENCE

Definition: ***At risk for behaviors in which an individual demonstrates that he or she can be physically, emotionally, and/or sexually harmful either to self or to others.***

Related/Risk Factors ("related to")

[Lack of trust (suspiciousness of others)]
[Panic level of anxiety]
[Catatonic excitement]
[Negative role modeling]
[Rage reactions]
[Command hallucinations]
[Delusional thinking]
Body language—rigid posture, clenching of fists and jaw, hyperactivity, pacing, breathlessness, and threatening stances.
[History or threats of violence toward self or others or of destruction of the property of others]
Impulsivity
Suicidal ideation, plan, available means
[Perception of the environment as threatening]
[Receiving auditory or visual "suggestions" of a threatening nature]

Goals/Objectives

Short-Term Goals

1. Within [a specified time], client will recognize signs of increasing anxiety and agitation and report to staff for assistance with intervention.
2. Client will not harm self or others.

Long-Term Goal

Client will not harm self or others.

Interventions with *Selected Rationales*

1. Maintain low level of stimuli in client's environment (low lighting, few people, simple decor, low noise level). ***Anxiety level rises in a stimulating environment. A suspicious, agitated client may perceive individuals as threatening.***
2. Observe client's behavior frequently (every 15 minutes). Do this in a manner of carrying out routine activities ***so as to avoid creating suspiciousness in the individual. Close observation is necessary so that intervention can occur if required to ensure client (and others') safety.***
3. Remove all dangerous objects from client's environment ***so that in his or her agitated, confused state client may not use them to harm self or others.***
4. Try to redirect the violent behavior to physical outlets for the client's anxiety (e.g., punching bag). ***Physical exercise is a safe and effective way of relieving pent-up tension.***
5. Staff should maintain and convey a calm attitude toward client. ***Anxiety is contagious and can be transmitted from staff to client.***
6. Have sufficient staff available to indicate a show of strength to client if it becomes necessary. ***This shows the client evidence of control over the situation and provides some physical security for staff.***
7. Administer tranquilizing medications as ordered by physician. Monitor medication for its effectiveness and for any adverse side effects. ***The avenue of the "least restrictive alternative" must be selected when planning interventions for a client.***
8. If client is not calmed by "talking down" or by medication, use of mechanical restraints may be necessary. Be sure to have sufficient staff available to assist. Follow protocol established by the institution. The Joint Commission on Accreditation of Healthcare Organizations requires that the physician reissue a new order for restraints every 4 hours for adults and every 1 to 2 hours for children and adolescents. If client has previously refused medication, administer after restraints have been applied. Most states consider this intervention appropriate in emergency situations or in the event that a client would likely harm self or others.
9. Observe client in restraints every 15 minutes (or according to institutional policy). Ensure that circulation to extremities is not compromised (check temperature, color, and pulses). Assist client with needs related to nutrition, hydration, and elimination. Position client so that comfort is facilitated and aspiration can be prevented. ***Client safety is a nursing priority.***
10. As agitation decreases, assess client's readiness for restraint re-

moval or reduction. Remove one restraint at a time while assessing client's response. ***This minimizes risk of injury to client and staff.***

Outcome Criteria

1. Anxiety is maintained at a level at which client feels no need for aggression.
2. Client demonstrates trust of others in his or her environment.
3. Client maintains reality orientation.
4. Client causes no harm to self or others.

SOCIAL ISOLATION

Definition: *Aloneness experienced by the individual and perceived as imposed by others and as a negative or threatened state.*

Possible Etiologies ("related to")

[Lack of trust]
[Panic level of anxiety]
[Regression to earlier level of development]
[Delusional thinking]
[Past experiences of difficulty in interactions with others]
[Weak ego development]
[Repressed fears]

Defining Characteristics ("evidenced by")

[Staying alone in room]
Uncommunicative, withdrawn, no eye contact, [mutism, autism]
Sad; dull affect
[Lying on bed in fetal position with back to door]
Inappropriate or immature interests and activities for developmental age or stage
Preoccupation with own thoughts; repetitive, meaningless actions
[Approaching staff for interaction, then refusing to respond to staff's acknowledgment]
Expression of feelings of rejection or of aloneness imposed by others

Goals/Objectives

Short-Term Goal

Client will willingly attend therapy activities accompanied by trusted staff member within 1 week.

Long-Term Goal

Client will voluntarily spend time with other clients and staff members in group activities in the unit by time of discharge.

Interventions with *Selected Rationales*

1. Convey an accepting attitude by making brief, frequent contacts. ***An accepting attitude increases feelings of self-worth and facilitates trust.***
2. Show unconditional positive regard. ***This conveys your belief in the client as a worthwhile human being.***
3. Be with the client to offer support during group activities that may be frightening or difficult for him or her. ***The presence of a trusted individual provides emotional security for the client.***
4. Be honest, and keep all promises. ***Honesty and dependability promote a trusting relationship.***
5. Orient client to time, person, and place, as necessary.
6. Be cautious with touch. Allow client extra space and an avenue for exit if he or she becomes too anxious. ***A suspicious client may perceive touch as a threatening gesture.***
7. Administer tranquilizing medications as ordered by physician. Monitor for effectiveness and for adverse side effects. ***Antipsychotic medications help to reduce psychotic symptoms in some individuals, thereby facilitating interactions with others.***
8. Discuss with client the signs of increasing anxiety and techniques for interrupting the response (e.g., relaxation exercises, thought stopping). ***Maladaptive behaviors such as withdrawal and suspiciousness are manifested during times of increased anxiety.***
9. Give recognition and positive reinforcement for client's voluntary interactions with others. ***Positive reinforcement enhances self-esteem and encourages repetition of acceptable behaviors.***

Outcome Criteria

1. Client demonstrates willingness and desire to socialize with others.
2. Client voluntarily attends group activities.
3. Client approaches others in appropriate manner for one-to-one interaction.

INEFFECTIVE COPING

Definition: *Inability to form a valid appraisal of the stressors, inadequate choices of practiced responses, and/or inability to use available resources.*

Possible Etiologies ("related to")

[Inability to trust]
[Panic level of anxiety]
[Personal vulnerability]
[Low self-esteem]
[Inadequate support systems]

[Negative role model]
[Repressed fears]
[Underdeveloped ego]
[Possible hereditary factor]
[Dysfunctional family system]

Defining Characteristics ("evidenced by")

[Suspiciousness of others, resulting in:
Alteration in societal participation
Inability to meet basic needs
Inappropriate use of defense mechanisms]

Goals/Objectives

Short-Term Goal

Client will develop trust in at least one staff member within 1 week.

Long-Term Goal

Client will demonstrate use of more adaptive coping skills as evidenced by appropriateness of interactions and willingness to participate in the therapeutic community.

Interventions with *Selected Rationales*

1. Encourage same staff to work with client as much as possible ***in order to promote development of trusting relationship.***
2. Avoid physical contact. ***Suspicious clients may perceive touch as a threatening gesture.***
3. Avoid laughing, whispering, or talking quietly where client can see but not hear what is being said. ***Suspicious clients often believe others are discussing them, and secretive behaviors reinforce paranoid feelings.***
4. Be honest, and keep all promises. ***Honesty and dependability promote a trusting relationship.***
5. A creative approach may have to be used to encourage food intake (e.g., canned food and own can opener or family-style meals). ***Suspicious clients may believe they are going to be poisoned and refuse to eat food from the individually prepared tray.***
6. Mouth checks may be necessary following medication administration ***to verify whether client is swallowing the tablets or capsules. Suspicious clients may believe they are being poisoned with their medication and attempt to discard the pills.***
7. Activities should never include anything competitive. Activities that encourage a one-to-one relationship with the nurse or therapist are best. ***Competitive activities are very threatening to suspicious clients.***
8. Encourage client to verbalize true feelings. The nurse should avoid becoming defensive when angry feelings are directed at him or her. ***Verbalization of feelings in a nonthreatening environment may help client come to terms with long-unresolved issues.***

9. An assertive, matter-of-fact, yet genuine approach is least threatening and most therapeutic. ***A suspicious person does not have the capacity to relate to an overly friendly, overly cheerful attitude.***

Outcome Criteria

1. Client is able to appraise situations realistically and refrain from projecting own feelings onto the environment.
2. Client is able to recognize and clarify possible misinterpretations of the behaviors and verbalizations of others.
3. Client eats food from tray and takes medications without evidence of mistrust.
4. Client appropriately interacts and cooperates with staff and peers in therapeutic community setting.

DISTURBED SENSORY PERCEPTION: AUDITORY/VISUAL

Definition: *Change in the amount or patterning of incoming stimuli [either internally or externally initiated] accompanied by a diminished, exaggerated, distorted, or impaired response to such stimuli.*

Possible Etiologies ("related to")

[Panic level of anxiety]
[Withdrawal into self]
[Stress sufficiently severe to threaten an already weak ego]

Defining Characteristics ("evidenced by")

[Talking and laughing to self]
[Listening pose (tilting head to one side as if listening)]
[Stops talking in middle of sentence to listen]
[Disorientation]
[Poor concentration]
[Rapid mood swings]
[Disordered thought sequencing]
[Inappropriate responses]

Goals/Objectives

Short-Term Goal

Client will discuss content of hallucinations with nurse or therapist within 1 week.

Long-Term Goal

Client will be able to define and test reality, eliminating the occurrence of hallucinations. (This goal may not be realistic for the individual with chronic illness who has experienced auditory hallucinations for many years.) A more realistic goal may be: Client will verbalize understanding that the voices are a result of his or her illness and demonstrate ways to interrupt the hallucination.

Interventions with *Selected Rationales*

1. Observe client for signs of hallucinations (listening pose, laughing or talking to self, stopping in mid-sentence). ***Early intervention may prevent aggressive responses to command hallucinations.***
2. Avoid touching client before warning him or her that you are about to do so. ***Client may perceive touch as threatening and respond in an aggressive manner.***
3. An attitude of acceptance will encourage client to share the content of the hallucination with you. ***This is important in order to prevent possible injury to client or others from command hallucinations.***
4. Do not reinforce the hallucination. Use "the voices" instead of words like "they," which implies validation. Let client know that you do not share the perception. Say, "Even though I realize that the voices are real to you, I do not hear any voices speaking." ***The nurse must be honest with client so that he or she may realize that the hallucinations are not real.***
5. Try to connect the times of the hallucinations to times of increased anxiety. Help client to understand this connection. ***If client can learn to interrupt escalating anxiety, hallucinations may be prevented.***
6. Try to distract client from the hallucination. ***Involvement in interpersonal activities and explanation of the actual situation will help bring client back to reality.***
7. For some clients, auditory hallucinations persist after the acute psychotic episode has subsided. Listening to the radio or watching television helps distract some clients from attention to the voices. Others have benefited from an intervention called ***voice dismissal.*** With this technique, the client is taught to say loudly, "Go away!" or "Leave me alone!" thereby exerting some conscious control over the behavior.

Outcome Criteria

1. Client is able to recognize that hallucinations occur at times of extreme anxiety.
2. Client is able to recognize signs of increasing anxiety and employ techniques to interrupt the response.

DISTURBED THOUGHT PROCESSES

Definition: *Disruption in cognitive operations and activities.*

Possible Etiologies ("related to")

[Inability to trust]
[Panic level of anxiety]
[Repressed fears]
[Stress sufficiently severe to threaten an already weak ego]
[Possible hereditary factor]

Defining Characteristics ("evidenced by")

[Delusional thinking (false ideas)]
[Inability to concentrate]
Hypervigilance
[Altered attention span]—distractibility
Inaccurate interpretation of the environment
[Impaired ability to make decisions, problem-solve, reason, abstract or conceptualize, calculate]
[Inappropriate social behavior (reflecting inaccurate thinking)]
Inappropriate nonreality-based thinking

Goals/Objectives

Short-Term Goal

By the end of 2 weeks, client will recognize and verbalize that false ideas occur at times of increased anxiety.

Long-Term Goal

Depending on chronicity of disease process, choose the most realistic long-term goal for the client:

1. By time of discharge from treatment, client will experience (verbalize evidence of) no delusional thoughts.
2. By time of discharge from treatment, client will be able to differentiate between delusional thinking and reality.

Interventions with *Selected Rationales*

1. Convey your acceptance of client's need for the false belief, while letting him or her know that you do not share the belief. ***It is important to communicate to client that you do not accept the delusion as reality.***
2. Do not argue or deny the belief. Use *reasonable doubt* as a therapeutic technique: "I find that hard to believe." ***Arguing with client or denying the belief serves no useful purpose, because delusional ideas are not eliminated by this approach, and the development of a trusting relationship may be impeded.***
3. Help client try to connect the false beliefs to times of increased anxiety. Discuss techniques that could be used to control anxiety (e.g., deep-breathing exercises, other relaxation exercises, thought-stopping techniques). ***If client can learn to interrupt escalating anxiety, delusional thinking may be prevented.***

4. Reinforce and focus on reality. Discourage long ruminations about the irrational thinking. Talk about real events and real people. ***Discussions that focus on the false ideas are purposeless and useless and may even aggravate the psychosis.***
5. Assist and support client in his or her attempt to verbalize feelings of anxiety, fear, or insecurity. ***Verbalization of feelings in a nonthreatening environment may help client come to terms with long-unresolved issues.***

Outcome Criteria

1. Verbalizations reflect thinking processes oriented in reality.
2. Client is able to maintain activities of daily living (ADLs) to his or her maximal ability.
3. Client is able to refrain from responding to delusional thoughts, should they occur.

IMPAIRED VERBAL COMMUNICATION

Definition: *Decreased, delayed, or absent ability to receive, process, transmit, and use a system of symbols.*

Possible Etiologies ("related to")

[Inability to trust]
[Panic level of anxiety]
[Regression to earlier level of development]
[Withdrawal into self]
[Disordered, unrealistic thinking]

Defining Characteristics ("evidenced by")

[Loose association of ideas]
[Use of words that are symbolic to the individual (neologisms)]
[Use of words in a meaningless, disconnected manner (word salad)]
[Use of words that rhyme in a nonsensical fashion (clang association)]
[Repetition of words that are heard (echolalia)]
[Does not speak (mutism)]
[Verbalizations reflect concrete thinking (inability to think in abstract terms)]
[Poor eye contact (either no eye contact or continuous staring into the other person's eyes)]

Goals/Objectives

Short-Term Goal

Client will demonstrate ability to remain on one topic, using appropriate, intermittent eye contact for 5 minutes with nurse or therapist.

Long-Term Goal

By time of discharge from treatment, client will demonstrate ability to carry on a verbal communication in a socially acceptable manner with staff and peers.

Interventions with *Selected Rationales*

1. Use the techniques of *consensual validation* and *seeking clarification* to decode communication patterns. (Examples: "Is it that you mean ...?" or "I don't understand what you mean by that. Would you please explain it to me?") ***These techniques reveal to the client how he or she is being perceived by others, and the responsibility for not understanding is accepted by the nurse.***
2. Maintain consistency of staff assignment over time ***to facilitate trust and the ability to understand client's actions and communication.***
3. In a nonthreatening manner, explain to client how his or her behavior and verbalizations are viewed by and may alienate others.
4. If client is unable or unwilling to speak (mutism), use of the technique of *verbalizing the implied* is therapeutic. (Example: "That must have been very difficult for you when . . .") ***This may help to convey empathy, develop trust, and eventually encourage client to discuss painful issues.***
5. Anticipate and fulfill client's needs until satisfactory communication patterns return. ***Client comfort and safety are nursing priorities.***

Outcome Criteria

1. Client is able to communicate in a manner that is understood by others.
2. Client's nonverbal messages are congruent with verbalizations.
3. Client is able to recognize that disorganized thinking and impaired verbal communication occur at times of increased anxiety and intervene to interrupt the process.

■ SELF-CARE DEFICIT (IDENTIFY SPECIFIC AREA)

Definition: *Impaired ability to perform or complete [activities of daily living].*

Possible Etiologies ("related to")

[Withdrawal into self]
[Regression to an earlier level of development]
[Panic level of anxiety]
Perceptual or cognitive impairment
[Inability to trust]

Defining Characteristics ("evidenced by")

[Difficulty in bringing or] inability to bring food from receptacle to mouth
Inability [or refusal] to wash body or body parts
[Impaired ability or lack of interest in selecting appropriate clothing to wear, dressing, grooming, or maintaining appearance at a satisfactory level]
[Inability or unwillingness to carry out toileting procedures without assistance]

Goals/Objectives

Short-Term Goal

Client will verbalize a desire to perform ADLs by end of 1 week.

Long-Term Goal

Client will be able to perform ADLs in an independent manner and demonstrate a willingness to do so by discharge from treatment.

Interventions with *Selected Rationales*

1. Encourage client to perform normal ADLs to his or her level of ability. ***Successful performance of independent activities enhances self-esteem.***
2. Encourage independence, but intervene when client is unable to perform. ***Client comfort and safety are nursing priorities.***
3. Offer recognition and positive reinforcement for independent accomplishments. (Example: "Mrs. J., I see you have put on a clean dress and combed your hair.") ***Positive reinforcement enhances self-esteem and encourages repetition of desirable behaviors.***
4. Show client, on concrete level, how to perform activities with which he or she is having difficulty. (Example: If client is not eating, place spoon in his or her hand, scoop some food into it, and say, "Now, eat a bite of mashed potatoes (or other food).") ***Because concrete thinking prevails, explanations must be provided at the client's concrete level of comprehension.***
5. Keep strict records of food and fluid intake. ***This information is necessary to acquire an accurate nutritional assessment.***
6. Offer nutritious snacks and fluids between meals. ***Client may be unable to tolerate large amounts of food at mealtimes and may therefore require additional nourishment at other times during the day to receive adequate nutrition.***
7. If client is not eating because of suspiciousness and fears of being poisoned, provide canned foods, and allow client to open them, or, if possible, suggest that food be served family-style ***so that client may see everyone eating from the same servings.***
8. If client is soiling self, establish routine schedule for toileting needs. Assist client to bathroom on hourly or bi-hourly schedule,

as need is determined, until he or she is able to fulfill this need without assistance.

Outcome Criteria

1. Client feeds self without assistance.
2. Client selects appropriate clothing, dresses and grooms self daily without assistance.
3. Client maintains optimal level of personal hygiene by bathing daily and carrying out essential toileting procedures without assistance.

DISTURBED SLEEP PATTERN

Definition: *Time-limited disruption of sleep (natural, periodic suspension of consciousness) amount and quality*

Possible Etiologies ("related to")

[Panic level of anxiety]
[Repressed fears]
[Hallucinations]
[Delusional thinking]

Defining Characteristics ("evidenced by")

[Difficulty falling asleep]
[Waking very early in the morning]
[Pacing; other signs of increasing irritability caused by lack of sleep]
[Frequent yawning, nodding off to sleep]

Goals/Objectives

Short-Term Goal

Within first week of treatment, client will fall asleep within 30 minutes of retiring and sleep 5 hours without waking, with use of sedative if needed.

Long-Term Goal

By time of discharge from treatment, client will be able to fall asleep within 30 minutes of retiring and sleep 6 to 8 hours without a sleeping aid.

Interventions with *Selected Rationales*

1. Keep strict records of sleeping patterns. ***Accurate baseline data are important in planning care to assist client with this problem.***
2. Discourage sleep during the day ***to promote more restful sleep at night.***

3. Administer antipsychotic medication at bedtime ***so client does not become drowsy during the day.***
4. Assist with measures that promote sleep, such as warm, nonstimulating drinks; light snacks; warm baths; and back rubs.
5. Performing relaxation exercises to soft music may be helpful before sleep.
6. Limit intake of caffeinated drinks such as tea, coffee, and colas. ***Caffeine is a CNS stimulant and may interfere with the client's achievement of rest and sleep.***

Outcome Criteria

1. Client is able to fall asleep within 30 minutes after retiring.
2. Client sleeps at least 6 consecutive hours without waking.
3. Client does not require a sedative to fall asleep.

■ INTERNET REFERENCES

Additional information about schizophrenia is located at the following websites:

- http://www.schizophrenia.com
- http://www.nimh.nih.gov
- http://schizophrenia.nami.org
- http://mentalhealth.com
- http://www2.health-center.com

Additional information about medications to treat schizophrenia is located at the following websites:

- http://www.mentalhealth.com/fr30.html/
- http://www.fadavis.com/townsend
- http://www.nlm.nih.gov/medlineplus

CHAPTER 6

Mood Disorders

BACKGROUND ASSESSMENT DATA

Mood is defined as an individual's sustained emotional tone, which significantly influences behavior, personality, and perception. A disturbance in mood is the predominant feature of the mood disorders (APA, 2000). Mood disorders are classified as depressive or bipolar.

Depressive Disorders*

296.xx Major Depressive Disorder

Major depressive disorder is described as a disturbance of mood involving depression or loss of interest or pleasure in the usual activities and pastimes. There is evidence of interference in social and occupational functioning for at least 2 weeks. There is no history of manic behavior, and the symptoms cannot be attributed to use of substances or a general medical condition. The following specifiers may be used to further describe the depressive episode:

1. **Single Episode or Recurrent:** This specifier identifies whether the individual has experienced prior episodes of depression.
2. **Mild, Moderate, or Severe:** These categories are identified by the number and severity of symptoms.
3. **With Psychotic Features:** Impairment of reality testing is evident. The individual experiences hallucinations and/or delusions.
4. **With Catatonic Features:** This category identifies the presence of psychomotor disturbances, such as severe psychomotor retardation, with or without the presence of waxy flexibility or stupor or excessive motor activity. The client also may manifest symptoms of negativism, mutism, echolalia, or echopraxia.
5. **With Melancholic Features:** This is a typically severe form of major depressive episode. Symptoms are exaggerated. There is a loss

* Classification and criteria for this and all subsequent diagnoses in this chapter marked with an asterisk are from the *Diagnostic and Statistical Manual of Mental Disorders, Fourth Edition, Text Revision, 2000.* Used with permission from the American Psychiatric Association.

of interest in all activities. Depression is regularly worse in the morning. There is a history of major depressive episodes that have responded well to somatic antidepressant therapy.

6. **Chronic:** This classification applies when the current episode of depressed mood has been evident continuously for at least the past 2 years.
7. **With Seasonal Pattern:** This diagnosis indicates the presence of depressive symptoms during the fall or winter months. This diagnosis is made when the number of seasonal depressive episodes substantially outnumbers the nonseasonal depressive episodes that have occurred over the individual's lifetime (APA, 2000). This disorder has previously been identified in the literature as seasonal affective disorder.
8. **With Postpartum Onset:** This specifier is used when symptoms of major depression occur within 4 weeks postpartum.

300.4 Dysthymic Disorder

A mood disturbance with characteristics similar to, if somewhat milder than, those ascribed to major depressive disorder. There is no evidence of psychotic symptoms.

Bipolar Disorders*

These disorders are characterized by mood swings from profound depression to extreme euphoria (mania), with intervening periods of normalcy.

During an episode of *mania*, the mood is elevated, expansive, or irritable. Motor activity is excessive and frenzied. Psychotic features may be present. A somewhat milder form is called *hypomania*. It is usually not severe enough to require hospitalization, and it does not include psychotic features.

The diagnostic picture for *bipolar depression* is identical to that described for major depressive disorder, with one addition. The client must have a history of one or more manic episodes.

When the symptom presentation includes rapidly alternating moods (sadness, irritability, euphoria) accompanied by symptoms associated with both depression and mania, the individual is given a diagnosis of *bipolar disorder, mixed.*

296.xx Bipolar I Disorder

Bipolar I disorder is the diagnosis given to an individual who is experiencing or has experienced a full syndrome of manic or mixed symptoms. The client may also have experienced episodes of depression.

296.89 Bipolar II Disorder

Bipolar II disorder is characterized by recurrent bouts of major depression with the episodic occurrence of hypomania. This individual has never experienced a full syndrome of manic or mixed symptoms.

301.13 Cyclothymic Disorder

The essential feature is a chronic mood disturbance of at least 2 years' duration, involving numerous periods of depression and hypomania but not of sufficient severity and duration to meet the criteria for either bipolar I or II disorder. There is an absence of psychotic features.

293.83 Mood Disorder due to General Medical Condition

This disorder is characterized by a prominent and persistent disturbance in mood (either depression or mania) that is judged to be the direct result of the physiological effects of a general medical condition (APA, 2000).

Substance-Induced Mood Disorder (Refer to Substance-Related Disorders for substance-specific codes.)

The disturbance of mood (depression or mania) associated with this disorder is considered to be the direct result of the physiological effects of a substance (e.g., use or abuse of a drug or a medication, or toxin exposure).

■ MAJOR DEPRESSIVE DISORDER; DYSTHYMIC DISORDER

Predisposing Factors

1. **Physiological**
   a. *Genetic:* Numerous studies have been conducted that support the involvement of heredity in depressive illness. The disorder is 1.5 to 3 times more common among first-degree relatives of individuals with the disorder than among the general population.
   b. *Biochemical:* A biochemical theory implicates the biogenic amines norepinephrine, dopamine, and serotonin. The levels of these chemicals have been found to be deficient in individuals with depressive illness.
   c. *Neuroendocrine Disturbances:* Elevated levels of serum cortisol and decreased levels of thyroid-stimulating hormone have been associated with depressed mood in some individuals.
   d. *Medication Side Effects:* A number of drugs can produce a depressive syndrome as a side effect. Examples include anxiolytics, antipsychotics, and sedative-hypnotics. Antihypertensive medications such as propranolol and reserpine also have been known to produce depressive symptoms.
   e. *Other Physiological Conditions:* Depressive symptoms may occur in the presence of electrolyte disturbances, nutritional deficiencies, and with certain physical disorders, such as cardiovascular accident, systemic lupus erythematosus (SLE), hepatitis, and diabetes mellitus.
2. **Psychosocial**
   a. *Psychoanalytical:* Freud observed that melancholia occurs after the loss of a loved object, either actually by death or emo-

tionally by rejection, or the loss of some other abstraction of value to the individual. Freud indicated that in clients with melancholia, the depressed person's rage is internally directed because of identification with the lost object (Kaplan and Sadock, 1998).

b. *Cognitive:* These theorists (Beck et al, 1979) believe that depressive illness occurs as a result of impaired cognition. Disturbed thought processes foster a negative evaluation of self by the individual. The perceptions are of inadequacy and worthlessness. Outlook for the future is one of pessimism and hopelessness.
c. *Learning Theory:* This theory (Seligman, 1973) proposes that depressive illness is predisposed by the individual's belief that there is a lack of control over his or her life situations. It is thought that this belief arises out of experiences that result in failure (either perceived or real). Following numerous failures, the individual feels helpless to succeed at any endeavor and therefore gives up trying. This "learned helplessness" is viewed as a predisposition to depressive illness.
d. *Object Loss Theory:* The theory of object loss suggests that depressive illness occurs as a result of having been abandoned by, or otherwise separated from, a significant other during the first 6 months of life. Because during this period the mother represents the child's main source of security, she is the "object." The response occurs not only with a physical loss. This absence of attachment, which may be either physical or emotional, leads to feelings of helplessness and despair that contribute to lifelong patterns of depression in response to loss.

Symptomatology (Subjective and Objective Data)

1. The affect of a depressed person is one of sadness, dejection, helplessness, and hopelessness. The outlook is gloomy and pessimistic. A feeling of worthlessness prevails.
2. Thoughts are slowed, and concentration is difficult. Obsessive ideas and rumination of negative thoughts are common. In severe depression (major depressive disorder or bipolar depression), psychotic features such as hallucinations and delusions may be evident, reflecting misinterpretations of the environment.
3. Physically, there is evidence of weakness and fatigue—very little energy to carry on activities of daily living (ADLs). The individual may express an exaggerated concern over bodily functioning, seemingly experiencing heightened sensitivity to somatic sensations. Some individuals may be inclined toward excessive eating and drinking, whereas others may experience anorexia and weight loss. In response to a general slowdown of the body, digestion is often sluggish, constipation is common, and urinary retention is possible. Sleep disturbances are common, either insomnia or hypersomnia. At the less severe level (dysthymic disorder), individu-

als tend to feel their best early in the morning, then continually feel worse as the day progresses. The opposite is true of persons experiencing severe depression. The exact cause of this phenomenon is unknown, but it is thought to be related to the circadian rhythm of the hormones and their effects on the body.

4. A general slowdown of motor activity commonly accompanies depression (psychomotor retardation). Energy level is depleted, movements are lethargic, and performance of ADLs is extremely difficult. Regression is common, evidenced by withdrawal into the self and retreat to the fetal position. Severely depressed persons may manifest psychomotor activity through symptoms of agitation. These are constant, rapid, purposeless movements, out of touch with the environment.
5. Verbalizations are limited. When depressed persons do speak, the content may be either ruminations regarding their own life regrets or, in psychotic clients, a reflection of their delusional thinking.
6. Social participation is diminished. The depressed client has an inclination toward egocentrism and narcissism—an intense focus on the self. This discourages others from pursuing a relationship with the individual, which increases his or her feelings of worthlessness and penchant for isolation.

Common Nursing Diagnoses and Interventions for Depression

(Interventions are applicable to various health-care settings, such as inpatient and partial hospitalization, community outpatient clinic, home health, and private practice.)

RISK FOR SUICIDE

Definition: *At risk for self-inflicted, life-threatening injury.*

Related/Risk Factors ("related to")

[Depressed mood]
[Feelings of worthlessness]
[Anger turned inward]
[Punitive superego and irrational feelings of guilt]
[Numerous failures (learned helplessness)]
[Feelings of abandonment by significant other]
Hopelessness
[Misinterpretations of reality]
[Making direct or indirect statements indicating a desire to commit suicide]
History of prior suicide attempt
[Has suicide plan and means to carry it out]

[Putting business affairs in order; writing a will; giving away prized possessions]
[Hallucinations]
[Delusional thinking]
[Suicidal ideation, plan, available means]

Goals/Objectives

Short-Term Goals

1. Client will seek out staff when feeling urge to harm self.
2. Client will make short-term verbal (or written) contract with nurse not to harm self.
3. Client will not harm self.

Long-Term Goal

Client will not harm self.

Interventions with *Selected Rationales*

1. Ask client directly, "Have you thought about killing yourself? If so, what do you plan to do? Do you have the means to carry out this plan?" ***The risk of suicide is greatly increased if the client has developed a plan and particularly if means exist for the client to execute the plan.***
2. Create a safe environment for the client. Remove all potentially harmful objects from client's access (sharp objects, straps, belts, ties, glass items). ***Client safety is a nursing priority.***
3. Formulate a short-term verbal contract with the client that he or she will not harm self during specific time period. When that contract expires, make another, and so forth. ***Discussion of suicidal feelings with a trusted individual provides some relief to the client. A contract gets the subject out in the open and places some of the responsibility for the client's safety with the client. An attitude of acceptance of the client as a worthwhile individual is conveyed.***
4. Secure promise from client that he or she will seek out a staff member or support person if thoughts of suicide emerge. ***Suicidal clients are often very ambivalent about their feelings. Discussion of feelings with a trusted individual may provide assistance before the client experiences a crisis situation.***
5. Encourage verbalizations of honest feelings. Through exploration and discussion, help client to identify symbols of hope in his or her life.
6. Encourage client to express angry feelings within appropriate limits. Provide safe method of hostility release. Help client to identify true source of anger and to work on adaptive coping skills for use outside the hospital. ***Depression and suicidal behaviors may be viewed as anger turned inward on the self. If this anger can be verbalized in a nonthreatening environment, the client***

may be able to resolve these feelings, regardless of the discomfort involved.

7. Identify community resources that client may use as support system and from which he or she may request help if feeling suicidal. ***Having a concrete plan for seeking assistance during a crisis may discourage or prevent self-destructive behaviors.***
8. Orient client to reality, as required. Point out sensory misperceptions or misinterpretations of the environment. Take care not to belittle client's fears or indicate disapproval of verbal expressions.
9. Most important, spend time with client. ***This provides a feeling of safety and security, while also conveying the message, "I want to spend time with you because I think you are a worthwhile person."***

Outcome Criteria

1. Client verbalizes no thoughts of suicide.
2. Client commits no acts of self-harm.
3. Client is able to verbalize names of resources outside the hospital from which he or she may request help if feeling suicidal.

DYSFUNCTIONAL GRIEVING

Defined: *Extended, unsuccessful use of intellectual and emotional responses by which individuals, families, or communities attempt to work through the process of modifying self-concept based upon the perception of [actual or potential] loss.*

Possible Etiologies ("related to")

[Real or perceived loss of any concept of value to the individual]
[Bereavement overload (cumulative grief from multiple unresolved losses)]
[Thwarted grieving response to a loss]
[Absence of anticipatory grieving]
[Feelings of guilt generated by ambivalent relationship with lost concept]

Defining Characteristics ("evidenced by")

Idealization of lost [concept]
Denial of loss
[Excessive anger, expressed inappropriately]
[Obsessions with past experiences]
[Ruminations of guilt feelings, excessive and exaggerated out of proportion to the situation]
Developmental regression
Difficulty in expressing loss
Repetitive use of ineffectual behaviors associated with attempts to reinvest in relationships

Reliving of past experiences with little or no reduction of intensity of the grief
Prolonged interference with life functioning, with onset or exacerbation of somatic or psychosomatic responses
Labile affect
Alterations in eating habits, sleep patterns, dream patterns, activity level, libido

Goals/Objectives

Short-Term Goal

Client will express anger toward lost concept.

Long-Term Goal

1. Client will be able to verbalize behaviors associated with the normal stages of grief.
2. Client will be able to recognize own position in grief process as he or she progresses at own pace toward resolution.

Interventions with *Selected Rationales*

1. Determine stage of grief in which client is fixed. Identify behaviors associated with this stage. ***Accurate baseline assessment data are necessary to effectively plan care for the grieving client.***
2. Develop trusting relationship with client. Show empathy and caring. Be honest, and keep all promises. ***Trust is the basis for a therapeutic relationship.***
3. Convey an accepting attitude, and enable the client to express feelings openly. ***An accepting attitude conveys to the client that you believe he or she is a worthwhile person. Trust is enhanced.***
4. Encourage client to express anger. Do not become defensive if initial expression of anger is displaced on nurse or therapist. Help client explore angry feelings so that they may be directed toward the intended object or person. ***Verbalization of feelings in a nonthreatening environment may help client come to terms with unresolved issues.***
5. Help client discharge pent-up anger through participation in large-motor activities (e.g., brisk walks, jogging, physical exercises, volleyball, punching bag, exercise bike). ***Physical exercise provides a safe and effective method for discharging pent-up tension.***
6. Teach the normal stages of grief and behaviors associated with each stage. Help client understand that feelings such as guilt and anger toward the lost concept are appropriate and acceptable during the grief process. ***Knowledge of acceptability of the feelings associated with normal grieving may help to relieve some of the guilt that these responses generate.***
7. Encourage client to review relationship with the lost concept. With support and sensitivity, point out reality of the situation in

areas where misrepresentations are expressed. ***Client must give up an idealized perception and be able to accept both positive and negative aspects about the lost concept before the grief process is complete.***

8. Communicate to client that crying is acceptable. Use of touch is therapeutic and appropriate with most clients. Knowledge of cultural influences specific to the client is important before using this technique.
9. Help client in problem solving as he or she attempts to determine methods for more adaptive coping with the experienced loss. Provide positive feedback for strategies identified and decisions made. ***Positive feedback increases self-esteem and encourages repetition of desirable behaviors.***
10. Encourage client to reach out for spiritual support during this time in whatever form is desirable to him or her. Assess spiritual needs of client, and assist as necessary in the fulfillment of those needs.

Outcome Criteria

1. Client is able to verbalize normal stages of the grief process and behaviors associated with each stage.
2. Client is able to identify own position within the grief process and express honest feelings related to the lost concept.
3. Client is no longer manifesting exaggerated emotions and behaviors related to dysfunctional grieving and is able to carry out ADLs independently.

LOW SELF-ESTEEM

Definition: *Negative self-evaluation and feelings about self or self-capabilities.*

Possible Etiologies ("related to")

[Lack of positive feedback]
[Feelings of abandonment by significant other]
[Numerous failures (learned helplessness)]
[Underdeveloped ego and punitive superego]
[Impaired cognition fostering negative view of self]

Defining Characteristics ("evidenced by")

[Difficulty accepting positive reinforcement]
[Withdrawal into social isolation]
[Being highly critical and judgmental of self and others]
[Expressions of worthlessness]
[Fear of failure]

[Inability to recognize own accomplishments]
[Setting self up for failure by establishing unrealistic goals]
[Unsatisfactory interpersonal relationships]
[Negative, pessimistic outlook]
[Hypersensitive to slight or criticism]
[Grandiosity]

Goals/Objectives

Short-Term Goals

1. Within reasonable period, client will discuss fear of failure with nurse.
2. Within reasonable period, client will verbalize areas he or she likes about self.

Long-Term Goals

1. By time of discharge from treatment, client will exhibit increased feelings of self-worth as evidenced by verbal expression of positive aspects of self, past accomplishments, and future prospects.
2. By time of discharge from treatment, client will exhibit increased feelings of self-worth by setting realistic goals and trying to reach them, thereby demonstrating a decrease in fear of failure.

Interventions with *Selected Rationales*

1. Be accepting of client and his or her negativism. ***An attitude of acceptance enhances feelings of self-worth.***
2. Spend time with client ***to convey acceptance and contribute toward feelings of self-worth.***
3. Help client recognize and focus on strengths and accomplishments. Minimize attention given to past (real or perceived) failures. ***Lack of attention may help to eliminate negative ruminations.***
4. Encourage participation in group activities ***from which client may receive positive feedback and support from peers.***
5. Help client identify areas he or she would like to change about self, and assist with problem solving toward this effort. ***Low self-worth may interfere with client's perception of own problem-solving ability. Assistance may be required.***
6. Ensure that client is not becoming increasingly dependent and that he or she is accepting responsibility for own behaviors. ***Client must be able to function independently if he or she is to be successful within the less structured community environment.***
7. Ensure that therapy groups offer client simple methods of achievement. Offer recognition and positive feedback for actual accomplishments. ***Successes and recognition increase self-esteem.***
8. Teach assertiveness techniques: the ability to recognize the differences among passive, assertive, and aggressive behaviors and the importance of respecting the human rights of others while pro-

tecting one's own basic human rights. ***Self-esteem is enhanced by the ability to interact with others in an assertive manner.***

9. Teach effective communication techniques, such as the use of "I" messages. Emphasize ways to avoid making judgmental statements.
10. Help client in performing aspects of self-care when required. Offer positive feedback for tasks performed independently. ***Positive feedback enhances self-esteem and encourages repetition of desirable behaviors.***

Outcome Criteria

1. Client is able to verbalize positive aspects of self.
2. Client is able to communicate assertively with others.
3. Client expresses some optimism and hope for the future.
4. Client sets realistic goals for self and demonstrates willing attempt to reach them.

SOCIAL ISOLATION/IMPAIRED SOCIAL INTERACTION

Definition: *Social isolation is the condition of aloneness experienced by the individual and perceived as imposed by others and as a negative or threatened state; impaired social interaction is an insufficient or excessive quantity or ineffective quality of social exchange.*

Possible Etiologies ("related to")

[Developmental regression]
[Egocentric behaviors (which offend others and discourage relationships)]
Altered thought processes [delusional thinking]
[Fear of rejection or failure of the interaction]
[Impaired cognition fostering negative view of self]
[Unresolved grief]
Absence of available significant others or peers

Defining Characteristics ("evidenced by")

Sad, dull affect
Being uncommunicative, withdrawn; lacking eye contact
Preoccupation with own thoughts; performance of repetitive, meaningless actions
Seeking to be alone
[Assuming fetal position]
Expression of feelings of aloneness or rejection
Verbalization or observation of discomfort in social situations
Dysfunctional interaction with peers, family, and others

Goals/Objectives

Short-Term Goal

Client will develop trusting relationship with nurse or counselor within reasonable period.

Long-Term Goals

1. Client will voluntarily spend time with other clients and nurse or therapist in group activities by time of discharge from treatment.
2. Client will refrain from using egocentric behaviors that offend others and discourage relationships by time of discharge from treatment.

Interventions with *Selected Rationales*

1. Spend time with client. This may mean just sitting in silence for a while. ***Your presence may help improve client's perception of self as a worthwhile person.***
2. Develop a therapeutic nurse-client relationship through frequent, brief contacts and an accepting attitude. Show unconditional positive regard. ***Your presence, acceptance, and conveyance of positive regard enhance the client's feelings of self- worth.***
3. After client feels comfortable in a one-to-one relationship, encourage attendance in group activities. May need to attend with client the first few times to offer support. Accept client's decision to remove self from group situation if anxiety becomes too great. ***The presence of a trusted individual provides emotional security for the client.***
4. Verbally acknowledge client's absence from any group activities. ***Knowledge that his or her absence was noticed may reinforce the client's feelings of self-worth.***
5. Teach assertiveness techniques. Interactions with others may be discouraged by client's use of passive or aggressive behaviors. ***Knowledge of the use of assertive techniques could improve client's relationships with others.***
6. Provide direct feedback about client's interactions with others. Do this in a nonjudgmental manner. Help client learn how to respond more appropriately in interactions with others. Teach client skills that may be used to approach others in a more socially acceptable manner. Practice these skills through role-play. ***Client may not realize how he or she is being perceived by others. Direct feedback from a trusted individual may help to alter these behaviors in a positive manner. Having practiced these skills in role-play facilitates their use in real situations.***
7. The depressed client must have much structure in his or her life because of the impairment in decision-making and problem-solving ability. Devise a plan of therapeutic activities, and provide client with a written time schedule. ***Remember:*** The client who is

moderately depressed feels best early in the day, whereas later in the day is a better time for the severely depressed individual to participate in activities. ***It is important to plan activities at a time when the client has more energy and is more likely to gain from the experience.***

8. Provide positive reinforcement for client's voluntary interactions with others. ***Positive reinforcement enhances self-esteem and encourages repetition of desirable behaviors.***

Outcome Criteria

1. Client demonstrates willingness and desire to socialize with others.
2. Client voluntarily attends group activities.
3. Client approaches others in appropriate manner for one-to-one interaction.

POWERLESSNESS

Definition: *Perception that one's own action will not significantly affect an outcome; a perceived lack of control over a current situation or immediate happening.*

Possible Etiologies ("related to")

Lifestyle of helplessness
Health-care environment
[Dysfunctional grieving process]
[Lack of positive feedback]
[Consistent negative feedback]

Defining Characteristics ("evidenced by")

Verbal expressions of having no control or influence over situation, outcome, or self-care
Nonparticipation in care or decision-making when opportunities are provided
Expression of doubt regarding role performance
Reluctance to express true feelings, fearing alienation from caregivers
Apathy
Dependence on others that may result in irritability, resentment, anger, and guilt
Passivity

Goals/ Objectives

Short-Term Goal

Client will participate in decision-making regarding own care within 5 days.

Long-Term Goal

Client will be able to effectively problem-solve ways to take control of his or her life situation by time of discharge from treatment, thereby decreasing feelings of powerlessness.

Interventions with *Selected Rationales*

1. Encourage client to take as much responsibility as possible for own self-care practices. ***Providing client with choices will increase his or her feelings of control.***
   a. Include client in setting the goals of care he or she wishes to achieve.
   b. Allow client to establish own schedule for self-care activities.
   c. Provide client with privacy as need is determined.
   d. Provide positive feedback for decisions made. Respect client's right to make those decisions independently, and refrain from attempting to influence him or her toward those that may seem more logical.
2. Help client set realistic goals. ***Unrealistic goals set the client up for failure and reinforce feelings of powerlessness.***
3. Help client identify areas of life situation that he or she can control. ***Client's emotional condition interferes with his or her ability to solve problems. Assistance is required to perceive the benefits and consequences of available alternatives accurately.***
4. Help client identify areas of life situation that are not within his or her ability to control. Encourage verbalization of feelings related to this inability ***in an effort to deal with unresolved issues and accept what cannot be changed.***
5. Identify ways in which client can achieve. Encourage participation in these activities, and provide positive reinforcement for participation as well as for achievement. ***Positive reinforcement enhances self-esteem and encourages repetition of desirable behaviors.***

Outcome Criteria

1. Client verbalizes choices made in a plan to maintain control over his or her life situation.
2. Client verbalizes honest feelings about life situations over which he or she has no control.
3. Client is able to verbalize system for problem solving as required for adequate role performance.

DISTURBED THOUGHT PROCESSES

Definition: *Disruption in cognitive operations and activities.*

Possible Etiologies ("related to")

[Withdrawal into the self]
[Underdeveloped ego; punitive superego]
[Impaired cognition fostering negative perception of self and the environment]

Defining Characteristics ("evidenced by")

Inaccurate interpretation of environment
[Delusional thinking]
Hypovigilance
[Altered attention span]—distractibility
Egocentricity
[Impaired ability to make decisions, problem-solve, reason]
[Negative ruminations]

Goals/Objectives

Short-Term Goal

Client will recognize and verbalize when interpretations of the environment are inaccurate within 1 week.

Long-Term Goal

Client will experience no delusional or distorted thinking by time of discharge from treatment.

Interventions with *Selected Rationales*

1. Convey your acceptance of client's need for the false belief, while letting him or her know that you do not share the delusion. ***A positive response would convey to the client that you accept the delusion as reality.***
2. Do not argue or deny the belief. Use *reasonable doubt* as a therapeutic technique: "I find that hard to believe." ***Arguing with the client or denying the belief serves no useful purpose, as delusional ideas are not eliminated by this approach, and the development of a trusting relationship may be impeded.***
3. Use the techniques of *consensual validation* and *seeking clarification* when communication reflects alteration in thinking. (Examples: "Is it that you mean . . . ?" or "I don't understand what you mean by that. Would you please explain?") ***These techniques reveal to the client how he or she is being perceived by others, while the responsibility for not understanding is accepted by the nurse.***
4. Reinforce and focus on reality. Talk about real events and real people. Use real situations and events to divert client away from long, purposeless, repetitive verbalizations of false ideas.
5. Give positive reinforcement as client is able to differentiate between reality-based and nonreality-based thinking. ***Positive reinforcement enhances self-esteem and encourages repetition of desirable behaviors.***

6. Teach client to intervene, using thought-stopping techniques, when irrational or negative thoughts prevail. ***Thought stopping*** involves using the command "Stop!" or a loud noise (such as hand clapping) to interrupt unwanted thoughts. ***This noise or command distracts the individual from the undesirable thinking that often precedes undesirable emotions or behaviors.***
7. Use touch cautiously, particularly if thoughts reveal ideas of persecution. ***Clients who are suspicious may perceive touch as threatening and may respond with aggression.***

Outcome Criteria

1. Client's thinking processes reflect accurate interpretation of the environment.
2. Client is able to recognize negative or irrational thoughts and intervene to "stop" their progression.

IMBALANCED NUTRITION, LESS THAN BODY REQUIREMENTS

Definition: *Intake of nutrients insufficient to meet metabolic needs.*

Possible Etiologies ("related to")

Inability to ingest food because of:
[Depressed mood]
[Loss of appetite]
[Energy level too low to meet own nutritional needs]
[Regression to lower level of development]
[Ideas of self-destruction]

Defining Characteristics ("evidenced by")

Loss of weight
Lack of interest in food
Pale conjunctiva and mucous membranes
Poor muscle tone
[Amenorrhea]
[Poor skin turgor]
[Edema of extremities]
[Electrolyte imbalances]
[Weakness]
[Constipation]
[Anemias]

Goals/Objectives

Short-Term Goal

Client will gain 2 pounds per week for the next 3 weeks.

Long-Term Goal

Client will exhibit no signs or symptoms of malnutrition by time of discharge from treatment (e.g., electrolytes and blood counts will be within normal limits; a steady weight gain will be demonstrated; constipation will be corrected; client will exhibit increased energy in participation in activities).

Interventions with *Selected Rationales*

1. In collaboration with dietitian, determine number of calories required to provide adequate nutrition and realistic (according to body structure and height) weight gain.
2. To prevent constipation, ensure that diet includes foods high in fiber content. Encourage client to increase fluid consumption and physical exercise to promote normal bowel functioning. ***Depressed clients are particularly vulnerable to constipation because of psychomotor retardation. Constipation is also a common side effect of many antidepressant medications.***
3. Keep strict documentation of intake, output, and calorie count. ***This information is necessary to make an accurate nutritional assessment and maintain client safety.***
4. Weigh client daily. ***Weight loss or gain is important assessment information.***
5. Determine client's likes and dislikes, and collaborate with dietitian to provide favorite foods. ***Client is more likely to eat foods that he or she particularly enjoys.***
6. Ensure that client receives small, frequent feedings, including a bedtime snack, rather than three larger meals. ***Large amounts of food may be objectionable, or even intolerable, to the client.***
7. Administer vitamin and mineral supplements and stool softeners or bulk extenders, as ordered by physician.
8. If appropriate, ask family members or significant others to bring in special foods that client particularly enjoys.
9. Stay with client during meals ***to assist as needed and to offer support and encouragement.***
10. Monitor laboratory values, and report significant changes to physician. ***Laboratory values provide objective data regarding nutritional status.***
11. Explain the importance of adequate nutrition and fluid intake. ***Client may have inadequate or inaccurate knowledge regarding the contribution of good nutrition to overall wellness.***

Outcome Criteria

1. Client has shown a slow, progressive weight gain during hospitalization.
2. Vital signs, blood pressure, and laboratory serum studies are within normal limits.

3. Client is able to verbalize importance of adequate nutrition and fluid intake.

DISTURBED SLEEP PATTERN

Definition: *Time-limited disruption of sleep (natural, periodic suspension of consciousness) amount and quality.*

Possible Etiologies ("related to")

Depression
[Repressed fears]
[Feelings of hopelessness]
Anxiety
[Hallucinations]
[Delusional thinking]

Defining Characteristics ("evidenced by")

Verbal complaints of difficulty falling asleep
Awakening earlier or later than desired
[Interrupted sleep]
Verbal complaints of not feeling well rested
Sleep onset more than 30 minutes
[Awakening very early in the morning and being unable to go back to sleep]
[Excessive yawning and desire to nap during the day]
[Hypersomnia; using sleep as an escape]

Goals/Objectives

Short-Term Goal

Client will be able to sleep 4 to 6 hours with the aid of a sleeping medication within 5 days.

Long-Term Goal

Client will be able to fall asleep within 30 minutes of retiring and obtain 6 to 8 hours of uninterrupted sleep each night without medication by time of discharge from treatment.

Interventions with *Selected Rationales*

1. Keep strict records of sleeping patterns. *Accurate baseline data are important in planning care to assist client with this problem.*
2. Discourage sleep during the day *to promote more restful sleep at night.*
3. Administer antidepressant medication at bedtime *so client does not become drowsy during the day.*

4. Assist with measures that may promote sleep, such as warm, non-stimulating drinks; light snacks, warm baths, back rubs.
5. Performing relaxation exercises to soft music may be helpful prior to sleep.
6. Limit intake of caffeinated drinks, such as tea, coffee, and colas. ***Caffeine is a central nervous system (CNS) stimulant that may interfere with the client's achievement of rest and sleep.***
7. Administer sedative medications, as ordered, ***to help client achieve sleep until normal sleep pattern is restored.***
8. For client experiencing hypersomnia, set limits on time spent in room. Plan stimulating diversionary activities on a structured, daily schedule. Explore fears and feelings that sleep is helping to suppress.

Outcome Criteria

1. Client is sleeping 6 to 8 hours per night without medication.
2. Client is able to fall asleep within 30 minutes of retiring.
3. Client is dealing with fears and feelings rather than escaping from them through excessive sleep.

BIPOLAR DISORDER, MANIA

Predisposing Factors

1. Biological
   a. Genetics. Studies indicate that there is a higher incidence of bipolar disorder in first-degree relatives of individuals with the disorder than in the general population. If one identical twin has bipolar disorder, the possibility is as high as 80 percent that the other will also develop the disorder (Kelsoe, 1991). Bipolar disorder appears to be equally common in men and women (APA, 2000). Increasing evidence continues to support the role of genetics in the predisposition to bipolar disorder.
   b. Biochemical. Just as there is an indication of lowered levels of norepinephrine and dopamine during an episode of depression, the opposite appears to be true of an individual experiencing a manic episode. Thus, the behavioral responses of elation and euphoria may be caused by an excess of these biogenic amines in the brain. It has also been suggested that manic individuals have increased intracellular sodium and calcium. These electrolyte imbalances may be related to abnormalities in cellular membrane function in bipolar disorder.
2. Physiological
   a. Brain Lesions. Studies have shown that lesions in the left frontotemporal or right parieto-occipital quadrants tend to be associated with depression (Goodwin and Jamison, 1990). The most common affective sequelae of brain lesions involve post-stroke depressions, the severity of which increases the closer

the damage is to the left frontal pole. Secondary manic-like symptoms appear to be associated with right frontotemporal or left parieto-occipital lesions.

b. Medication Side Effects. Certain medications used to treat somatic illnesses have been known to trigger a manic response. The most common of these are the steroids frequently used to treat chronic illnesses such as multiple sclerosis and SLE. Some clients whose first episode of mania occurred during steroid therapy have reported spontaneous recurrence of manic symptoms years later. Amphetamines and tricyclic antidepressants also have the potential for initiating a manic episode.

Symptomatology (Subjective and Objective Data)

1. The affect of a manic individual is one of elation and euphoria—a continuous "high." However, the affect is very labile and may change quickly to hostility, particularly in response to attempts at limit setting, or to sadness, ruminating about past failures.
2. Alterations in thought processes and communication patterns are manifested by the following:
   a. Flight of Ideas. There is a continuous, rapid shift from one topic to another.
   b. Loquaciousness. The pressure of the speech is so forceful and strong that it is difficult to interrupt maladaptive thought processes.
   c. Delusions of Grandeur. The individual believes he or she is all-important and all-powerful, with feelings of greatness and magnificence.
   d. Delusions of Persecution. The individual believes someone or something desires to harm or violate him or her in some way.
3. Motor activity is constant. The individual is literally moving at all times.
4. Dress is often inappropriate: bright colors that do not match; clothing inappropriate for age or stature; excessive makeup and jewelry.
5. The individual has a meager appetite, despite excessive activity level. He or she is unable or unwilling to stop moving in order to eat.
6. Sleep patterns are disturbed. Client becomes oblivious to feelings of fatigue, and rest and sleep are abandoned for days or weeks.
7. Spending sprees are common. Individual spends large amounts of money, which is not available, on numerous items, which are not needed.
8. Usual inhibitions are discarded in favor of sexual and behavioral indiscretions.
9. Manipulative behavior and limit testing are common in the attempt to fulfill personal desires. Verbal or physical hostility may follow failure in these attempts.

10. Projection is a major defense mechanism. The individual refuses to accept responsibility for the negative consequences of personal behavior.
11. There is an inability to concentrate because of a limited attention span. The individual is easily distracted by even the slightest stimulus in the environment.
12. Alterations in sensory perception may occur, and the individual may experience hallucinations.
13. As agitation increases, symptoms intensify. Unless the client is placed in a protective environment, death can occur from exhaustion or injury.

Common Nursing Diagnoses and Interventions for Mania

(Interventions are applicable to various health-care settings, such as inpatient and partial hospitalization, community outpatient clinic, home health, and private practice.)

RISK FOR INJURY

Definition: ***At risk of injury as a result of environmental conditions interacting with the individual's adaptive and defensive resources.***

Related/Risk Factors ("related to")

[Extreme hyperactivity]
[Destructive behaviors]
[Anger directed at the environment]
[Hitting head (hand, arm, foot, etc.) against wall when angry]
[Temper tantrums—becomes destructive of inanimate objects]
[Increased agitation and lack of control over purposeless, and potentially injurious, movements]

Goals/Objectives

Short-Term Goal

Client will no longer exhibit potentially injurious movements after 24 hours with administration of tranquilizing medication.

Long-Term Goal

Client will experience no physical injury.

Interventions with *Selected Rationales*

1. Reduce environmental stimuli. Assign private room, if possible, with soft lighting, low noise level, and simple room decor. ***In hyperactive state, client is extremely distractible, and responses to even the slightest stimuli are exaggerated.***

2. Assign to quiet unit, if possible. ***Milieu unit may be too distracting.***
3. Limit group activities. Help client try to establish one or two close relationships. ***Client's ability to interact with others is impaired. He or she feels more secure in a one-to-one relationship that is consistent over time.***
4. Remove hazardous objects and substances from client's environment (including smoking materials). ***Client's rationality is impaired, and he or she may harm self inadvertently. Client safety is a nursing priority.***
5. Stay with the client ***to offer support and provide a feeling of security*** as agitation grows and hyperactivity increases.
6. Provide structured schedule of activities that includes established rest periods throughout the day. ***A structured schedule provides a feeling of security for the client.***
7. Provide physical activities as a substitution for purposeless hyperactivity. (Examples: brisk walks, housekeeping chores, dance therapy, aerobics.) ***Physical exercise provides a safe and effective means of relieving pent-up tension.***
8. Administer tranquilizing medication, as ordered by physician. Antipsychotic drugs, such as chlorpromazine (Thorazine), haloperidol (Haldol), or olanzapine (Zyprexa) are commonly prescribed for rapid relief of agitation and hyperactivity. Observe for effectiveness and evidence of adverse side effects.

Outcome Criteria

1. Client is no longer exhibiting signs of physical agitation.
2. Client exhibits no evidence of physical injury obtained while experiencing hyperactive behavior.

RISK FOR SELF-DIRECTED OR OTHER-DIRECTED VIOLENCE

Definition: ***At risk for behaviors in which an individual demonstrates that he/she can be physically, emotionally, and/or sexually harmful either to self or to others.***

Related/Risk Factors ("related to")

[Manic excitement]
[Dysfunctional grieving—denial of depression]
[Hereditary factors]
[Biochemical alterations]
[Threat to self-concept]
[Suspicion of others]
[Paranoid ideation]
[Delusions]

[Hallucinations]
[Rage reactions]
Body language—rigid posture, clenching of fists and jaw, hyperactivity, pacing, breathlessness, and threatening stances
[History or threats of violence toward self or others or of destruction to the property of others]
Impulsivity
Suicidal ideation, plan, available means
[Repetition of verbalizations (continuous complaints, requests, and demands)]

Goals/Objectives

Short-Term Goal

Client's agitation will be maintained at manageable level with the administration of tranquilizing medication during first week of treatment (decreasing risk of violence to self or others).

Long-Term Goal

Client will not harm self or others.

Interventions with *Selected Rationales*

1. Maintain low level of stimuli in client's environment (low lighting, few people, simple decor, low noise level). ***Anxiety and agitation rise in a stimulating environment. Individuals may be perceived as threatening by a suspicious, agitated client.***
2. Observe client's behavior frequently (every 15 minutes). ***Close observation is required so that intervention can occur if required to ensure client's (and others') safety.***
3. Remove all dangerous objects from client's environment (sharp objects, glass or mirrored items, belts, ties, smoking materials) ***so that in his or her agitated, hyperactive state client may not use them to harm self or others.***
4. Try to redirect the violent behavior with physical outlets for the client's hostility (e.g., punching bag). ***Physical exercise is a safe and effective way of relieving pent-up tension.***
5. Staff should maintain and convey a calm attitude to the client. Respond matter-of-factly to verbal hostility. ***Anxiety is contagious and can be transmitted from staff to client.***
6. Have sufficient staff available to indicate a show of strength to client if necessary. ***This conveys to the client evidence of control over the situation and provides some physical security for staff.***
7. Administer tranquilizing medications as ordered by physician. Monitor medication for effectiveness and for adverse side effects.
8. If the client is not calmed by "talking down" or by medication, use mechanical restraints as necessary. Be sure to have sufficient staff available to assist. Follow protocol established by the institu-

tion. The Joint Commission on Accreditation of Healthcare Organizations requires that the physician reissue a new order for restraints every 4 hours for adults and every 1 to 2 hours for children and adolescents. If the client has refused medication, administer medication after restraints have been applied. Most states consider this intervention appropriate in emergency situations or in the event that a client would likely harm self or others.

9. Observe the client in restraints every 15 minutes (or according to institutional policy). Ensure that circulation to extremities is not compromised (check temperature, color, pulses). Assist client with needs related to nutrition, hydration, and elimination. Position client so that comfort is facilitated and aspiration can be prevented. ***Client safety is a nursing priority.***
10. As agitation decreases, assess client's readiness for restraint removal or reduction. Remove one restraint at a time while assessing client's response. ***This procedure minimizes the risk of injury to client and staff.***

Outcome Criteria

1. Client is able to verbalize anger in an appropriate manner.
2. There is no evidence of violent behavior to self or others.
3. Client is no longer exhibiting hyperactive behaviors.

IMBALANCED NUTRITION, LESS THAN BODY REQUIREMENTS

Definition: ***Intake of nutrients insufficient to meet metabolic needs.***

Possible Etiologies ("related to")

[Refusal or inability to sit still long enough to eat meals]
[Lack of appetite]
[Excessive physical agitation]
[Physical exertion in excess of energy produced through caloric intake]
[Lack of interest in food]

Defining Characteristics ("evidenced by")

Loss of weight
Pale conjunctiva and mucous membranes
Poor muscle tone
[Amenorrhea]
[Poor skin turgor]
[Anemias]
[Electrolyte imbalances]

Goals/ Objectives

Short-Term Goal

Client will consume sufficient finger foods and between-meal snacks to meet recommended daily allowances of nutrients.

Long-Term Goal

Client will exhibit no signs or symptoms of malnutrition.

Interventions with *Selected Rationales*

1. In collaboration with dietitian, determine number of calories required to provide adequate nutrition for maintenance or realistic (according to body structure and height) weight gain.
2. Provide client with high-protein, high-calorie, nutritious finger foods and drinks that can be consumed "on the run." ***Because of hyperactive state, client has difficulty sitting still long enough to eat a meal. The likelihood is greater that he or she will consume food and drinks that can be carried around and eaten with little effort.***
3. Have juice and snacks available in the unit at all times. ***Nutritious intake is required on a regular basis to compensate for increased caloric requirements due to hyperactivity.***
4. Maintain accurate record of intake, output, and calorie count. ***This information is necessary to make an accurate nutritional assessment and maintain client's safety.***
5. Weigh client daily. ***Weight loss or gain is important nutritional assessment information.***
6. Determine client's likes and dislikes, and collaborate with dietitian to provide favorite foods. ***Client is more likely to eat foods that he or she particularly enjoys.***
7. Administer vitamin and mineral supplements, as ordered by physician, ***to improve nutritional state.***
8. Pace or walk with client as finger foods are taken. As agitation subsides, sit with client during meals. Offer support and encouragement. Assess and record amount consumed. ***Presence of a trusted individual may provide feeling of security and decrease agitation. Encouragement and positive reinforcement increase self-esteem and foster repetition of desired behaviors.***
9. Monitor laboratory values, and report significant changes to physician. ***Laboratory values provide objective nutritional assessment data.***
10. Explain the importance of adequate nutrition and fluid intake. ***Client may have inadequate or inaccurate knowledge regarding the contribution of good nutrition to overall wellness.***

Outcome Criteria

1. Client has gained (maintained) weight during hospitalization.
2. Vital signs, blood pressure, and laboratory serum studies are within normal limits.
3. Client is able to verbalize importance of adequate nutrition and fluid intake.

DISTURBED THOUGHT PROCESSES

Definition: *Disruption in cognitive operations and activities.*

Possible Etiologies ("related to")

[Hereditary factors]
[Biochemical alterations]
[Unmet dependency needs]
[Unresolved grief—denial of depression]

Defining Characteristics ("evidenced by")

Inaccurate interpretation of environment
Hypervigilance
[Altered attention span]—distractibility
Egocentricity
[Decreased ability to grasp ideas]
[Impaired ability to make decisions, problem-solve, reason]
[Delusions of grandeur]
[Delusions of persecution]
[Suspiciousness]

Goals/Objectives

Short-Term Goal

Within 1 week, client will be able to recognize and verbalize when thinking is nonreality-based.

Long-Term Goal

Client will experience no delusional thinking by time of discharge from treatment.

Interventions with *Selected Rationales*

1. Convey your acceptance of client's need for the false belief, while letting him or her know that you do not share the delusion. ***A positive response would convey to the client that you accept the delusion as reality.***

2. Do not argue or deny the belief. Use *reasonable doubt* as a therapeutic technique: "I find that hard to believe." ***Arguing with the client or denying the belief serves no useful purpose, because delusional ideas are not eliminated by this approach, and the development of a trusting relationship may be impeded.***
3. Use the techniques of *consensual validation* and *seeking clarification* when communication reflects alteration in thinking. (Examples: "Is it that you mean . . . ?" or "I don't understand what you mean by that. Would you please explain?") ***These techniques reveal to the client how he or she is being perceived by others, and the responsibility for not understanding is accepted by the nurse.***
4. Reinforce and focus on reality. Talk about real events and real people. Use real situations and events to divert client away from long, tedious, repetitive verbalizations of false ideas.
5. Give positive reinforcement as client is able to differentiate between reality-based and nonreality-based thinking. ***Positive reinforcement enhances self-esteem and encourages repetition of desirable behaviors.***
6. Teach client to intervene, using thought-stopping techniques, when irrational thoughts prevail. Thought stopping involves using the command "Stop!" or a loud noise (such as hand clapping) to interrupt unwanted thoughts. ***This noise or command distracts the individual from the undesirable thinking, which often precedes undesirable emotions or behaviors.***
7. Use touch cautiously, particularly if thoughts reveal ideas of persecution. ***Clients who are suspicious may perceive touch as threatening and may respond with aggression.***

Outcome Criteria

1. Thought processes reflect an accurate interpretation of environment.
2. Client is able to recognize thoughts that are not based in reality and intervene to stop their progression.

DISTURBED SENSORY PERCEPTION

Definition: *Change in the amount or patterning of incoming stimuli [either internally or externally initiated] accompanied by a diminished, exaggerated, distorted, or impaired response to such stimuli.*

Possible Etiologies ("related to")

[Hereditary factors]
Biochemical imbalance

Electrolyte imbalance
[Unmet dependency needs]
[Unresolved grief—denial of depression]
[Sleep deprivation]

Defining Characteristics ("evidenced by")

Change in usual response to stimuli
Hallucinations
Disorientation
[Inappropriate responses]
[Rapid mood swings]
[Exaggerated emotional responses]
[Visual and auditory distortions]
[Talking and laughing to self]
[Listening pose (tilting head to one side as if listening)]
[Stops talking in middle of sentence to listen]

Goals/Objectives

Short-Term Goal

Client will be able to recognize and verbalize when he or she is interpreting the environment inaccurately.

Long-Term Goal

Client will be able to define and test reality, eliminating the occurrence of sensory misperceptions.

Interventions with *Selected Rationales*

1. Observe client for signs of hallucinations (listening pose, laughing or talking to self, stopping in midsentence). ***Early intervention may prevent aggressive responses to command hallucinations.***
2. Avoid touching the client before warning him or her that you are about to do so. ***Client may perceive touch as threatening and respond in an aggressive manner.***
3. An attitude of acceptance will encourage the client to share the content of the hallucination with you. ***This is important in order to prevent possible injury to the client or others from command hallucinations.***
4. Do not reinforce the hallucination. Use "the voices" instead of words like "they" that imply validation. Let the client know that you do not share the perception. Say, "Even though I realize that the voices are real to you, I do not hear any voices speaking." ***The nurse must be honest with the client so that client may realize that the hallucinations are not real.***
5. Try to connect the times of the misperceptions to times of increased anxiety. Help client understand this connection. ***If client can learn to interrupt the escalating anxiety, reality orientation may be maintained.***

6. Try to distract the client away from the misperception. ***Involvement in interpersonal activities and explanation of the actual situation may bring the client back to reality.***

Outcome Criteria

1. Client is able to differentiate between reality and unrealistic events or situations.
2. Client is able to refrain from responding to false sensory perceptions.

IMPAIRED SOCIAL INTERACTION

Definition: *Insufficient or excessive quantity or ineffective quality of social exchange.*

Possible Etiologies ("related to")

Altered thought processes
[Strong dependency needs]
[Delusions of grandeur]
[Delusions of persecution]
[Underdeveloped ego]
[Low self-esteem]

Defining Characteristics ("evidenced by")

Verbalized or observed discomfort in social situations
Verbalized or observed inability to receive or communicate a satisfying sense of belonging, caring, interest, or shared history
Observed use of unsuccessful social interaction behaviors
Dysfunctional interaction with peers, family, and others
[Excessive use of projection—does not accept responsibility for own behavior]
[Verbal manipulation]
[Inability to delay gratification]

Goals/Objectives

Short-Term Goal

Client will verbalize which of his or her interaction behaviors are appropriate and which are inappropriate within 1 week.

Long-Term Goal

Client will demonstrate use of appropriate interaction skills as evidenced by lack of, or marked decrease in, manipulation of others to fulfill own desires.

Interventions with *Selected Rationales*

1. Recognize the purpose these behaviors serve for the client: to reduce feelings of insecurity by increasing feelings of power

and control. ***Understanding the motivation behind the manipulation may facilitate acceptance of the individual and his or her behavior.***

2. Set limits on manipulative behaviors. Explain to client what you expect and what the consequences are if the limits are violated. Limits must be agreed upon by all staff who will be working with the client. ***Client is unable to establish own limits, so this must be done for him or her. Unless administration of consequences for violation of limits is consistent, manipulative behavior will not be eliminated.***
3. Do not argue, bargain, or try to reason with the client. Merely state the limits and expectations. Be sure to follow through with consequences if limits are violated. ***Consistency is essential for success of this intervention.*** Do not let this "charmer" talk you out of it. ***Ignoring these attempts may work to decrease manipulative behaviors.***
4. Provide positive reinforcement for nonmanipulative behaviors. Explore feelings, and help the client seek more appropriate ways of dealing with them. ***Positive reinforcement enhances self-esteem and promotes repetition of desirable behaviors.***
5. Help client recognize consequences of own behaviors and refrain from attributing them to others. ***Client must accept responsibility for own behaviors before adaptive change can occur.***
6. Help client identify positive aspects of self, recognize accomplishments, and feel good about them. ***As self-esteem is increased, client will feel less need to manipulate others for own gratification.***

Outcome Criteria

1. Client is able to verbalize positive aspects of self.
2. Client accepts responsibility for own behaviors.
3. Client does not manipulate others for gratification of own needs.

DISTURBED SLEEP PATTERN

Definition: *Time-limited disruption of sleep (natural, periodic suspension of consciousness) amount and quality.*

Possible Etiologies ("related to")

[Excessive hyperactivity]
[Agitation]
[Biochemical alterations]

Defining Characteristics ("evidenced by")

[Pacing in hall during sleeping hours]
Sleep onset greater than 30 minutes
[Sleeping only short periods at a time]

[Numerous periods of wakefulness during the night]
[Awakening and rising extremely early in the morning; exhibiting signs of restlessness]

Goals/Objectives

Short-Term Goal

Within 3 days, with the aid of a sleeping medication, client will sleep 4 to 6 hours without awakening.

Long-Term Goal

By time of discharge from treatment, client will be able to acquire 6 to 8 hours of uninterrupted sleep without medication.

Interventions with *Selected Rationales*

1. Provide a quiet environment with a low level of stimulation. ***Hyperactivity increases and ability to achieve sleep and rest are hindered in a stimulating environment.***
2. Monitor sleep patterns. Provide structured schedule of activities that includes established times for naps or rest. ***Accurate baseline data are important in planning care to help client with this problem. A structured schedule, including time for naps, will help the hyperactive client achieve much-needed rest.***
3. Assess client's activity level. Client may ignore or be unaware of feelings of fatigue. Observe for signs such as increasing restlessness; fine tremors; slurred speech; and puffy, dark circles under eyes. ***Client can collapse from exhaustion if hyperactivity is uninterrupted and rest is not achieved.***
4. Before bedtime, provide nursing measures that promote sleep, such as back rub; warm bath; warm, nonstimulating drinks; soft music; and relaxation exercises.
5. Prohibit intake of caffeinated drinks, such as tea, coffee, and colas. ***Caffeine is a CNS stimulant and may interfere with the client's achievement of rest and sleep.***
6. Administer sedative medications, as ordered, to help client achieve sleep until normal sleep pattern is restored.

Outcome Criteria

1. Client is sleeping 6 to 8 hours per night without medication.
2. Client is able to fall asleep within 30 minutes of retiring.
3. Client is dealing openly with fears and feelings rather than manifesting denial of them through hyperactivity.

■ INTERNET REFERENCES

Additional information about mood disorders, including psychosocial and pharmacological treatment of these disorders, may be located at the following websites:

- http://www.pslgroup.com/depression.htm
- http://depression.miningco.com/
- http://www.ndmda.org
- http://www.fadavis.com/townsend
- http://www.laurus.com
- www.mentalhealth.com/p.html
- www.mhsource.com/bipolar
- www.mhsource.com/depression
- text.nlm.nih.gov/nih/cdc/www/44.html
- www.mental-health-matters.com/mood.html
- www.mentalhelp.net

CHAPTER 7

*Anxiety Disorders**

BACKGROUND ASSESSMENT DATA

The characteristic features of this group of disorders are symptoms of anxiety and avoidance behavior. Anxiety disorders are categorized in the following manner:

Panic Disorder

300.01 Without Agoraphobia
300.21 With Agoraphobia

Panic disorder is characterized by recurrent panic attacks, the onset of which are unpredictable, and manifested by intense apprehension, fear, or terror, often associated with feelings of impending doom and accompanied by intense physical discomfort. The attacks usually last minutes or, more rarely, hours. If accompanied by agoraphobia, there is a fear of being in places or situations from which escape might be difficult or in which help might not be available in the event of a panic attack (APA, 2000). Common agoraphobic situations include being outside the home alone, being in a crowd or standing in a line, being on a bridge, and traveling in a bus, train, or car.

300.22 Agoraphobia Without History of Panic Disorder

The *Diagnostic and Statistical Manual of Mental Disorders, Fourth Edition, Text Revision (DSM-IV-TR)* identifies the essential feature of this disorder as fear of being in places or situations from which escape might be difficult or in which help might not be available in the event of suddenly developing a symptom(s) that could be incapacitating or extremely embarrassing. Travel is restricted, or the individual may require a companion when away from home.

---

* Classification and criteria for all diagnoses in this chapter are from the *Diagnostic and Statistical Manual of Mental Disorders, Fourth Edition, Text Revision, 2000.* Used with permission from the American Psychiatric Association.

300.23 Social Phobia

Social phobia is characterized by a persistent fear of behaving or performing in the presence of others in a way that will be humiliating or embarrassing to the individual. The individual has extreme concerns about being exposed to possible scrutiny by others and fears social or performance situations in which embarrassment may occur (APA, 2000). Exposure to the phobic situation is avoided, or it is endured with intense anxiety. Common social phobias include speaking or writing in front of a group of people, eating in the presence of others, and using public restrooms.

300.29 Specific Phobia

Formerly called simple phobia, this disorder is characterized by persistent fears of specific objects or situations. These phobias are fairly widespread among the general population, the most common being fear of animals (zoophobia), fear of closed places (claustrophobia), and fear of heights (acrophobia). Exposure to the phobic stimulus is avoided or endured with intense anxiety.

300.3 Obsessive-Compulsive Disorder

This disorder is characterized by involuntary recurring thoughts or images that the individual is unable to ignore and by recurring impulses to perform a seemingly purposeless activity. These obsessions and compulsions serve to prevent the individual's extreme anxiety.

309.81 Posttraumatic Stress Disorder

Posttraumatic stress disorder (PTSD) is characterized by the development of physiological and behavioral symptoms following a psychologically traumatic event that is generally outside the range of usual human experience. The stressor, which would be considered markedly distressing to almost anyone, has usually been experienced with intense fear, terror, and helplessness. If duration of the symptoms is 3 months or more, the diagnosis is specified as "chronic." If there is a delay of 6 months or more in the onset of symptoms, the diagnosis is specified as "delayed onset."

308.3 Acute Stress Disorder

Acute stress disorder is characterized by the development of physiological and behavioral symptoms similar to those of PTSD. The major difference in the diagnoses lies in the length of time the symptoms exist. With acute stress disorder, the symptoms must subside within 4 weeks of occurrence of the stressor. If they last longer than 4 weeks, the individual is given the diagnosis of PTSD.

300.02 Generalized Anxiety Disorder

This disorder is characterized by chronic, unrealistic, and excessive anxiety and worry. The symptoms must have occurred more days than not for at least 6 months and must cause clinically significant distress or impairment in social, occupational, or other important areas of functioning. Symptoms include restlessness, feeling "on edge," becoming easily fatigued, difficulty concentrating, and irritability.

293.84 Anxiety Disorder due to a General Medical Condition

The symptoms of this disorder are considered the direct physiological consequence of a general medical condition. Symptoms may include prominent generalized anxiety symptoms, panic attacks, or obsessions or compulsions (APA, 2000). Medical conditions that have been known to cause anxiety disorders include endocrine, cardiovascular, respiratory, metabolic, and neurological disorders.

Substance-Induced Anxiety Disorder (Refer to Substance-Related Disorders for substance-specific codes)

The *DSM-IV-TR* (APA, 2000) describes the essential features of this disorder as prominent anxiety symptoms that are judged to be caused by the direct physiological effects of a substance (i.e., a drug of abuse, a medication, or toxin exposure). The symptoms may occur during substance intoxication or withdrawal and may involve prominent anxiety, panic attacks, phobias, or obsessions or compulsions.

Predisposing Factors

1. **Physiological**
   a. ***Biochemical:*** Increased levels of norepinephrine have been noted in panic and generalized anxiety disorders. Abnormal elevations of blood lactate have also been noted in clients with panic disorder. Decreased levels of serotonin have been implicated in the etiology of obsessive-compulsive disorder.
   b. ***Genetic:*** Studies suggest that anxiety disorders are prevalent within the general population. It has been shown that they are more common among first-degree biological relatives of people with the disorders than among the general population (APA, 2000).
   c. ***Medical or Substance-Induced:*** Anxiety disorders may be caused by a variety of medical conditions or the ingestion of various substances. (Refer to the previous section on categories of anxiety disorders.)
2. **Psychosocial**
   a. ***Psychodynamic Theory:*** The psychodynamic view focuses on the inability of the ego to intervene when conflict occurs between the id and the superego, producing anxiety. For various reasons (unsatisfactory parent-child relationship, conditional love, or provisional gratification), ego development is delayed. When developmental defects in ego functions compromise the

capacity to modulate anxiety, the individual resorts to unconscious mechanisms to resolve the conflict. Overuse or ineffective use of ego defense mechanisms results in maladaptive responses to anxiety.

b. ***Cognitive Theory:*** The main thesis of the cognitive view is that faulty, distorted, or counterproductive thinking patterns accompany or precede maladaptive behaviors and emotional disorders (Kaplan & Sadock, 1998). When there is a disturbance in this central mechanism of cognition, there is a consequent disturbance in feeling and behavior. Because of distorted thinking, anxiety is maintained by erroneous or dysfunctional appraisal of a situation. There is a loss of ability to reason regarding the problem, whether it is physical or interpersonal. The individual feels vulnerable in a given situation, and the distorted thinking results in an irrational appraisal, fostering a negative outcome.

Symptomatology (Subjective and Objective Data)

An individual may experience a panic attack under any of the following conditions:

- As the predominant disturbance, with no apparent precipitant
- When exposed to a phobic stimulus
- When attempts are made to curtail ritualistic behavior
- Following a psychologically traumatic event

Symptoms include the following (APA, 2000):

- Palpitations, pounding heart, or accelerated heart rate
- Sweating
- Trembling or shaking
- Sensations of shortness of breath or smothering
- Feeling of choking
- Chest pain or discomfort
- Nausea or abdominal distress
- Feeling dizzy, unsteady, lightheaded, or faint
- Derealization (feelings of unreality) or depersonalization (being detached from oneself)
- Fear of losing control or going crazy
- Fear of dying
- Paresthesias (numbness or tingling sensations)
- Chills or hot flashes

Other symptoms of anxiety disorders include the following:

1. Restlessness, feeling "on edge," excessive worry, being easily fatigued, difficulty concentrating, irritability, muscle tension, and sleep disturbances (generalized anxiety disorder).
2. Recurrent and intrusive recollections or dreams about the traumatic event, feeling of reliving the trauma (flashback episodes), difficulty feeling emotion (a "numbing" affect), insomnia, irritability, or outbursts of anger (PTSD).

3. Repetitive, obsessive thoughts, common ones being related to violence, contamination, and doubt; repetitive, compulsive performance of purposeless activity, such as handwashing, counting, checking, touching (obsessive-compulsive disorder).
4. Marked and persistent fears of specific objects or situations (specificphobia), social or performance situations (social phobia), or being in a situation from which one has difficulty escaping (agoraphobia).

Common Nursing Diagnoses and Interventions

(Interventions are applicable to various health-care settings, such as inpatient and partial hospitalization, community outpatient clinic, home health, and private practice.)

ANXIETY (PANIC)

Definition: ***Vague uneasy feeling of discomfort or dread accompanied by an autonomic response (the source often nonspecific or unknown to the individual); a feeling of apprehension caused by anticipation of danger. It is an alerting signal that warns of impending danger and enables the individual to take measures to deal with threat.***

Possible Etiologies ("related to")

Unconscious conflict about essential values and goals of life
Situational and maturational crises
[Real or perceived] threat to self-concept
[Real or perceived] threat of death
Unmet needs
[Being exposed to a phobic stimulus]
[Attempts at interference with ritualistic behaviors]
[Traumatic experience]

Defining Characteristics ("evidenced by")

Increased respiration
Increased pulse
Decreased or increased blood pressure
Nausea
Confusion
Increased perspiration
Faintness
Trembling or shaking
Restlessness
Insomnia
[Nightmares or visual perceptions of traumatic event]
[Fear of dying, going crazy, or doing something uncontrolled during an attack]

Goals/Objectives

Short-Term Goal

Client will verbalize ways to intervene in escalating anxiety within 1 week.

Long-Term Goal

Client will be able to recognize symptoms of onset of anxiety and intervene before reaching panic stage by time of discharge from treatment.

Interventions with *Selected Rationales*

1. Maintain a calm, nonthreatening manner while working with client. ***Anxiety is contagious and may be transferred from staff to client or vice versa. Client develops feeling of security in presence of calm staff person.***
2. Reassure client of his or her safety and security. This can be conveyed by physical presence of nurse. Do not leave client alone at this time. ***Client may fear for his or her life. Presence of a trusted individual provides client with feeling of security and assurance of personal safety.***
3. Use simple words and brief messages, spoken calmly and clearly, to explain hospital experiences to client. ***In an intensely anxious situation, client is unable to comprehend anything but the most elementary communication.***
4. Keep immediate surroundings low in stimuli (dim lighting, few people, simple decor). ***A stimulating environment may increase level of anxiety.***
5. Administer tranquilizing medication, as ordered by physician. Assess medication for effectiveness and for adverse side effects.
6. When level of anxiety has been reduced, explore with client possible reasons for occurrence. ***Recognition of precipitating factor(s) is the first step in teaching the client to interrupt escalation of the anxiety.***
7. Encourage client to talk about traumatic experience under nonthreatening conditions. Help client work through feelings of guilt related to the traumatic event. Help client understand that this was an event to which most people would have responded in like manner. Support client during flashbacks of the experience. ***Verbalization of feelings in a nonthreatening environment may help client come to terms with unresolved issues.***
8. Teach signs and symptoms of escalating anxiety and ways to interrupt its progression (e.g., relaxation techniques, deep breathing exercises, physical exercises, brisk walks, jogging, meditation).

Outcome Criteria

1. Client is able to maintain anxiety at level in which problem solving can be accomplished.
2. Client is able to verbalize signs and symptoms of escalating anxiety.
3. Client is able to demonstrate techniques for interrupting the progression of anxiety to the panic level.

FEAR

Definition: ***Response to perceived threat that is consciously recognized as a danger.***

Possible Etiologies ("related to")

Phobic stimulus
[Being in place or situation from which escape might be difficult]
[Causing embarrassment to self in front of others]

Defining Characteristics ("evidenced by")

[Refuses to leave own home alone]
[Refuses to eat in public]
[Refuses to speak or perform in public]
[Refuses to expose self to (specify phobic object or situation)]
Identifies object of fear
[Symptoms of apprehension or sympathetic stimulation in presence of phobic object or situation]

Goals/Objectives

Short-Term Goal

Client will discuss phobic object or situation with nurse or therapist within 5 days.

Long-Term Goal

Client will be able to function in presence of phobic object or situation without experiencing panic anxiety by time of discharge from treatment.

Interventions with *Selected Rationales*

1. Reassure client of his or her safety and security. ***At panic level of anxiety, client may fear for own life.***
2. Explore client's perception of threat to physical integrity or threat to self-concept. ***It is important to understand the client's perception of the phobic object or situation in order to assist with the desensitization process.***

3. Discuss the reality of the situation with client in order to recognize aspects that can be changed and those that cannot. ***Client must accept the reality of the situation (aspects that cannot change) before the work of reducing the fear can progress.***
4. Include client in making decisions related to selection of alternative coping strategies. (Example: Client may choose either to avoid the phobic stimulus or to attempt to eliminate the fear associated with it.) ***Allowing the client choices provides a measure of control and serves to increase feelings of self-worth.***
5. If the client elects to work on elimination of the fear, techniques of desensitization may be employed. This is a systematic plan of behavior modification, designed to expose the individual gradually to the situation or object (either in reality or through fantasizing) until the fear is no longer experienced. This is also sometimes accomplished through implosion therapy, in which the individual is "flooded" with stimuli related to the phobic situation or object (rather than in gradual steps) until anxiety is no longer experienced in relation to the object or situation. ***Fear is decreased as the physical and psychological sensations diminish in response to repeated exposure to the phobic stimulus under nonthreatening conditions.***
6. Encourage client to explore underlying feelings that may be contributing to irrational fears. Help client understand how facing these feelings, rather than suppressing them, can result in more adaptive coping abilities. ***Verbalization of feelings in a nonthreatening environment may help client come to terms with unresolved issues.***

Outcome Criteria

1. Client does not experience disabling fear when exposed to phobic object or situation

   or
2. Client verbalizes ways in which he or she will be able to avoid the phobic object or situation with minimal change in lifestyle.
3. Client is able to demonstrate adaptive coping techniques that may be used to maintain anxiety at a tolerable level.

INEFFECTIVE COPING

Definition: *Inability to form a valid appraisal of the stressors, inadequate choices of practiced responses, and/or inability to use available resources*

Possible Etiologies ("related to")

[Underdeveloped ego; punitive superego]
[Fear of failure]
[Unmet dependency needs]
Situational crises
[Personal vulnerability]
[Inadequate support systems]
Maturational crises

Defining Characteristics ("evidenced by")

[Ritualistic behavior]
[Obsessive thoughts]
Inability to meet basic needs
Inability to meet role expectations
Inability to problem-solve
[Alteration in societal participation]

Goals/Objectives

Short-Term Goal

Within 1 week, client will decrease participation in ritualistic behavior by half.

Long-Term Goal

By time of discharge from treatment, client will demonstrate ability to cope effectively without resorting to obsessive-compulsive behaviors or increased dependency.

Interventions with *Selected Rationales*

1. Assess client's level of anxiety. Try to determine the types of situations that increase anxiety and result in ritualistic behaviors. ***Recognition of precipitating factors is the first step in teaching the client to interrupt the escalating anxiety.***
2. Initially meet client's dependency needs as required. Encourage independence, and give positive reinforcement for independent behaviors. ***Sudden and complete elimination of all avenues for dependency would create intense anxiety in client. Positive reinforcement enhances self-esteem and encourages repetition of desired behaviors.***
3. In the beginning of treatment, allow plenty of time for rituals. Do not be judgmental or verbalize disapproval of the behavior. ***To deny client ritual behavior may precipitate panic level of anxiety.***
4. Support client's efforts to explore the meaning and purpose of the behavior. ***Client may be unaware of the relationship between emotional problems and compulsive behaviors. Recognition is important before change can occur.***

5. Provide structured schedule of activities for the client, including adequate time for completion of rituals. ***Structure provides a feeling of security for the anxious client.***
6. Gradually begin to limit amount of time allotted for ritualistic behavior as client becomes more involved in unit activities. ***Anxiety is minimized when client is able to replace ritualistic behaviors with more adaptive ones.***
7. Give positive reinforcement for nonritualistic behaviors. ***Positive reinforcement enhances self-esteem and encourages repetition of desired behaviors.***
8. Encourage recognition of situations that provoke obsessive thoughts or ritualistic behaviors. Explain ways of interrupting these thoughts and patterns of behavior (e.g., thought-stopping techniques, relaxation techniques, physical exercise, or other constructive activity with which client feels comfortable).

Outcome Criteria

1. Client is able to verbalize signs and symptoms of increasing anxiety and is able to intervene to maintain anxiety at manageable level.
2. Client demonstrates ability to interrupt obsessive thoughts and to refrain from ritualistic behaviors in response to stressful situations.

POWERLESSNESS

Definition: *The perception that one's own action will not significantly affect an outcome; a perceived lack of control over a current situation or immediate happening.*

Possible Etiologies ("related to")

Lifestyle of helplessness
[Fear of disapproval from others]
[Unmet dependency needs]
[Lack of positive feedback]
[Consistent negative feedback]

Defining Characteristics ("evidenced by")

Verbal expressions of having no control or influence over situation, outcome, or self-care.
Nonparticipation in care or decision making when opportunities are provided
Expression of doubt regarding role performance
Reluctance to express true feelings, fearing alienation from caregivers
Apathy

Dependence on others that may result in irritability, resentment, anger, and guilt
Passivity

Goals/Objectives

Short-Term Goal

Client will participate in decision making regarding own care within 5 days.

Long-Term Goal

Client will be able to effectively problem-solve ways to take control of his or her life situation by time of discharge from treatment, thereby decreasing feelings of powerlessness.

Interventions with *Selected Rationales*

1. Allow client to take as much responsibility as possible for own self-care practices. ***Providing client with choices will increase his or her feelings of control.*** Examples are as follows:
   a. Include client in setting the goals of care he or she wishes to achieve.
   b. Allow client to establish own schedule for self-care activities.
   c. Provide client with privacy as need is determined.
   d. Provide positive feedback for decisions made. Respect client's right to make those decisions independently, and refrain from attempting to influence him or her toward those that may seem more logical.
2. Help client set realistic goals. ***Unrealistic goals set the client up for failure and reinforce feelings of powerlessness.***
3. Help identify areas of life situation that client can control. ***Client's emotional condition interferes with his or her ability to solve problems. Assistance is required to perceive the benefits and consequences of available alternatives accurately.***
4. Help client identify areas of life situation that are not within his or her ability to control. Encourage verbalization of feelings related to this inability ***in an effort to deal with unresolved issues and accept what cannot be changed.***
5. Identify ways in which client can achieve. Encourage participation in these activities, and provide positive reinforcement for participation as well as for achievement. ***Positive reinforcement enhances self-esteem and encourages repetition of desirable behaviors.***

Outcome Criteria

1. Client verbalizes choices made in a plan to maintain control over his or her life situation.

2. Client verbalizes honest feelings about life situations over which he or she has no control.
3. Client is able to verbalize system for problem solving as required for adequate role performance.

SOCIAL ISOLATION

Definition: *Aloneness experienced by the individual and perceived as imposed by others and as a negative or threatening state.*

Possible Etiologies ("related to")

[Panic level of anxiety]
[Past experiences of difficulty in interactions with others]
[Need to engage in ritualistic behavior in order to keep anxiety under control]
[Repressed fears]

Defining Characteristics ("evidenced by")

[Stays alone in room]
Inability to communicate, withdrawal, lack of eye contact
Inappropriate or immature interests and activities for developmental age or stage
Preoccupation with own thoughts; repetitive, meaningless actions
Expression of feelings of rejection or of aloneness imposed by others
Experiencing feelings of difference from others
Insecurity in public

Goals/Objectives

Short-Term Goal

Client will willingly attend therapy activities accompanied by trusted support person within 1 week.

Long-Term Goal

Client will voluntarily spend time with other clients and staff members in group activities by time of discharge from treatment.

Interventions with *Selected Rationales*

1. Convey an accepting attitude by making brief, frequent contacts. ***An accepting attitude increases feelings of self-worth and facilitates trust.***
2. Show unconditional positive regard. ***Convey your belief in the client as a worthwhile human being.***
3. Be with the client to offer support during group activities that may

be frightening or difficult for him or her. ***The presence of a trusted individual provides emotional security for the client.***

4. Be honest, and keep all promises. ***Honesty and dependability promote a trusting relationship.***
5. Be cautious with touch. Allow client extra space and an avenue for exit if he or she becomes too anxious. ***A person in panic anxiety may perceive touch as a threatening gesture.***
6. Administer tranquilizing medications as ordered by physician. Monitor for effectiveness as well as for adverse side effects. ***Short-term use of antianxiety medications, such as diazepam, chlordiazepoxide, or alprazolam, helps to reduce level of anxiety in most individuals, thereby facilitating interactions with others.***
7. Discuss with client the signs of increasing anxiety and techniques for interrupting the response (e.g., relaxation exercises, thought stopping). ***Maladaptive behaviors, such as withdrawal and suspiciousness, are manifested during times of increased anxiety.***
8. Give recognition and positive reinforcement for client's voluntary interactions with others. ***Positive reinforcement enhances self-esteem and encourages repetition of acceptable behaviors.***

Outcome Criteria

1. Client demonstrates willingness or desire to socialize with others.
2. Client voluntarily attends group activities.
3. Client approaches others in appropriate manner for one-to-one interaction.

SELF-CARE DEFICIT (Identify Specific Area)

Definition: *Impaired ability to perform or complete [activities of daily living (ADLs) independently]*

Possible Etiologies ("related to")

[Withdrawal; isolation from others]
[Unmet dependency needs]
[Excessive ritualistic behavior]
[Disabling anxiety]
[Irrational fears]

Defining Characteristics ("evidenced by")

[Unwillingness to bathe regularly]
[Uncombed hair; dirty clothes; offensive body and breath odor; disheveled appearance]
[Eating only a few bites of food from meal tray]

[Lack of interest in selecting appropriate clothing to wear, dressing, grooming, or maintaining appearance at a satisfactory level]
[Incontinence]

Goals/Objectives

Short-Term Goal

Client will verbalize desire to take control of self-care activities within 5 days.

Long-Term Goal

Client will be able to take care of own ADLs and demonstrate a willingness to do so by time of discharge from treatment.

Interventions with *Selected Rationales*

1. Urge client to perform normal ADLs to his or her level of ability. ***Successful performance of independent activities enhances self-esteem.***
2. Encourage independence, but intervene when client is unable to perform. ***Client comfort and safety are nursing priorities.***
3. Offer recognition and positive reinforcement for independent accomplishments. (Example: "Mrs. J., I see you have put on a clean dress and combed your hair.") ***Positive reinforcement enhances self-esteem and encourages repetition of desired behaviors.***
4. Show client how to perform activities with which he or she is having difficulty. ***When anxiety is high, client may require simple, concrete demonstrations of activities that would be performed without difficulty under normal conditions.***
5. Keep strict records of food and fluid intake. ***This information is necessary to formulate an accurate nutritional assessment.***
6. Offer nutritious snacks and fluids between meals. ***Client may be unable to tolerate large amounts of food at mealtimes and may therefore require additional nourishment at other times during the day to receive adequate nutrition.***
7. If client is incontinent, establish routine schedule for toileting needs. Assist client to bathroom on hourly or bi-hourly schedule, as need is determined, until he or she is able to fulfill this need without assistance.

Outcome Criteria

1. Client feeds self, leaving no more than a few bites of food on food tray.
2. Client selects appropriate clothing and dresses and grooms self daily.
3. Client maintains optimal level of personal hygiene by bathing daily and carrying out essential toileting procedures without assistance.

INTERNET REFERENCES

Additional information about anxiety disorders and medications to treat these disorders may be located at the following websites:

- http://www.adaa.org
- http://www.mentalhealth.com
- http://www.psychweb.com/disorders/index.htm
- http://www.nimh.nih.gov
- http://www.anxietynetwork.com/pdhome.html
- http://www.ocdresource.com
- http://www.psychiatrymatters.md/index.asp?sec=sres&criteria=anxiolytics
- http://www.fadavis.com/townsend

CHAPTER 8

*Somatoform and Sleep Disorders**

BACKGROUND ASSESSMENT DATA

Somatoform disorders are identified by the presence of physical symptoms for which there are no demonstrable organic findings or known physiological mechanisms and for which there is evidence, or a strong presumption, that the symptoms are linked to psychological factors or conflicts. Disordered sleep is a problem that identifies abnormalities in the amount, quality, or timing of sleep and abnormal behavioral and physiological events occurring in association with sleep, specific sleep stages, or sleep-wake transitions. The *Diagnostic and Statistical Manual of Mental Disorders, Fourth Edition, Text Revision, 2000 (DSM-IV-TR)* (APA, 2000) identifies the following categories of somatoform and sleep disorders:

SOMATOFORM DISORDERS

300.81 Somatization Disorder

Somatization disorder is a chronic syndrome of multiple somatic symptoms that cannot be explained medically and are associated with psychosocial distress and long-term seeking of assistance from health-care professionals. Symptoms can represent any organ system but commonly are expressed as neurological, gastrointestinal, psychosexual, or cardiopulmonary disorders. Onset of the disorder is usually in adolescence or early adulthood and is more common in women than in men. The disorder usually runs a fluctuating course, with periods of remission and exacerbation.

---

* Classification and criteria for this and all subsequent diagnoses in this chapter marked with an asterisk are from the *Diagnostic and Statistical Manual of Mental Disorders, Fourth Edition, Text Revision, 2000.* Used with permission from the American Psychiatric Association.

307.xx Pain Disorder

The essential feature of pain disorder is severe and prolonged pain that causes clinically significant distress or impairment in social, occupational, or other important areas of functioning (APA, 2000). This diagnosis is made when psychological factors have been judged to have a major role in the onset, severity, exacerbation, or maintenance of the pain, even when the physical examination reveals organic pathology that is associated with the pain.

300.7 Hypochondriasis

Hypochondriasis is an unrealistic preoccupation with the fear of having a serious illness. The *DSM-IV-TR* suggests that this fear arises out of an unrealistic interpretation of physical signs and symptoms. Occasionally, medical disease may be present, but in the hypochondriacal individual, the symptoms are grossly disproportionate to the extent of organic pathology. Individuals with hypochondriasis often have a long history of "doctor shopping" and are convinced that they are not receiving the proper care.

300.11 Conversion Disorder

Conversion disorder is a loss of or change in body function resulting from a psychological conflict, the physical symptoms of which cannot be explained by any known medical disorder or pathophysiological mechanism. The most common conversion symptoms are those that suggest neurological disease such as paralysis, aphonia, seizures, coordination disturbance, akinesia, dyskinesia, blindness, tunnel vision, anosmia, anesthesia, and paresthesia.

300.7 Body Dysmorphic Disorder

This disorder, formerly called dysmorphophobia, is characterized by the exaggerated belief that the body is deformed or defective in some specific way. The most common complaints involve imagined or slight flaws of the face or head, such as thinning hair, acne, wrinkles, scars, vascular markings, facial swelling or asymmetry, and excessive facial hair (APA, 2000).

■ SLEEP DISORDERS

307.42 Insomnia

Insomnia is defined as difficulty with initiating or maintaining sleep. It is identified as *primary* when it is not associated with any physical or mental illness and *secondary* when it is associated with another physical or mental illness.

307.44 Hypersomnia

Hypersomnia (sometimes called *somnolence*) is defined as excessive sleepiness or seeking excessive amounts of sleep. Primary hypersomnia refers to the condition when no other cause for the symptom can be found. With this disorder, individuals have difficulty staying awake during what would be considered the waking hours of the sleep-wake cycle.

347 Narcolepsy

Narcolepsy is a disorder similar to hypersomnia in that both produce excessive sleepiness. The characteristic manifestation of narcolepsy, however, is sleep attacks. When the attack occurs, the individual cannot prevent falling asleep, sometimes in the middle of a task or even in the middle of a sentence. Also associated with the sleep attack in 50 to 70 percent of the cases is *cataplexy*, a sudden loss of muscle tone, such as jaw drop, head drop, weakness of the knees, or paralysis of all skeletal muscles with collapse (Kaplan & Sadock, 1998).

307.47 Nightmare Disorder

Nightmares are frightening dreams that lead to awakenings from sleep (APA, 2000). Nightmare disorder is diagnosed when there is a repeated occurrence of the frightening dreams, which interferes with social or occupational functioning.

307.46 Sleep Terror Disorder

The manifestations of sleep terrors include abrupt arousal from sleep with a piercing scream or cry. The individual is difficult to awaken or comfort, and if wakefulness does occur, the individual is usually disoriented and expresses a sense of intense fear but cannot recall the dream episode. On awakening in the morning, the individual has amnesia for the whole experience.

307.46 Sleepwalking

The disorder of sleepwalking is characterized by the performance of motor activity initiated during sleep in which the individual may leave the bed and walk about, dress, go to the bathroom, talk, scream, or even drive (Kaplan & Sadock, 1998). Episodes may last from a few minutes to a half hour. Most often, the person returns to bed and has no memory of the event on awakening. Should the individual awaken during the episode, he or she may experience several minutes of confusion and disorientation.

307.45 Circadian Rhythm Sleep Disorder

Sleep-wake schedule disturbances can be described as a misalignment between sleep and wake behaviors. *Circadian rhythm sleep disorder* occurs when the normal sleep-wake schedule is disrupted from its usual circadian rhythm. The individual is unable to sleep (or be awake) when he or she wants to sleep (or be awake) but can do so at other times. Sleep-wake schedule disturbances are common among shift workers and airplane travelers (commonly called *jet lag*).

Predisposing Factors

1. **Physiological**
   a. ***Genetic.*** Studies have shown an increased incidence of somatization disorder and hypochondriasis in first-degree relatives, implying a possible inheritable predisposition (Kaplan & Sadock, 1998). Genetic or familial patterns are thought to play a contributing role in primary insomnia, primary hypersomnia, narcolepsy, sleep terror disorder, and sleepwalking.
   b. ***Biochemical.*** Decreased levels of serotonin and endorphins may play a role in the etiology of pain disorder.
   c. ***Medical Conditions.*** A number of medical conditions, including sleep apnea, endocrine or metabolic disorders, infectious or neoplastic disease, and central nervous system (CNS) lesions, have been associated with insomnia and/or hypersomnia. Neurological abnormalities, particularly in the temporal lobe, may be related to precipitation of night terrors.
2. **Psychosocial**
   a. ***Psychodynamic.*** Some psychodynamicists view hypochondriasis as an ego defense mechanism. They hypothesize that physical complaints are the expression of low self-esteem and feelings of worthlessness and that the individual believes it is easier to feel something is wrong with the body than to feel something is wrong with the self. The psychodynamic theory of conversion disorder proposes that emotions associated with a traumatic event that the individual cannot express because of moral or ethical unacceptability are "converted" into physical symptoms. The unacceptable emotions are repressed and converted to a somatic hysterical symptom that is symbolic in some way of the original emotional trauma.
   b. ***Family Dynamics.*** Some families have difficulty expressing emotions openly and resolving conflicts verbally. When this occurs, the child may become ill, and a shift in focus is made from the open conflict to the child's illness, leaving unresolved the underlying issues that the family cannot confront openly. Thus, somatization by the child brings some stability to the family, as harmony replaces discord, and the child's welfare becomes the common concern. The child in turn receives positive reinforcement for the illness.
   c. ***Sociocultural/Familial Factors.*** Somatic complaints are often reinforced when the sick role relieves the individual from the need to deal with a stressful situation, whether it be within society or within the family. When the sick person is allowed to avoid stressful obligations and postpone unwelcome challenges, is excused from troublesome duties, or becomes the prominent focus of attention because of the illness, positive reinforcement guarantees repetition of the response.

d. ***Past Experience with Physical Illness.*** Personal experience, or the experience of close family members, with serious or life-threatening illness can predispose an individual to hypochondriasis. Once an individual has experienced a threat to biological integrity, he or she may develop a fear of recurrence. The fear of recurring illness generates an exaggerated response to minor physical changes, leading to hypochondriacal behaviors.

e. ***Cultural and Environmental Factors.*** Some cultures and religions carry implicit sanctions against verbalizing or directly expressing emotional states, thereby indirectly encouraging "more acceptable" somatic behaviors. Cross-cultural studies have shown that the somatization symptoms associated with depression are relatively similar, but the "cognitive" or emotional symptoms such as guilt are predominantly seen in Western societies. In Middle Eastern and Asian cultures, depression is almost exclusively manifested by somatic or vegetative symptoms. Environmental influences may be significant in the predisposition to somatization disorder. Some studies have suggested that a tendency toward somatization appears to be more common in individuals who have low socioeconomic, occupational, and educational status (Cloninger, 1994).

Symptomatology (Subjective and Objective Data)

1. Any physical symptom for which there is no organic basis but for which there is evidence of psychological factors.
2. Depressed mood is common.
3. Loss or alteration in physical functioning, with no organic basis. Examples include the following:
   a. Blindness or tunnel vision
   b. Paralysis
   c. Anosmia (inability to smell)
   d. Aphonia (inability to speak)
   e. Seizures
   f. Coordination disturbances
   g. Pseudocyesis (false pregnancy)
   h. Akinesia or dyskinesia
   i. Anesthesia or paresthesia
4. "La belle indifference"—a relative lack of concern regarding the severity of the symptoms just described (e.g., a person is suddenly blind but shows little anxiety over the situation).
5. "Doctor shopping."
6. Excessive use of analgesics.
7. Requests for surgery.
8. Assumption of an invalid role.
9. Impairment in social or occupational functioning because of preoccupation with physical complaints.

10. Psychosexual dysfunction (impotence, dyspareunia [painful coitus experienced by women], sexual indifference).
11. Excessive dysmenorrhea.
12. Excessive preoccupation with physical defect that is out of proportion to the actual condition.
13. Difficulty initiating or maintaining sleep.
14. Excessive sleepiness or seeking excessive amounts of sleep.
15. Sleep attacks.
16. Persistent, frightening nightmares.
17. Sleep terrors (abrupt arousal from sleep with a piercing scream or cry).
18. Physical motor activity initiated during sleep.
19. Inability to sleep (or be awake) when desiring to sleep (or be awake).

Common Nursing Diagnoses and Interventions

(Interventions are applicable to various health-care settings, such as inpatient and partial hospitalization, community outpatient clinic, home health, and private practice.)

CHRONIC PAIN

Definition: ***Unpleasant sensory and emotional experience arising from actual or potential tissue damage or described in terms of such damage (International Association for the Study of Pain); sudden or slow onset of any intensity from mild to severe, constant or recurring without an anticipated or predictable end and a duration of longer than 6 months.***

Possible Etiologies ("related to")

[Severe level of anxiety, repressed]
[Low self-esteem]
[Unmet dependency needs]
[Secondary gains from the sick role]

Defining Characteristics ("evidenced by")

[Verbal complaints of pain, in the absence of pathophysiological evidence]
[Social withdrawal]
[Facial mask of pain]
[Guarding behaviors]
[Demanding behaviors]
[Refuses to attend therapeutic activities because of pain]
[History of seeking assistance from numerous health-care professionals]

[Excessive use of analgesics, without relief of pain]
[Self-focusing]

Goals/Objectives

Short-Term Goal

Within 2 weeks, client will verbalize understanding of correlation between pain and psychological problems.

Long-Term Goal

By time of discharge from treatment, client will verbalize a noticeable, if not complete, relief from pain.

Interventions with *Selected Rationales*

1. Monitor physician's ongoing assessments and laboratory reports ***to ascertain that organic pathology is clearly ruled out.***
2. Recognize and accept that the pain is real to the individual, even though no organic cause can be identified. ***Denying the client's feelings is nontherapeutic and hinders the development of a trusting relationship.***
3. Observe and record the duration and intensity of the pain. Note factors that precipitate the onset of pain. ***Identification of the precipitating stressor is important for assessment purposes. This information will be used to develop a plan for assisting the client to cope more adaptively.***
4. Provide pain medication as prescribed by physician. ***Client comfort and safety are nursing priorities.***
5. Assist with comfort measures, such as back rub, warm bath, and heating pad. Be careful, however, not to respond in a way that reinforces the behavior. ***Secondary gains from physical symptoms may prolong maladaptive behaviors.***
6. Offer your attention at times when client is not focusing on pain. ***Positive reinforcement encourages repetition of adaptive behaviors.***
7. Identify activities that serve to distract client from focus on self and pain. ***These distractors serve in a therapeutic manner as a transition from focus on self or physical manifestations to focus on unresolved psychological issues.***
8. Encourage verbalization of feelings. Explore meaning that pain holds for client. Help client connect symptoms of pain to times of increased anxiety and to identify specific situations that cause anxiety to rise. ***Verbalization of feelings in a nonthreatening environment facilitates expression and resolution of disturbing emotional issues.***
9. Encourage client to identify alternative methods of coping with stress. ***These may avert the physical pain as a maladaptive response to stress.***

10. Explore ways to intervene as symptoms begin to intensify so that pain does not become disabling. (e.g., visual or auditory distractions, mental imagery, deep-breathing exercises, application of hot or cold compresses, relaxation exercises).
11. Provide positive reinforcement for adaptive behaviors. ***Positive reinforcement enhances self-esteem and encourages repetition of desired behaviors.***

Outcome Criteria

1. Client verbalizes that pain does not interfere with completion of daily activities.
2. Client verbalizes an understanding of the relationship between pain and emotional problems.
3. Client demonstrates ability to intervene as anxiety rises, to prevent the onset or increase in severity of pain.

INEFFECTIVE COPING

Definition: *Inability to form a valid appraisal of the stressors, inadequate choices of practiced responses, and/or inability to use available resources.*

Possible Etiologies ("related to")

[Severe level of anxiety, repressed]
[Low self-esteem]
[Unmet dependency needs]
[History of self or loved one having experienced a serious illness or disease]
[Regression to, or fixation in, an earlier level of development]
[Retarded ego development]
[Inadequate coping skills]

Defining Characteristics ("evidenced by")

[Numerous physical complaints verbalized in the absence of any pathophysiological evidence]
[Total focus on the self and physical symptoms]
[History of doctor shopping]
[Demanding behaviors]
[Refuses to attend therapeutic activities]
[Does not correlate physical symptoms with psychological problems]
Inability to meet basic needs
Inability to meet role expectations
Inability to problem-solve
Sleep disturbance

Goals/Objectives

Short-Term Goal

Within 2 weeks, client will verbalize understanding of correlation between physical symptoms and psychological problems.

Long-Term Goal

By time of discharge from treatment, client will demonstrate ability to cope with stress by means other than preoccupation with physical symptoms.

Interventions with *Selected Rationales*

1. Monitor physician's ongoing assessments, laboratory reports, and other data to maintain assurance that possibility of organic pathology is clearly ruled out. ***Knowledge of these data is vital for the provision of adequate and appropriate client care.***
2. Recognize and accept that the physical complaint is real to the individual, even though no organic cause can be identified. ***Denial of the client's feelings is nontherapeutic and interferes with establishment of a trusting relationship.***
3. Identify gains that the physical symptom is providing for the client: increased dependency, attention, distraction from other problems. ***These are important assessment data to be used in assisting the client with problem resolution.***
4. Initially, fulfill client's most urgent dependency needs. ***Failure to do this may cause client to become extremely anxious, with an increase in maladaptive behaviors.***
5. Gradually withdraw attention to physical symptoms. Minimize time given in response to physical complaints. ***Lack of positive response will discourage repetition of undesirable behaviors.***
6. Explain to client that any new physical complaints will be referred to the physician, and give no further attention to them. Be sure to note physician's assessment of the complaint. ***The possibility of organic pathology must always be taken into consideration. Failure to do so could jeopardize client's safety.***
7. Encourage client to verbalize fears and anxieties. Explain that attention will be withdrawn if rumination about physical complaints begins. Follow through. ***Without consistency of limit setting, change will not occur.***
8. Help client observe that physical symptoms occur because of, or are exacerbated by, specific stressors. Discuss alternative coping responses to these stressors. Give positive reinforcement for adaptive coping strategies. ***Positive reinforcement encourages repetition of desired behaviors.***
9. Help client identify ways to achieve recognition from others without resorting to physical symptoms. ***Positive recognition from***

others enhances self-esteem and minimizes the need for attention through maladaptive behaviors.

10. Discuss how interpersonal relationships are affected by client's narcissistic behavior. Explain how this behavior alienates others. ***Client may not realize how he or she is perceived by others.***
11. Provide instruction in relaxation techniques and assertiveness skills. ***These approaches decrease anxiety and increase self-esteem, which facilitate adaptive responses to stressful situations.***

Outcome Criteria

1. Client is able to demonstrate techniques that may be used in response to stress to prevent the occurrence or exacerbation of physical symptoms.
2. Client verbalizes an understanding of the relationship between emotional problems and physical symptoms.

DISTURBED BODY IMAGE

Definition: *Confusion in mental picture of one's physical self.*

Possible Etiologies ("related to")

[Severe level of anxiety, repressed]
[Low self-esteem]
[Unmet dependency needs]

Defining Characteristics ("evidenced by")

[Preoccupation with real or imagined change in bodily structure or function]
[Verbalizations about physical appearance that are out of proportion to any actual physical abnormality that may exist]
Fear of rejection or of reaction by others
Negative feelings about body
Change in social involvement

Goals/Objectives

Short-Term Goal

Client will verbalize understanding that changes in bodily structure or function are exaggerated out of proportion to the change that actually exists. (Time frame for this goal must be determined according to individual client's situation.)

Long-Term Goal

Client will verbalize perception of own body that is realistic to actual structure or function by discharge from treatment.

Interventions with *Selected Rationales*

1. Establish trusting relationship with client. ***Trust enhances therapeutic interactions between nurse and client.***
2. If there is actual change in body structure or function, encourage client to progress through stages of grieving. Assess level of knowledge, and provide information regarding normal grieving process and associated feelings. ***Knowledge of acceptable feelings facilitates progression through the grieving process.***
3. Identify misperceptions or distortions client has regarding body image. Correct inaccurate perceptions in a matter-of-fact, nonthreatening manner. Withdraw attention when preoccupation with distorted image persists. ***Lack of attention may encourage elimination of undesirable behaviors.***
4. Help client recognize personal body boundaries. ***Use of touch may help him or her recognize acceptance of the individual by others and reduce fear of rejection because of changes in bodily structure or function.***
5. Encourage independent self-care activities, providing assistance as required. ***Self-care activities accomplished independently enhance self-esteem and also create the necessity for client to confront reality of his or her bodily condition.***
6. Provide positive reinforcement for client's expressions of realistic bodily perceptions. ***Positive reinforcement enhances self-esteem and encourages repetition of desired behaviors.***

Outcome Criteria

1. Client verbalizes realistic perception of bodily condition.
2. Client demonstrates acceptance of changes in bodily structure or function, as evidenced by expression of positive feelings about body, ability or willingness to perform self-care activities independently, and a focus on personal achievements rather than preoccupation with distorted body image.

DISTURBED SENSORY PERCEPTION

Definition: *Change in the amount or patterning of incoming stimuli [either internally or externally initiated] accompanied by a diminished, exaggerated, distorted, or impaired response to such stimuli.*

Possible Etiologies ("related to")

[Severe level of anxiety, repressed]
[Low self-esteem]
[Unmet dependency needs]
[Regression to, or fixation in, an earlier level of development]
[Retarded ego development]

[Inadequate coping skills]
Psychological stress [narrowed perceptual fields caused by anxiety]

Defining Characteristics ("evidenced by")

[Loss or alteration in physical functioning suggesting a physical disorder (often neurological in nature) but for which organic pathology is not evident. Common alterations include paralysis, anosmia, aphonia, deafness, and blindness]
[La belle indifference]

Goals/Objectives

Short-Term Goal

Client will verbalize understanding of emotional problems as a contributing factor to alteration in physical functioning within 10 days.

Long-Term Goal

Client will demonstrate recovery of lost function.

Interventions with *Selected Rationales*

1. Monitor physician's ongoing assessments, laboratory reports, and other data to maintain assurance that possibility of organic pathology is clearly ruled out. ***Failure to do so may jeopardize client's safety.***
2. Identify gains that the physical symptom is providing for the client: increased dependency, attention, distraction from other problems. ***These are important assessment data to be used in assisting the client with problem resolution.***
3. Fulfill client's needs related to activities of daily living (ADLs) with which the physical symptom is interfering. ***Client comfort and safety are nursing priorities.***
4. Do not focus on the disability, and allow client to be as independent as possible. Intervene only when client requires assistance. ***Positive reinforcement would encourage continual use of the maladaptive response for secondary gains, such as dependency.***
5. Encourage client to participate in therapeutic activities to the best of his or her ability. Do not allow client to use the disability as a manipulative tool. Withdraw attention if client continues to focus on physical limitation. Reinforce reality as required, but ensure maintenance of a nonthreatening environment.
6. Encourage client to verbalize fears and anxieties. Help client recognize that the physical symptom appears at a time of extreme stress and is a mechanism used for coping. ***Client may be unaware of the relationship between physical symptom and emotional stress.***

7. Help client identify coping mechanisms that he or she could use when faced with stressful situations rather than retreating from reality with a physical disability.
8. Explain assertiveness techniques, and practice use of same through role playing. ***Use of assertiveness techniques enhances self-esteem and minimizes anxiety in interpersonal relationships.***
9. Help client identify a satisfactory support system within the community from which he or she may seek assistance as needed to cope with overwhelming stress.

Outcome Criteria

1. Client is no longer experiencing symptoms of altered physical functioning.
2. Client verbalizes an understanding of the relationship between extreme psychological stress and loss of physical functioning.
3. Client is able to verbalize adaptive ways of coping with stress and identify community support systems to which he or she may go for help.

SELF-CARE DEFICIT (Identify Specific Area)

Definition: *Impaired ability to perform or complete [ADLs independently].*

Possible Etiologies ("related to")

[Paralysis of body part]
[Inability to see]
[Inability to hear]
[Inability to speak]
Pain, discomfort

Defining Characteristics ("evidenced by")

Inability to bring food from a receptacle to the mouth
Inability to wash body or body parts; obtain or get to water sources; regulate temperature or flow
Impaired ability to put on or take off necessary items of clothing, obtain or replace articles of clothing, fasten clothing, maintain appearance at a satisfactory level
Inability to get to toilet or commode [impaired mobility]
Inability to manipulate clothing for toileting
Inability to flush toilet or commode
Inability to sit on or rise from toilet or commode
Inability to carry out proper toilet hygiene

Goals/Objectives

Short-Term Goal

Client will perform self-care needs independently, to the extent that physical ability will allow, within 5 days.

Long-Term Goal

By discharge from treatment, client will be able to perform ADLs independently and demonstrate a willingness to do so.

Interventions with *Selected Rationales*

1. Assess client's level of disability; note areas of strength and impairment. ***This knowledge is required to develop adequate plan of care for client.***
2. Encourage client to perform normal ADLs to his or her level of ability. ***Successful performance of independent activities enhances self-esteem.***
3. Encourage independence, but intervene when client is unable to perform. ***Client comfort and safety are nursing priorities.***
4. Ensure that nonjudgmental attitude is conveyed as nursing assistance with self-care activities is provided. Remember that the physical symptom is real to the client. It is not within the client's conscious control. ***A judgmental attitude interferes with the nurse's ability to provide therapeutic care for this client.***
5. Feed client, if necessary, and provide assistance with containers, positioning, and other matters, as required. ***Client comfort and safety are nursing priorities.***
6. Bathe client, or assist with bath, depending on his or her level of ability. ***Client comfort and safety are nursing priorities.***
7. Assist client with dressing, oral hygiene, combing hair, and applying makeup, as required. ***Client comfort and safety are nursing priorities.***
8. Provide bedpan, commode, or assistance to bathroom as determined by client's level of ability. ***Client comfort and safety are nursing priorities.***
9. Provide positive reinforcement for ADLs performed independently. ***Positive reinforcement enhances self-esteem and encourages repetition of desired behaviors.***
10. Take precautions against fostering dependency by intervening when client is capable of performing independently. Allow ample time for client to complete these activities to the best of his or her ability without assistance.
11. Encourage client to discuss feelings regarding the disability and the need for dependency it creates. Help client see the purpose this disability is serving for him or her. ***Self-disclosure and exploration of feelings with a trusted individual may help client fulfill unmet needs and confront unresolved issues.***

Outcome Criteria

1. Client feeds self without assistance.
2. Client selects appropriate clothing and dresses and grooms self daily.
3. Client maintains optimal level of personal hygiene by bathing daily and carrying out essential toileting procedures without assistance.

DEFICIENT KNOWLEDGE (Psychological Causes for Physical Symptoms)

Definition: *Absence or deficiency of cognitive information related to a specific topic.*

Possible Etiologies ("related to")

Lack of interest in learning
[Severe level of anxiety]

Defining Characteristics ("evidenced by")

[Denial of emotional problems]
[Statements such as, "I don't know why the doctor put me in the psychiatric unit. I have a physical problem."]
[History of "shopping" for a doctor who will substantiate symptoms as pathophysiological]
[Noncompliance with psychiatric treatment plan]

Goals/Objectives

Short-Term Goal

Client will verbalize an understanding that no pathophysiological condition exists to substantiate physical symptoms.

Long-Term Goal

By time of discharge from treatment, client will be able to verbalize psychological cause(s) for physical symptoms.

Interventions with *Selected Rationales*

1. Assess client's level of knowledge regarding effects of psychological problems on the body. ***An adequate database is necessary for the development of an effective teaching plan.***
2. Assess client's level of anxiety and readiness to learn. ***Learning does not occur beyond the moderate level of anxiety.***
3. Discuss physical examinations and laboratory tests that have been conducted. Explain purpose and results of each.
4. Explore feelings and fears held by client. Go slowly. These feelings

may have been suppressed or repressed for a very long time, and their disclosure will undoubtedly be a painful experience. Be supportive. ***Verbalization of feelings in a nonthreatening environment may help client come to terms with long-unresolved issues.***

5. Have client keep a diary of appearance, duration, and intensity of physical symptoms. A separate record of situations that the client finds especially stressful should also be kept. ***Comparison of these records may provide objective data from which to observe the relationship between physical symptoms and stress.***
6. Help client identify needs that are being met through the sick role. Together, formulate a more adaptive means for fulfilling these needs. Practice by role-playing. ***Change cannot occur until the client realizes that physical symptoms are used to fulfill unmet needs. Anxiety is relieved by role-playing, because the client is able to anticipate responses to stressful situations.***
7. Explain assertiveness techniques to the client. Discuss the importance of recognizing the differences among passive, assertive, and aggressive behaviors and of respecting the human rights of others while protecting one's own basic human rights. ***Use of these techniques enhances self-esteem and facilitates client's interpersonal relationships.***
8. Discuss adaptive methods of stress management: relaxation techniques, physical exercise, meditation, breathing exercises, and mental imagery. ***These techniques may be employed in an attempt to relieve anxiety and discourage the use of physical symptoms as a maladaptive response.***

Outcome Criteria

1. Client verbalizes an understanding of the relationship between psychological stress and physical symptoms.
2. Client demonstrates the ability to use therapeutic techniques in the management of stress.

DISTURBED SLEEP PATTERN

Definition: *Time-limited disruption of sleep (natural, periodic suspension of consciousness) amount and quality.*

Possible Etiologies ("related to")

[A specific medical condition]
[Use of, or withdrawal from, substances]
Anxiety
Depression

Circadian asynchrony
Frequently changing sleep-wake schedule
[Familial patterns]

Defining Characteristics ("evidenced by")

[Insomnia]
[Hypersomnia]
[Nightmares]
[Sleep terrors]
[Sleepwalking]

Goals/Objectives

Short-Term Goal

Client will verbalize causal relationship of sleep disorder.

Long-Term Goals

Client will be able to achieve adequate, uninterrupted sleep. Client will report feeling rested and demonstrate a sense of well-being.

Interventions with *Selected Rationales*

1. To promote sleep:
   a. Encourage activities that prepare one for sleep: soft music, relaxation exercises, warm bath. ***These activities promote relaxation.***
   b. Discourage strenuous exercise within 1 hour of bedtime. ***Strenuous exercise can be stimulating and keep one awake.***
   c. Control intake of caffeine-containing substances within 4 hours of bedtime (e.g., coffee, tea, colas, chocolate, and certain analgesic medications). ***Caffeine is a CNS stimulant and can interfere with the promotion of sleep.***
   d. Provide a high-carbohydrate snack before bedtime. Carbohydrates increase the levels of the amino acid tryptophan, a precursor to the neurotransmitter serotonin. ***Serotonin is thought to play a role in the promotion of sleep.***
   e. Keep the temperature of the room between 68° and 72°F. ***This range provides the temperature most conducive to sleep.***
   f. Instruct the client not to use alcoholic beverages to relax. ***Although alcohol may initially induce drowsiness and promote falling asleep, a rebound stimulation occurs in the CNS within several hours after drinking alcohol. The individual may fall asleep, only to be wide awake a few hours later.***
   g. Discourage smoking and the use of other tobacco products near sleep time. ***These products produce a stimulant effect on the CNS.***

h. Discourage daytime napping. Increase program of activities to keep the person busy. ***Sleeping during the day can interfere with the ability to achieve sleep at night.***
i. Individuals with chronic insomnia should use sleeping medications judiciously. ***Sedatives and hypnotics have serious side effects and are highly addicting. Life-threatening symptoms can occur with abrupt withdrawal, and discontinuation should be tapered under a physician's supervision. Long-term use can result in rebound insomnia.***

2. To prevent "jet lag" (circadian rhythm disruption):
   a. If time permits, use a preventive strategy of altering mealtimes and sleep times in the appropriate direction ***to prepare the body for the oncoming change.***
   b. If preventive measures are impossible, increasing the amount of sleep on arrival sometimes helps ***to reduce fatigue and restore the rested feeling.***
   c. Short-term use of sleep medication may be helpful.

Outcome Criteria

1. Client verbalizes a decrease in problems with sleep.
2. Client reports feeling rested and demonstrates a sense of well-being.

RISK FOR INJURY

Definition: *At risk of injury as a result of environmental conditions interacting with the individual's adaptive and defensive resources.*

Related/Risk Factors ("related to")

[Excessive sleepiness]
[Sleep terrors]
[Sleepwalking]
[Sleep deprivation]

Goals/Objectives

Short-Term and Long-Term Goal

Client will not experience injury.

Interventions with *Selected Rationales*

1. Ensure that side rails are up on the bed. ***An individual who experiences serious nightmares or night terrors can fall from the bed during an episode.***
2. Keep the bed in a low position ***to diminish the risk of injury by the person who gets out of bed during a sleepwalking episode.***

3. Equip the bed with a bell (or other noisemaker) that is activated when the bed is exited. ***This may alert the caretaker so that supervision to prevent accidental injury can be instituted.***
4. Keep a night light on, and arrange the furniture in the bedroom in a manner that promotes safety ***to provide a safe environment for the individual who awakens (fully or partially) during the night.***
5. Administer drug therapy as ordered. ***Insomnia and parasomnias have been treated effectively with benzodiazepines. The usual treatment for hypersomnia and narcolepsy has been with CNS stimulants such as amphetamines. In some instances, the serotonin-specific reuptake inhibitors have also been helpful for these problems.***
6. For the child who experiences nightmares, encourage him or her to talk about the dream. Tell the child that all people have dreams. Validate his or her feeling of fearfulness while ensuring safety. Keep a light on in the room, or give the child a flashlight. ***Talking about the dream helps to promote the unreality of the dream and to differentiate between what is real and what is not real. Light gives the child a feeling of control over the darkness within the room.***

Outcome Criteria

1. Client has not experienced injury from behaviors associated with sleep disorders.
2. Client is following medication regimen and is experiencing no adverse effects.

INTERNET REFERENCES

Additional information about somatoform disorders may be located at the following websites:

- http://www.psyweb.com/Mdisord/somatd.html
- http://www.uib.no/med/avd/med_a/gastro/wilhelms/hypochon.html
- http://www.mc.vanderbilt.edu/peds/pidl/adolesc/convreac.htm
- http://www.emedicine.com/EMERG/topic112.Htm
- http://www.findarticles.com/cf_dls/g2601/0012/2601001276/p1/article.jhtml

Additional information about sleep disorders may be located at the following websites:

- http://www.sleepnet.com/disorder.htm
- http://www.asda.org/
- http://www.sleepmedservices.com/
- http://sleepdisorderscenter.com/

Information about medications for sleep disorders may be located at the following websites:

- http://www.rxmed.com/rxmed/b.main/b2.pharmaceutical/b2.prescribe.html
- http://www.mentalhealth.com/drug/
- http://www.nlm.nih.gov/medlineplus
- http://www.fadavis.com/townsend

CHAPTER 9

*Dissociative Disorders**

BACKGROUND ASSESSMENT DATA

The essential feature of the dissociative disorders is a disruption in the usually integrated functions of consciousness, memory, identity, or perception (APA, 2000). During periods of intolerable stress, the individual blocks off part of his or her life from consciousness. The stressful emotion becomes a separate entity, as the individual "splits" from it and mentally drifts into a fantasy state. The following categories are defined in the *Diagnostic and Statistical Manual of Mental Disorders, Fourth Edition, Text Revision, 2000 (DSM-IV-TR)* (APA, 2000):

1. **300.12 Dissociative Amnesia.** An inability to recall important personal information, usually of a traumatic or stressful nature. The extent of the disturbance is too great to be explained by ordinary forgetfulness. Types of impairment in recall include the following:
   a. ***Localized Amnesia.*** Inability to recall all incidents associated with a traumatic event for a specific period following the event (usually a few hours to a few days).
   b. ***Selective Amnesia.*** Inability to recall only certain incidents associated with a traumatic event for a specific period following the event.
   c. ***Generalized Amnesia.*** Failure of recall encompassing one's entire life.
   d. ***Continuous Amnesia.*** Inability to recall events subsequent to a specific time up to and including the present. (The memory does not return after a short period, as in localized amnesia. The individual is unable to form new memories.)

* Classification and criteria for all diagnoses in this chapter are from the *Diagnostic and Statistical Manual of Mental Disorders, Fourth Edition, Text Revision, 2000.* Used with permission from the American Psychiatric Association.

e. ***Systematized Amnesia.*** Inability to remember events that relate to a specific category of information, such as one's family, or to one particular person or event.

2. **300.13 Dissociative Fugue.** A sudden, unexpected travel away from home or customary work locale along with assumption of a new identity and an inability to recall the previous identity. Following recovery, there is no recollection of events that took place during the fugue. Course is typically brief—hours to days, rarely months. Recurrences are rare.
3. **300.14 Dissociative Identity Disorder.** The existence within the individual of two or more distinct personalities, each of which is dominant at a particular time. The original personality is usually not aware (at least initially) of the existence of subpersonalities. When there are more than two subpersonalities, however, they are usually aware of each other. Transition from one personality to another is usually sudden and often associated with psychosocial stress. The course tends to be more chronic than in the other dissociative disorders.
4. **300.6 Depersonalization Disorder.** Characterized by a temporary change in the quality of self-awareness, which often takes the form of feelings of unreality, changes in body image, feelings of detachment from the environment, or a sense of observing oneself from outside the body.

Predisposing Factors

1. **Physiological**
   a. ***Genetics.*** The *DSM-IV-TR* suggests that dissociative identity disorder (DID) is more common in first-degree relatives of people with the disorder than in the general population. The disorder is often seen in more than one generation of a family.
   b. ***Neurobiological.*** Some clinicians have suggested a possible correlation between neurological alterations and dissociative disorders. Although available information is inadequate, it is possible that dissociative amnesia and dissociative fugue may be related to alterations in certain areas of the brain that have to do with memory. These include the hippocampus, the mammillary bodies, the dorsomedial thalamus, and the inferior temporal cortices (Waziri, 1994). Some studies have suggested a possible link between DID and certain neurological conditions, such as temporal lobe epilepsy, severe migraine headaches, cerebral cortical damage, and visual alterations. Electroencephalographic abnormalities have been observed in some clients with DID.
2. **Psychosocial**
   a. **Psychodynamic Theory.** Freud (1962) believed that dissociative behaviors occurred when individuals repressed distressing mental contents from conscious awareness. He believed that the unconscious was a dynamic entity in which repressed men-

tal contents were stored and unavailable to conscious recall. Current psychodynamic explanations of dissociation are based on Freud's concepts.

b. **Psychological Trauma.** A growing body of evidence points to the cause of DID as a set of traumatic experiences that overwhelms the individual's capacity to cope by any means other than dissociation. These experiences usually take the form of severe physical, sexual, and/or psychological abuse by a parent or significant other in the child's life. DID is thought to serve as a survival strategy for the child in this traumatic environment, whereby he or she creates a new being who is able to experience the overwhelming pain of the cruel reality, while the primary self can then escape awareness of the pain. It has been suggested that the number of an individual's alternate personalities may be related to the number of different types of abuse he or she suffered as a child.

Symptomatology (Subjective and Objective Data)

1. Impairment in recall.
   a. Inability to remember specific incidents.
   b. Inability to recall any of one's past life, including one's identity.
2. Sudden travel away from familiar surroundings; assumption of new identity, with inability to recall past.
3. Assumption of additional identities within the personality; behavior involves transition from one identity to another as a method of dealing with stressful situations.
4. Feeling of unreality; detachment from a stressful situation—may be accompanied by dizziness, depression, obsessive rumination, somatic concerns, anxiety, fear of going insane, and a disturbance in the subjective sense of time.

Common Nursing Diagnoses and Interventions

(Interventions are applicable to various health-care settings, such as inpatient and partial hospitalization, community outpatient clinic, home health, and private practice.)

INEFFECTIVE COPING

Definition: *Inability to form a valid appraisal of the stressors, inadequate choices of practiced responses, and/or inability to use available resources.*

Possible Etiologies ("related to")

[Severe level of anxiety, repressed]
[Childhood trauma]

[Childhood abuse]
[Low self-esteem]
[Unmet dependency needs]
[Regression to, or fixation in, an earlier level of development]
[Retarded ego development]
[Inadequate coping skills]

Defining Characteristics ("evidenced by")

[Dissociating self from painful situation by experiencing:
- Memory loss (partial or complete)
- Sudden travel away from home with inability to recall previous identity
- The presence of more than one personality within the individual
- Detachment from reality]

Inability to problem-solve
Inability to meet role expectations
[Inappropriate use of defense mechanisms]

Goals/Objectives

Short-Term Goals

1. Client will verbalize understanding that he or she is employing dissociative behaviors in times of psychosocial stress.
2. Client will verbalize more adaptive ways of coping in stressful situations than resorting to dissociation.

Long-Term Goal

Client will demonstrate ability to cope with stress (employing means other than dissociation).

Interventions with *Selected Rationales*

1. Reassure client of safety and security by your presence. Dissociative behaviors may be frightening to the client. ***Presence of a trusted individual provides feeling of security and assurance of freedom from harm.***
2. Identify stressor that precipitated severe anxiety. ***This information is necessary to the development of an effective plan of client care and problem resolution.***
3. Explore feelings that client experienced in response to the stressor. Help client understand that the disequilibrium felt is acceptable—indeed, even expected—in times of severe stress. ***Client's self-esteem is preserved by the knowledge that others may experience these behaviors in similar circumstances.***
4. As anxiety level decreases (and memory returns), use exploration and an accepting, nonthreatening environment to encourage client to identify repressed traumatic experiences that contribute to chronic anxiety.
5. Have client identify methods of coping with stress in the past, and determine whether the response was adaptive or maladaptive. ***In times of extreme anxiety, client is unable to evaluate appropri-***

ateness of response. This information is necessary for client to develop a plan of action for the future.

6. Help client define more adaptive coping strategies. Make suggestions of alternatives that might be tried. Examine benefits and consequences of each alternative. Assist client in the selection of those that are most appropriate for him or her. ***Depending on current level of anxiety, client may require assistance with problem solving and decision making.***
7. Provide positive reinforcement for client's attempts to change. ***Positive reinforcement enhances self-esteem and encourages repetition of desired behaviors.***
8. Identify community resources to which the individual may go for support if past maladaptive coping patterns return.

Outcome Criteria

1. Client is able to demonstrate techniques that may be used in response to stress to prevent dissociation.
2. Client verbalizes an understanding of the relationship between severe anxiety and the dissociative response.

DISTURBED THOUGHT PROCESSES

Definition: *Disruption in cognitive operations and activities.*

Possible Etiologies ("related to")

[Severe level of anxiety, repressed]
[Childhood trauma]
[Childhood abuse]
[Threat to physical integrity]
[Threat to self-concept]

Defining Characteristics ("evidenced by")

[Memory loss—inability to recall selected events related to a stressful situation]
[Memory loss—inability to recall events associated with entire life]
[Memory loss—inability to recall own identity]

Goals/Objectives

Short-Term Goal

Client will verbalize understanding that loss of memory is related to stressful situation and begin discussing stressful situation with nurse or therapist.

Long-Term Goal

Client will recover deficits in memory and develop more adaptive coping mechanisms to deal with stressful situations.

Interventions with *Selected Rationales*

1. Obtain as much information as possible about client from family and significant others (likes, dislikes, important people, activities, music, pets). ***A baseline assessment is important for the development of an effective plan of care.***
2. Do not flood client with data regarding his or her past life. ***Individuals who are exposed to painful information from which the amnesia is providing protection may decompensate even further into a psychotic state.***
3. Instead, expose client to stimuli that represent pleasant experiences from the past, such as smells associated with enjoyable activities, beloved pets, and music known to have been pleasurable to client.
4. As memory begins to return, engage client in activities that may provide additional stimulation. ***Recall may occur during activities that simulate life experiences.***
5. Encourage client to discuss situations that have been especially stressful and to explore the feelings associated with those times. ***Verbalization of feelings in a nonthreatening environment may help client come to terms with unresolved issues that may be contributing to the dissociative process.***
6. Identify specific conflicts that remain unresolved, and help client identify possible solutions. ***Unless these underlying conflicts are resolved, any improvement in coping behaviors must be viewed as only temporary.***
7. Provide instruction regarding more adaptive ways to respond to anxiety ***so that dissociative behaviors are no longer needed.***

Outcome Criteria

1. Client is able to recall all events of past life.
2. Client is able to demonstrate adaptive coping strategies that may be used in response to severe anxiety to avert amnestic behaviors.

DISTURBED PERSONAL IDENTITY

Definition: *Inability to distinguish between self and nonself.*

Possible Etiologies ("related to")

[Severe level of anxiety, repressed]
[Childhood trauma]
[Childhood abuse]
[Threat to physical integrity]
[Threat to self-concept]
[Underdeveloped ego]

Defining Characteristics ("evidenced by")

[Presence of more than one personality within the individual]

Goals/Objectives

Short-Term Goal

Client will verbalize understanding of the existence of multiple personalities within the self and be able to recognize stressful situations that precipitate transition from one to another.

Long-Term Goal

Client will verbalize understanding of the need for, enter into, and cooperate with long-term therapy for this disorder, with the ultimate goal being integration into one personality.

Interventions with *Selected Rationales*

1. The nurse must develop a trusting relationship with the original personality and with each of the subpersonalities. ***Trust is the basis of a therapeutic relationship. Each of the personalities views itself as a separate entity and must initially be treated as such.***
2. Help the client understand the existence of the subpersonalities. ***Client may be unaware of this dissociative response to stressful situations.***
3. Help client identify the need each subpersonality serves in the personal identity of the individual. ***Knowledge of these unfulfilled needs is the first step toward integration of the personalities and the client's ability to face unresolved issues without dissociation.***
4. Help the client identify stressful situations that precipitate the transition from one personality to another. Carefully observe and record these transitions. ***This knowledge is required to assist the client in responding more adaptively and to eliminate the need for transition to another personality.***
5. Use nursing interventions necessary to deal with maladaptive behaviors associated with individual subpersonalities. For example, if one personality is suicidal, precautions must be taken to guard against client's self-harm. If another personality has a tendency toward physical hostility, precautions must be taken for the protection of others. ***Safety of the client and others is a nursing priority.***
6. Help subpersonalities understand that their "being" will not be destroyed but integrated into a unified identity within the individual. ***Because subpersonalities function as separate entities, the idea of total elimination generates fear and defensiveness.***
7. Provide support during disclosure of painful experiences and reassurance when the client becomes discouraged with lengthy treatment.

Outcome Criteria

1. Client recognizes the existence of more than one personality.
2. Client is able to verbalize the purpose these personalities serve.
3. Client verbalizes the intention of seeking long-term outpatient psychotherapy.

DISTURBED SENSORY PERCEPTION (Kinesthetic)

Definition: *Change in the amount or patterning of incoming stimuli [either internally or externally initiated] accompanied by a diminished, exaggerated, distorted, or impaired response to such stimuli.*

Possible Etiologies ("related to")

[Severe level of anxiety, repressed]
[Childhood trauma]
[Childhood abuse]
[Threat to physical integrity]
[Threat to self-concept]
[Underdeveloped ego]

Defining Characteristics ("evidenced by")

[Alteration in the perception or experience of the self]
[Loss of one's own sense of reality]
[Loss of the sense of reality of the external world]

Goals/Objectives

Short-Term Goal

Client will verbalize adaptive ways of coping with stress.

Long-Term Goal

By time of discharge from treatment, client will demonstrate the ability to perceive stimuli correctly and maintain a sense of reality during stressful situations.

Interventions with *Selected Rationales*

1. Provide support and encouragement during times of depersonalization. The client manifesting these symptoms may express fear and anxiety at experiencing such behaviors. They do not understand the response and may express a fear of "going insane." ***Support and encouragement from a trusted individual provide a feeling of security when fears and anxieties are manifested.***
2. Explain the depersonalization behaviors and the purpose they usually serve for the client. ***This knowledge may help to minimize fears and anxieties associated with their occurrence.***

3. Explain the relationship between severe anxiety and depersonalization behaviors. ***The client may be unaware that the occurrence of depersonalization behaviors is related to severe anxiety.***
4. Help client relate these behaviors to times of severe psychological stress that he or she has experienced personally.
5. Explore past experiences and possibly repressed painful situations such as trauma or abuse. ***It is thought that traumatic experiences predispose individuals to dissociative disorders.***
6. Discuss these painful experiences with the client and encourage him or her to deal with the feelings associated with these situations. Work to resolve the conflicts these repressed feelings have nurtured. ***These interventions serve to decrease the need for the dissociative response to anxiety.***
7. Discuss ways the client may more adaptively respond to stress, and role-play with him or her to practice using these new methods.

Outcome Criteria

1. Client perceives stressful situations correctly and is able to maintain a sense of reality.
2. Client demonstrates use of adaptive strategies for coping with stress.

■ INTERNET REFERENCES

Additional information about dissociative disorders may be located at the following websites:

- http://www.human-nature.com/odmh/dissociative.html
- http://www.nami.org/helpline/dissoc.htm
- http://www.voiceofwomen.com/VOW2_11950/center.html
- http://www.issd.org/
- http://www.findarticles.com/cf_dls/g2601/0004/2601000438/p1/article.jhtml
- http://www.healinghopes.org/library/dissociation.html

CHAPTER 10

*Sexual and Gender Identity Disorders**

BACKGROUND ASSESSMENT DATA

The *Diagnostic and Statistical Manual of Mental Disorders, Fourth Edition, Text Revision, 2000 (DSM-IV-TR)* (APA, 2000) identifies two categories of sexual disorders: paraphilias and sexual dysfunctions. Paraphilias are characterized by recurrent, intense sexual urges, fantasies, or behaviors that involve unusual objects, activities, or situations (APA, 2000). Sexual dysfunction disorders can be described as an impairment or disturbance in any of the phases of the sexual response cycle. These include disorders of desire, arousal, and orgasm, and disorders that relate to the experience of genital pain during intercourse. Gender identity disorders are characterized by strong and persistent cross-gender identification accompanied by persistent discomfort with one's assigned gender (APA, 2000).

Paraphilias

Kaplan and Sadock (1998) identify the term *paraphilia* as repetitive or preferred sexual fantasies or behaviors that involve any of the following:

1. The preference for use of a nonhuman object.
2. Repetitive sexual activity with humans involving real or simulated suffering or humiliation.
3. Repetitive sexual activity with nonconsenting partners.

Types of paraphilias include the following:

1. **302.4 Exhibitionism.** The major symptoms include recurrent, intense sexual urges or behaviors or sexually arousing fantasies, of at least 6 months' duration, involving the exposure of one's genitals

---

*Classification and criteria for all psychiatric diagnoses in this chapter are from the *Diagnostic and Statistical Manual of Mental Disorders, Fourth Edition, Text Revision, 2000.* Used with permission from the American Psychiatric Association.

to an unsuspecting stranger (APA, 2000). Masturbation may occur during the exhibitionism. The condition apparently only occurs in men, and the victims are women in 99 percent of the cases (Kaplan & Sadock, 1998)

2. **302.81 Fetishism.** Fetishism involves recurrent, intense sexual urges or behaviors or sexually arousing fantasies, of at least 6 months' duration, involving the use of nonliving objects (APA, 2000). Common fetish objects include bras, women's underpants, stockings, shoes, boots, or other wearing apparel. The fetish object is generally used during masturbation or incorporated into sexual activity with another person to produce sexual excitation. When the fetish involves cross-dressing, the disorder is called **transvestic fetishism (302.3).**
3. **302.89 Frotteurism.** This disorder is defined as the recurrent preoccupation with intense sexual urges or fantasies, of at least 6 months' duration, involving touching or rubbing against a nonconsenting person (APA, 2000). Sexual excitement is derived from the actual touching or rubbing, not from the coercive nature of the act.
4. **302.2 Pedophilia.** The *DSM-IV-TR* describes the essential feature of pedophilia as recurrent sexual urges or behaviors or sexually arousing fantasies, of at least 6 months' duration, involving sexual activity with a prepubescent child. The age of the molester is 16 or older and is at least 5 years older than the child. This category of paraphilia is the most common of sexual assaults.
5. **302.83 Sexual Masochism.** The identifying feature of this disorder is recurrent, intense sexual urges or behaviors or sexually arousing fantasies, of at least 6 months' duration, involving the act (real, not simulated) of being humiliated, beaten, bound, or otherwise made to suffer (APA, 2000). These masochistic activities may be fantasized or solitary or with a partner. Examples include becoming sexually aroused by self-inflicted pain or by being restrained, raped, or beaten by a sexual partner.
6. **302.84 Sexual Sadism**. The essential feature of sexual sadism is identified as recurrent, intense, sexual urges or behaviors or sexually arousing fantasies, of at least 6 months' duration, involving acts (real, not simulated) in which the psychological or physical suffering (including humiliation) of the victim is sexually exciting (APA, 2000). The sadistic activities may be fantasized or acted on with a consenting or nonconsenting partner. In all instances, sexual excitation occurs in response to the suffering of the victim. Examples include rape, beating, torture, or even killing.
7. **302.82 Voyeurism.** This disorder is identified by recurrent, intense sexual urges or behaviors or sexually arousing fantasies, of at least 6 months' duration, involving the act of observing an unsuspecting person who is naked, in the process of disrobing, or engaging in sexual activity (APA, 2000). Sexual excitement is

achieved through the act of looking, and no contact with the person is attempted. Masturbation usually accompanies the "window peeping" but may occur later as the individual fantasizes about the voyeuristic act.

Predisposing Factors (to Paraphilias)

1. **Physiological**
   a. ***Physical Factors.*** Various studies have implicated several organic factors in the causation of paraphilias. Destruction of parts of the limbic system in animals has been shown to cause hypersexual behavior (Becker & Kavoussi, 1994). Temporal lobe diseases, such as psychomotor seizures or temporal lobe tumors, have been implicated in some individuals with paraphilias. Abnormal levels of androgens also may contribute to inappropriate sexual arousal. The majority of studies involved violent sex offenders; therefore, the results cannot accurately be generalized.
2. **Psychosocial**
   a. ***Psychoanalytical Theory.*** The psychoanalytic approach defines a paraphiliac as one who has failed the normal developmental process toward heterosexual adjustment (Kaplan & Sadock, 1998). This occurs when the individual fails to resolve the Oedipal crisis and identifies with the parent of the opposite gender. This creates intense anxiety, which leads the individual to seek sexual gratification in ways that provide a "safe substitution" for the parent (Becker & Kavoussi, 1994).

Symptomatology (Subjective and Objective Data)

1. Exposure of one's genitals to a stranger.
2. Sexual arousal in the presence of nonliving objects.
3. Touching and rubbing one's genitals against an unconsenting person.
4. Sexual attraction to, or activity with, a prepubescent child.
5. Sexual arousal from being humiliated, beaten, bound, or otherwise made to suffer (through fantasy, self-infliction, or by a sexual partner).
6. Sexual arousal by inflicting psychological or physical suffering on another individual (either consenting or nonconsenting).
7. Sexual arousal from dressing in the clothes of the opposite gender.
8. Sexual arousal from observing unsuspecting people either naked or engaged in sexual activity.
9. Masturbation often accompanies the activities described when they are performed solitarily.
10. The individual is markedly distressed by these activities.

Sexual Dysfunctions

Sexual dysfunctions may occur in any phase of the sexual response cycle. Types of sexual dysfunctions include the following:

1. **Sexual Desire Disorders**
   a. ***302.71 Hypoactive Sexual Desire Disorder.*** This disorder is defined by the *DSM-IV-TR* (APA, 2000) as a persistent or recurrent deficiency or absence of sexual fantasies and desire for sexual activity. The complaint appears to be more common among women than men.
   b. ***302.79 Sexual Aversion Disorder.*** This disorder is characterized by a persistent or recurrent extreme aversion to, and avoidance of, all (or almost all) genital sexual contact with a sexual partner (APA, 2000).
2. **Sexual Arousal Disorders**
   a. ***302.72 Female Sexual Arousal Disorder.*** This disorder is identified in the *DSM-IV-TR* (APA, 2000) as a persistent or recurrent inability to attain, or to maintain until completion of the sexual activity, an adequate lubrication or swelling response of sexual excitement.
   b. ***302.72 Male Erectile Disorder.*** This disorder is characterized by a persistent or recurrent inability to attain, or to maintain until completion of the sexual activity, an adequate erection (APA, 2000).
3. **Orgasmic Disorders**
   a. ***302.73 Female Orgasmic Disorder (Anorgasmia).*** This disorder is defined by the *DSM-IV-TR* as a persistent or recurrent delay in, or absence of, orgasm following a normal sexual excitement phase.
   b. ***302.74 Male Orgasmic Disorder (Retarded Ejaculation).*** With this disorder, the man is unable to ejaculate, even though he has a firm erection and has had more than adequate stimulation. The severity of the problem may range from only occasional problems ejaculating to a history of never having experienced an orgasm.
   c. ***302.75 Premature Ejaculation.*** The *DSM-IV-TR* describes this disorder as persistent or recurrent ejaculation with minimal sexual stimulation before, on, or shortly after penetration and before the person wishes it.
4. **Sexual Pain Disorders**
   a. ***302.76 Dyspareunia.*** Dyspareunia is defined as recurrent or persistent genital pain associated with sexual intercourse, in either a man or a woman, that is not caused by vaginismus, lack of lubrication, other general medical condition, or the physiological effects of substance use (APA, 2000).
   b. ***306.51 Vaginismus.*** Vaginismus is characterized by an involuntary constriction of the outer third of the vagina, which prevents penile insertion and intercourse.

Predisposing Factors (to Sexual Dysfunctions)

1. **Physiological Factors**
   a. ***Hypoactive Sexual Desire Disorders.*** These disorders have

been linked to low levels of serum testosterone in men and to elevated levels of serum prolactin in both men and women. Various medications, such as antihypertensives, antipsychotics, antidepressants, anxiolytics, and anticonvulsants, as well as chronic use of drugs such as alcohol and cocaine have also been implicated in sexual desire disorders (Kaplan & Sadock, 1998).

b. ***Sexual Arousal Disorders.*** These may occur in response to decreased estrogen levels in postmenopausal women. Medications such as antihistamines and cholinergic blockers may produce similar results. Erectile dysfunctions in men may be attributed to arteriosclerosis, diabetes, temporal lobe epilepsy, multiple sclerosis, some medications (antihypertensives, tranquilizers), spinal cord injury, pelvic surgery, and chronic use of alcohol.

c. ***Orgasmic Disorders.*** In women, these may be attributed to some medical conditions (hypothyroidism, diabetes, and hyperprolactinemia) and certain medications (antihypertensives, antidepressants). Medical conditions that may interfere with male orgasm include genitourinary surgery (e.g., prostatectomy), Parkinson's disease, and diabetes. Various medications have also been implicated, including antihypertensives, antidepressants, and antipsychotics. Transient cases of the disorder may occur with excessive alcohol intake.

d. ***Sexual Pain Disorders.*** In women, these can be caused by disorders of the vaginal entrance, irritation or damage to the clitoris, vaginal or pelvic infections, endometriosis, tumors, or cysts. Painful intercourse in men may be attributed to penile infections, phimosis, urinary tract infections, or prostate problems.

2. **Psychosocial Factors**

a. ***Sexual Desire Disorders.*** Phillips (2000) has identified a number of individual and relationship factors that may contribute to hypoactive sexual desire disorder. Individual causes include religious orthodoxy; sexual identity conflicts; past sexual abuse; financial, family, or job problems; depression; and aging-related concerns (e.g., changes in physical appearance). Among the relationship causes are interpersonal conflicts; current physical, verbal, or sexual abuse; extramarital affairs; and desire or practices different from those of the partner.

b. ***Sexual Arousal Disorders.*** In women, these may be attributed to doubts, fears, guilt, anxiety, shame, conflict, embarrassment, tension, disgust, resentment, grief, anger toward the partner, and puritanical or moralistic upbringing. A history of sexual abuse may also be an important etiologic factor (Leiblum, 1999). The etiology of male erectile disorder may be related to chronic stress, anxiety, or depression (Kaplan & Sadock, 1998).

Early developmental factors that promote feelings of inadequacy and a sense of being unloving or unlovable may also result in impotence. Difficulties in the relationship may also be a contributing factor.

c. ***Orgasmic Disorders.*** A number of factors have been implicated in the cause of female orgasm disorders. They include fear of becoming pregnant, hostility toward men, negative cultural conditioning, childhood exposure to rigid relgious orthodoxy, and traumatic sexual experiences during childhood or adolescence. Orgasm disorders in men may be related to a rigid, puritanical background where sex was perceived as sinful and the genitals as dirty; or interpersonal difficulties such as ambivalence about commitment, fear of pregnancy, or unexpressed hostility may be implicated.
d. ***Sexual Pain Disorders.*** Vaginismus may occur after having experienced painful intercourse for any organic reason, after which involuntary constriction of the vagina occurs in anticipation and fear of recurring pain. Other psychosocial factors that have been implicated as causes of vaginismus include negative childhood conditioning of sex as dirty, sinful, and shameful; early childhood sexual trauma; homosexual orientation; traumatic experience with an early pelvic examination; pregnancy phobia; venereal disease phobia; or cancer phobia (Phillips, 2000; Leiblum, 1999; Kaplan & Sadock, 1998).

Symptomatology (Subjective and Objective Data)

1. Absence of sexual fantasies and desire for sexual activity.
2. Discrepancy between partners' levels of desire for sexual activity.
3. Feelings of disgust, anxiety, or panic responses to genital contact.
4. Inability to produce adequate lubrication for sexual activity.
5. Absence of a subjective sense of sexual excitement during sexual activity.
6. Failure to attain or maintain penile erection until completion of sexual activity.
7. Inability to achieve orgasm (in men, to ejaculate) following a period of sexual excitement judged adequate in intensity and duration to produce such a response.
8. Ejaculation occurs with minimal sexual stimulation or before, on, or shortly after penetration and before the individual wishes it.
9. Genital pain occurs before, during, or after sexual intercourse.
10. Constriction of the outer third of the vagina prevents penile penetration.

Common Nursing Diagnoses and Interventions

(Interventions are applicable to various health-care settings, such as inpatient and partial hospitalization, community outpatient clinic, home health, and private practice.)

SEXUAL DYSFUNCTION

Definition: ***Change in sexual function that is viewed as unsatisfying, unrewarding, or inadequate.***

Possible Etiologies ("related to")

Ineffectual or absent role models
Physical [or sexual] abuse
Psychosocial abuse
Values conflict
Lack of privacy
Lack of significant other
Altered body structure or function (pregnancy, recent childbirth, drugs, surgery, anomalies, disease process, trauma, radiation)
Misinformation or lack of knowledge
[Depression]
[Pregnancy phobia]
[Venereal disease phobia]
[Cancer phobia]
[Previous painful experience]
[Severe anxiety]
[Relationship difficulties]

Defining Characteristics ("evidenced by")

Verbalization of problem:

- [Absence of desire for sexual activity
- Feelings of disgust, anxiety, or panic responses to genital contact
- Absence of lubrication or subjective sense of sexual excitement during sexual activity
- Failure to attain or maintain penile erection during sexual activity
- Inability to achieve orgasm or ejaculation
- Premature ejaculation
- Genital pain during intercourse
- Constriction of the vagina that prevents penile penetration]

Inability to achieve desired satisfaction

Goals/Objectives

Short-Term Goals

1. Client will identify stressors that may contribute to loss of sexual function within 1 week *or*
2. Client will discuss pathophysiology of disease process that contributes to sexual dysfunction within 1 week.
3. (For client with permanent dysfunction due to disease process:)

Client will verbalize willingness to seek professional assistance from a sex therapist in order to learn alternative ways of achieving sexual satisfaction with partner by (time is individually determined).

Long-Term Goal

Client will resume sexual activity at level satisfactory to self and partner by (time is individually determined).

Interventions with *Selected Rationales*

1. Assess client's sexual history and previous level of satisfaction in sexual relationship. ***This establishes a database from which to work and provides a foundation for goal setting.***
2. Assess client's perception of the problem. ***Client's idea of what constitutes a problem may differ from the nurse's. It is the client's perception on which the goals of care must be established.***
3. Help client determine period associated with the onset of the problem, and discuss what was happening in life situation at that time. ***Stress in any areas of life can affect sexual functioning. Client may be unaware of correlation between stress and sexual dysfunction.***
4. Assess client's mood and level of energy. ***Depression and fatigue decrease desire and enthusiasm for participation in sexual activity.***
5. Review medication regimen; observe for side effects. ***Many medications can affect sexual functioning. Evaluation of drug and individual response is important to ascertain whether drug may be contributing to the problem.***
6. Encourage client to discuss disease process that may be contributing to sexual dysfunction. Ensure that client is aware that alternative methods of achieving sexual satisfaction exist and can be learned through sex counseling if he or she and partner desire to do so. ***Client may be unaware that satisfactory changes can be made in his or her sex life. He or she may also be unaware of the availability of sex counseling.***
7. Encourage client to ask questions regarding sexuality and sexual functioning that may be troubling him or her. ***Increasing knowledge and correcting misconceptions can decrease feelings of powerlessness and anxiety and facilitate problem resolution.***
8. Make referral to sex therapist, if necessary. Client may even request that an initial appointment be made for him or her. ***Complex problems are likely to require assistance from an individual who is specially trained to treat problems related to sexuality. Client and partner may be somewhat embarrassed to seek this kind of assistance. Support from a trusted nurse can provide the impetus for them to pursue the help they need.***

Outcome Criteria

1. Client is able to correlate physical or psychosocial factors that interfere with sexual functioning.
2. Client is able to communicate with partner about their sexual relationship without discomfort.
3. Client and partner verbalize willingness and desire to seek assistance from professional sex therapist *or*
4. Client verbalizes resumption of sexual activity at level satisfactory to self and partner.

INEFFECTIVE SEXUALITY PATTERNS

Definition: *Expressions of concern regarding own sexuality.*

Possible Etiologies ("related to")

Lack of significant other
Ineffective or absent role models
[Illness-related alterations in usual sexuality patterns]
Conflicts with sexual orientation or variant preferences
[Unresolved Oedipal conflict]
[Delayed sexual adjustment]

Defining Characteristics ("evidenced by")

Reported difficulties, limitations, or changes in sexual behaviors or activities
[Expressed dissatisfaction with sexual behaviors]
[Reports that sexual arousal can only be achieved through variant practices, such as pedophilia, fetishism, masochism, sadism, frotteurism, exhibitionism, voyeurism]
[Desires to experience satisfying sexual relationship with another individual without need for arousal through variant practices]

Goals/Objectives

(Time elements to be determined by individual situation)

Short-Term Goals

1. Client will verbalize aspects about sexuality that he or she would like to change.
2. Client and partner will communicate with each other ways in which each believes their sexual relationship could be improved.

Long-Term Goals

1. Client will express satisfaction with own sexuality pattern.
2. Client and partner will express satisfaction with sexual relationship.

Interventions with *Selected Rationales*

1. Take sexual history, noting client's expression of areas of dissatisfaction with sexual pattern. ***Knowledge of what client perceives as the problem is essential for providing the type of assistance he or she may need.***
2. Assess areas of stress in client's life, and examine relationship with sexual partner. ***Variant sexual behaviors are often associated with added stress in the client's life. Relationship with partner may deteriorate as individual eventually gains sexual satisfaction only from variant practices.***
3. Note cultural, social, ethnic, racial, and religious factors that may contribute to conflicts regarding variant sexual practices. ***Client may be unaware of the influence these factors exert in creating feelings of discomfort, shame, and guilt regarding sexual attitudes and behavior.***
4. Be accepting and nonjudgmental. ***Sexuality is a very personal and sensitive subject. The client is more likely to share this information if he or she does not fear being judged by the nurse.***
5. Assist therapist in plan of behavior modification to help client who desires to decrease variant sexual behaviors. ***Individuals with paraphilias are treated by specialists who have experience in modifying variant sexual behaviors. Nurses can intervene by providing assistance with implementation of the plan for behavior modification.***
6. If altered sexuality patterns are related to illness or medical treatment, provide information to client and partner regarding the correlation between the illness and the sexual alteration. Explain possible modifications in usual sexual patterns that client and partner may try in an effort to achieve a satisfying sexual experience in spite of the limitation. ***Client and partner may be unaware of alternate possibilities for achieving sexual satisfaction, or anxiety associated with the limitation may interfere with rational problem solving.***
7. Explain to client that sexuality is a normal human response and is not synonymous with any one sexual act; it involves complex interrelationships among one's self-concept, body image, personal history, family and cultural influences, and all interactions with others (VandeVusse & Simandl, 1992). ***If client feels "abnormal" or very unlike everyone else, the self-concept is likely to be very low—he or she may even feel worthless. To increase the client's feelings of self-worth and desire to change behavior, help him or her see that even though the behavior is variant, feelings and motivations are common.***

Outcome Criteria

1. Client is able to verbalize fears about abnormality and inappropriateness of sexual behaviors.

2. Client expresses desire to change variant sexual behavior and cooperates with plan of behavior modification.
3. Client and partner verbalize modifications in sexual activities in response to limitations imposed by illness or medical treatment.
4. Client expresses satisfaction with own sexuality pattern or satisfying sexual relationship with another.

Gender Identity Disorders

Gender identity is the sense of knowing to which gender one belongs—that is, the awareness of one's masculinity or femininity. Gender identity disorders occur when there is incongruity between anatomic sex and gender identity. An individual with gender identity disorder has an intense desire to be, or insists that he or she is of, the other gender. The *DSM-IV-TR* (APA, 2000) identifies two categories of the disorder:

1. **302.6 Gender Identity Disorder in Children**
2. **302.85 Gender Identity Disorder in Adolescents and Adults**

Kaplan, Sadock, and Grebb (1994) report that intervention with adolescents and adults with gender identity disorder is difficult. Adolescents commonly act out and rarely have the motivation required to alter their cross-gender roles. Adults generally seek therapy to learn how to cope with their altered sexual identity, not to correct it.

Treatment of children with the disorder is aimed at helping them to become more comfortable with their assigned sex and to avoid the possible development of gender dissatisfaction in adulthood.

Predisposing Factors (to Gender Identity Disorder)

1. **Physiological.** Studies of genetics and physiological alterations have been conducted in an attempt to determine whether a biological predisposition to gender identity disorder exists. To date, no clear evidence has been demonstrated.
2. **Psychosocial**
   a. ***Family Dynamics.*** It appears that family dynamics plays the most influential role in the cause of gender disorders. Kaplan and Sadock (1998) state, "Children develop a gender identity consonant with their sex of rearing (also known as assigned sex)." Gender roles are culturally determined, and parents encourage masculine or feminine behaviors in their children. Although "temperament" may play a role with certain behavioral characteristics being present at birth, mothers usually foster a child's pride in their gender. Kaplan and Sadock (1998) state: "The father's role is also important in the early years, and his presence normally helps the separation-individuation process. Without a father, mother and child may remain overly close. For a girl, the father is normally the prototype of future love objects; for a boy, the father is a model for male identification." (p. 712)

b. ***Psychoanalytical Theory.*** This theory suggests that gender identity problems begin during the struggle of the Oedipal conflict. Problems may reflect real family events and those created in the child's imagination. These conflicts, whether real or imagined, interfere with the child's loving of the opposite-gender parent and identifying with the same-gender parent and ultimately with normal gender identity.

Symptomatology (Subjective and Objective Data)

In children or adolescents:

1. Repeatedly stating intense desire to be of the opposite gender.
2. Insistence that one is of the opposite gender.
3. Preference in males for cross-dressing or simulating female attire.
4. Insistence by females on wearing only stereotypical masculine clothing.
5. Fantasies of being of the opposite gender.
6. Intense desire to participate in the stereotypical games and pastimes of the opposite gender.
7. Strong preference for playmates (peers) of the opposite gender.

In adults:

1. A stated desire to be of the opposite gender.
2. Frequently passing as the opposite gender.
3. Desire to live or be treated as the opposite gender.
4. Stated conviction that one has the typical feelings and reactions of the opposite gender.
5. Persistent discomfort with or sense of inappropriateness in the assigned gender role.
6. Request for opposite gender hormones or surgery to alter sexual characteristics.

Common Nursing Diagnoses and Interventions

(Interventions are applicable to various health-care settings, such as inpatient and partial hospitalization, community outpatient clinic, home health, and private practice.)

NOTE: Because adults and adolescents rarely have the desire or motivation to modify their gender identity, nursing interventions in this section are focused on working with gender-disordered children.

DISTURBED PERSONAL IDENTITY

Definition: *Inability to distinguish between self and nonself.*

Possible Etiologies ("related to")

[Parenting patterns that encourage culturally unacceptable behaviors for assigned gender]

[Unresolved Oedipal conflict]

Defining Characteristics ("evidenced by")

[Statements of desire to be opposite gender]
[Statements that one is the opposite gender]
[Cross-dressing, or passing as the opposite gender]
[Strong preference for playmates (peers) of the opposite gender]
[Stated desire to be treated as the opposite gender]
[Statements of having feelings and reactions of the opposite gender]

Goals/Objectives

Short-Term Goals

1. Client will verbalize knowledge of behaviors that are appropriate and culturally acceptable for assigned gender.
2. Client will verbalize desire for congruence between personal feelings and behavior and assigned gender.

Long-Term Goals

1. Client will demonstrate behaviors that are appropriate and culturally acceptable for assigned gender.
2. Client will express personal satisfaction and feelings of being comfortable in assigned gender.

Interventions with *Selected Rationales*

1. Spend time with client, and show positive regard. ***Trust and unconditional acceptance are essential to the establishment of a therapeutic nurse-client relationship.***
2. Be aware of own feelings and attitudes toward this client and his or her behavior. ***Attitudes influence behavior. The nurse must not allow negative attitudes to interfere with the effectiveness of interventions.***
3. Allow client to describe his or her perception of the problem. ***It is important to know how the client perceives the problem before attempting to correct misperceptions.***
4. Discuss with the client the types of behaviors that are more culturally acceptable. Practice these behaviors through role playing or with play therapy strategies (e.g., male and female dolls). Positive reinforcement or social attention may be given for use of appropriate behaviors. No response is given for stereotypical opposite-gender behaviors. ***The goal is to enhance culturally appropriate same-gender behaviors but not necessarily to extinguish all coexisting opposite-gender behaviors.***

Outcome Criteria

1. Client demonstrates behaviors that are culturally appropriate for assigned gender.
2. Client verbalizes and demonstrates self-satisfaction with assigned gender role.
3. Client demonstrates development of a close relationship with the parent of the same gender.

IMPAIRED SOCIAL INTERACTION

Definition: *Insufficient or excessive quantity or ineffective quality of social exchange.*

Possible Etiologies ("related to")

[Socially and culturally unacceptable behavior]
[Negative role modeling]
[Low self-esteem]

Defining Characteristics ("evidenced by")

Verbalized or observed discomfort in social situations
Verbalized or observed inability to receive or communicate a satisfying sense of belonging, caring, interest, or shared history
Observed use of unsuccessful social interaction behaviors
Dysfunctional interaction with peers, family, or others

Goals/Objectives

Short-Term Goal

Client will verbalize possible reasons for ineffective interactions with others.

Long-Term Goal

Client will interact with others using culturally acceptable behaviors.

Interventions with *Selected Rationales*

1. Once client feels comfortable with the new behaviors in role playing or one-to-one nurse-client interactions, the new behaviors may be tried in group situations. If possible, remain with the client during initial interactions with others. ***Presence of a trusted individual provides security for the client in a new situation. It also provides the potential for feedback to the client about his or her behavior.***
2. Observe client behaviors and the responses he or she elicits from others. Give social attention (e.g., smile, nod) to desired behaviors. Follow-up these "practice" sessions with one-to-one processing of the interaction. Give positive reinforcement for efforts. ***Positive reinforcement encourages repetition of desirable behaviors. One-to-one processing provides time for discussing the appropriateness of specific behaviors and why they should or should not be repeated.***
3. Offer support if client is feeling hurt from peer ridicule. Matter-of-factly discuss the behaviors that elicited the ridicule. Offer no personal reaction to the behavior. ***Personal reaction from the nurse would be considered judgmental. Validation of client's feelings is important, yet it is also important that client under-***

stand why his or her behavior was the subject of ridicule and how to avoid it in the future.

Outcome Criteria

1. Client interacts appropriately with others demonstrating culturally acceptable behaviors.
2. Client verbalizes and demonstrates comfort in assigned gender role in interactions with others.

LOW SELF-ESTEEM

Definition: *Negative self-evaluation and feelings about self or self-capabilities.*

Possible Etiologies ("related to")

[Rejection by peers]
[Lack of positive feedback]
[Repeated negative feedback, resulting in diminished self-worth]
[Dysfunctional family system]
[Lack of personal satisfaction with assigned gender]

Defining Characteristics ("evidenced by")

[Inability to form close, personal relationships]
[Negative view of self]
[Expressions of worthlessness]
[Social isolation]
[Hypersensitivity to slight or criticism]
Expressions of shame or guilt
Self-negating verbalizations
Lack of eye contact

Goals/Objectives

Short-Term Goal

Client will verbalize positive statements about self, including past accomplishments and future prospects.

Long-Term Goal

Client will verbalize and demonstrate behaviors that indicate self-satisfaction with assigned gender, ability to interact with others, and a sense of self as a worthwhile person.

Interventions with *Selected Rationales*

1. ***To enhance the child's self-esteem:***
   a. Encourage the child to engage in activities in which he or she is likely to achieve success.

b. Help the child focus on aspects of his or her life for which positive feelings exist. Discourage rumination about situations that are perceived as failures or over which the client has no control. Give positive feedback for these behaviors.

2. Help the client identify behaviors or aspects of life he or she would like to change. If realistic, assist the child in problem-solving ways to bring about the change. ***Having some control over his or her life may decrease feelings of powerlessness and increase feelings of self-worth.***
3. Offer to be available for support to the child when he or she is feeling rejected by peers. ***Having an available support person who does not judge the child's behavior and who provides unconditional acceptance assists the child to progress toward acceptance of self as a worthwhile person.***

Outcome Criteria

1. Client verbalizes positive perception of self.
2. Client verbalizes self-satisfaction about accomplishments and demonstrates behaviors that reflect self-worth.

INTERNET REFERENCES

Additional information about sexual disorders may be located at the following websites:

- http://www.sexualhealth.com/
- http://www-hsl.mcmaster.ca/tomflem/sexual.html
- http://www.priory.com/sex.htm

Additional information about gender identity disorders may be located at the following websites:

- http://www.avitale.com/
- http://eserver.org/gender/
- http://www.findarticles.com/cf_dis/g2699/0001/269900148/p1/article.jhtml

CHAPTER 11

Eating Disorders

BACKGROUND ASSESSMENT DATA

The *Diagnostic and Statistical Manual of Mental Disorders, Fourth Edition, Text Revision, 2000 (DSM-IV-TR)* (APA, 2000) identifies eating disorders as characterized by severe disturbances in eating behavior. Two such disorders are described in the *DSM-IV-TR:* anorexia nervosa and bulimia nervosa. Obesity is not classified as a psychiatric disorder per se; however, because of the strong emoional factors associated with it, obesity may be considered in the category of *Psychological Factors Affecting Medical Condition.*

307.1 Anorexia Nervosa*

Defined

Anorexia nervosa is a clinical syndrome in which the person has a morbid fear of obesity. It is characterized by the individual's gross distortion of body image, preoccupation with food, and refusal to eat. The *DSM-IV-TR* lists the following criteria, which must be present to confirm the diagnosis of anorexia nervosa:

1. Refusal to maintain body weight at or above a minimally normal weight for age and height (e.g., weight loss leading to maintenance of body weight less than 85 percent of that expected; or failure to make expected weight gain during period of growth, leading to body weight less than 85 percent of that expected).
2. Intense fear of gaining weight or becoming fat, even though underweight.
3. Disturbance in the way one's body weight or shape is experienced, undue influence of body weight or shape on self-evaluation, or denial of the seriousness of the current low body weight.
4. In postmenarcheal females, amenorrhea (i.e., the absence of at least three consecutive menstrual cycles).

---

*Classification and criteria for this and all subsequent psychiatric diagnoses in this chapter marked with an asterisk are from the *Diagnostic and Statistical Manual of Mental Disorders, Fourth Edition, Text Revision, 2000.* Used with permission from the American Psychiatric Association.

5. The disorder occurs predominantly in females age 12 to 30 years. Without intervention, death from starvation can occur.

Symptomatology (Subjective and Objective Data)

1. Morbid fear of obesity. Preoccupied with body size. Reports "feeling fat" even when in an emaciated condition.
2. Refusal to eat. Reports "not being hungry," although it is thought that the actual feelings of hunger do not cease until late in the disorder.
3. Preoccupation with food. Thinks and talks about food at great length. Prepares enormous amounts of food for friends and family members but refuses to eat any of it.
4. Amenorrhea is common, often appearing even before noticeable weight loss has occurred.
5. Delayed psychosexual development.
6. Compulsive behavior, such as excessive hand washing, may be present.
7. Extensive exercising is common.
8. Feelings of depression and anxiety often accompany this disorder.
9. May engage in the "binge-and-purge syndrome" from time to time (see following section on Bulimia Nervosa).

307.51 Bulimia Nervosa*

Defined

Bulimia nervosa is an eating disorder (commonly called the binge-and-purge syndrome) characterized by extreme overeating, followed by self-induced vomiting and abuse of laxatives and diuretics. Diagnostic criteria for bulimia, as identified by the *DSM-IV-TR*, include the following:

1. Recurrent episodes of binge eating that is characterized by the following:
   a. Eating, within a discrete time (e.g., within any 2-hour period), an amount of food that is definitely larger than most people would eat during a similar period and under similar circumstances.
   b. A sense of lack of control over eating during the episode (e.g., a feeling that one cannot stop eating or control what or how much one is eating).
2. Recurrent, inappropriate compensatory behavior intended to prevent weight gain, such as self-induced vomiting; misuse of laxatives, diuretics, enemas, or other medications; fasting; or excessive exercise.
3. The binge eating and inappropriate compensatory behaviors both occur, on average, at least twice a week for 3 months.
4. Self-evaluation is unduly influenced by body shape and weight.
5. The disturbance does not occur exclusively during episodes of anorexia nervosa.

6. The disorder occurs predominantly in females and begins in adolescence or early adult life.

Symptomatology (Subjective and Objective Data)

1. Binges are usually solitary and secret, and the individual may consume thousands of calories in one episode.
2. After the binge has begun, there is often a feeling of loss of control or inability to stop eating.
3. Eating binges may be viewed as pleasurable but are followed by intense self-criticism and depressed mood.
4. Individuals with bulimia are usually within normal weight range, some a few pounds underweight, some a few pounds overweight.
5. Obsession with body image and appearance is a predominant feature of this disorder. Individuals with bulimia display undue concern with sexual attractiveness and how they will appear to others.
6. Binges usually alternate with periods of normal eating and fasting.
7. Excessive vomiting may lead to problems with dehydration and electrolyte imbalance.
8. Gastric acid in the vomitus also may contribute to the erosion of tooth enamel.

Predisposing Factors to Anorexia Nervosa and Bulimia Nervosa

1. **Physiological Factors**
   a. ***Genetics.*** An hereditary predisposition to eating disorders has been hypothesized on the basis of family histories and an apparent association with other disorders for which the likelihood of genetic influences exist. Anorexia nervosa is more common among sisters and mothers of those with the disorder than among the general population.
   b. ***Neuroendocrine Abnormalities.*** Some speculation has occurred regarding a primary hypothalamic dysfunction in anorexia nervosa. Studies consistent with this theory revealed elevated cerebrospinal fluid cortisol levels and a possible impairment of dopaminergic regulation in individuals with anorexia (Eckert & Mitchell, 1994).
2. **Psychosocial Factors**
   a. ***Psychodynamic Theory.*** The psychodynamic theory suggests that behaviors associated with eating disorders reflect a developmental arrest in the very early years of childhood caused by disturbances in mother-infant interactions. The tasks of trust, autonomy, and separation-individuation go unfulfilled, and the individual remains in the dependent position. Ego development is retarded. The problem is compounded when the mother responds to the child's physical and emotional needs with food. Manifestations include a disturbance in body iden-

tity and a distortion in body image. When events occur that threaten the vulnerable ego, feelings emerge of lack of control over one's body (self). Behaviors associated with food and eating provide feelings of control over one's life.

b. ***Family Dynamics.*** This theory proposes that the issue of control becomes the overriding factor in the family of the individual with an eating disorder. These families often consist of a passive father, a domineering mother, and an overly dependent child. A high value is placed on perfectionism in this family, and the child feels he or she must satisfy these standards. Parental criticism promotes an increase in obsessive and perfectionistic behavior in the child, who continues to seek love, approval, and recognition. The child eventually begins to feel helpless and ambivalent toward the parents. In adolescence, these distorted eating patterns may represent a rebellion against the parents, viewed by the child as a means of gaining and remaining in control. The symptoms are often triggered by a stressor that the adolescent perceives as a loss of control in some aspect of his or her life.

Obesity

Defined

The following formula is used to determine the degree of obesity in an individual:

$$\text{Body mass index (BMI)} = \frac{\text{weight (kg)}}{\text{height (m)}^2}$$

The BMI range for normal weight is 20 to 24.9. Studies by the National Center for Health Statistics indicate that *overweight* is defined as a BMI of 25.0 to 29.9 (based on U.S. Dietary Guidelines for Americans), and *obesity* is defined as a BMI of 30.0 or greater (based on criteria of the World Health Organization). These guidelines, which were released by the National Heart, Lung, and Blood Institute in June 1998, have been received by the medical community with a great deal of controversy. This change in guidelines increased the number of individuals in the United States considered to be overweight from one third to approximately one half. The average American woman has a BMI of 26, and fashion models typically have BMIs of 18 (America's Health Network, 1998).

Obesity is known to contribute to a number of health problems, including hyperlipidemia, diabetes mellitus, osteoarthritis, and increased workload on the heart and lungs.

Predisposing Factors to Obesity

1. **Physiological Factors**
   a. ***Genetics.*** Genetics have been implicated in the development of obesity in that 80 percent of offspring of two obese parents are

obese (Halmi, 1994). This hypothesis has also been supported by studies of twins reared by normal and overweight parents.

b. ***Physical Factors.*** Overeating and/or obesity has also been associated with lesions in the appetite and satiety centers of the hypothalamus, hypothyroidism, decreased insulin production in diabetes mellitus, and increased cortisone production in Cushing's disease.

2. **Psychosocial Factors**

a. ***Psychoanalytical Theory.*** This theory suggests that obesity is the result of unresolved dependency needs, with the individual being fixed in the oral stage of psychosexual development. The symptoms of obesity are viewed as depressive equivalents, attempts to regain "lost" or frustrated nurturance and care.

Common Nursing Diagnoses and Interventions (for Anorexia and Bulimia)

(Interventions are applicable to various health-care settings, such as inpatient and partial hospitalization, community outpatient clinic, home health, and private practice.)

IMBALANCED NUTRITION: LESS THAN BODY REQUIREMENTS

Definition: ***Intake of nutrients insufficient to meet metabolic needs.***

Possible Etiologies ("related to")

[Refusal to eat]
[Ingestion of large amounts of food, followed by self-induced vomiting]
[Abuse of laxatives, diuretics, and/or diet pills]
[Physical exertion in excess of energy produced through caloric intake]

Defining Characteristics ("evidenced by")

[Loss of 15 percent of expected body weight (anorexia nervosa)]
Pale conjunctiva and mucous membranes
Poor muscle tone
Excessive loss of hair [or increased growth of hair on body (lanugo)]
[Amenorrhea]
[Poor skin turgor]
[Electrolyte imbalances]
[Hypothermia]
[Bradycardia]
[Hypotension]

[Cardiac irregularities]
[Edema]

Goals/Objectives

Short-Term Goal

Client will gain____ pounds per week (amount to be established by client, nurse, and dietitian).

Long-Term Goal

By discharge from treatment, client will exhibit no signs or symptoms of malnutrition.

Interventions with *Selected Rationales*

1. If client is unable or unwilling to maintain adequate oral intake, physician may order a liquid diet to be administered via nasogastric tube. Nursing care of the individual receiving tube feedings should be administered according to established hospital procedures. ***The client's physical safety is a nursing priority, and without adequate nutrition, a life-threatening situation exists.***

For oral diet:

1. In collaboration with dietitian, determine number of calories required to provide adequate nutrition and realistic (according to body structure and height) weight gain.
2. Explain to client details of behavior modification program as outlined by physician.
3. Explain benefits of compliance with prandial routine and consequences for noncompliance. ***Behavior modification bases privileges granted or restricted directly on weight gain and loss. Focus is placed on emotional issues rather than on food and eating specifically.***
4. Sit with client during mealtimes for support and to observe amount ingested. A limit (usually 30 minutes) should be imposed on time allotted for meals. ***Without a time limit, meals can become lengthy, drawn-out sessions, providing client with attention based on food and eating.***
5. Client should be observed for at least 1 hour following meals. ***Otherwise, this time may be used by client to discard food stashed from tray or to engage in self- induced vomiting.***
6. Client may need to be accompanied to bathroom if self-induced vomiting is suspected.
7. Strict documentation of intake and output. ***This information is required to promote client safety and plan nursing care.***
8. Weigh client daily immediately on arising and following first voiding. Always use same scale, if possible. ***Client care, privileges, and restrictions will be based on accurate daily weights.***
9. Do not discuss food or eating with client, once protocol has been established. Do, however, offer support and positive reinforce-

ment for obvious improvements in eating behaviors. ***Discussing food with client provides positive feedback for maladaptive behaviors.***

10. Client must understand that if, because of poor oral intake, nutritional status does not improve, tube feedings will be initiated ***to ensure client's safety.*** Staff must be consistent and firm with this action, using a matter-of-fact approach regarding the tube insertion and subsequent feedings.
11. As nutritional status improves and eating habits are established, begin to explore with client the feelings associated with his or her extreme fear of gaining weight. ***Emotional issues must be resolved if maladaptive responses are to be eliminated.***

Outcome Criteria

1. Client has achieved and maintained at least 85 percent of expected body weight.
2. Vital signs, blood pressure, and laboratory serum studies are within normal limits.
3. Client verbalizes importance of adequate nutrition.

DEFICIENT FLUID VOLUME

Definition: *Decreased intravascular, interstitial, and/or intracellular fluid. This refers to dehydration, water loss alone without change in sodium.*

Possible Etiologies ("related to")

[Decreased fluid intake]
[Abnormal fluid loss caused by self-induced vomiting]
[Excessive use of laxatives or enemas]
[Excessive use of diuretics]
[Electrolyte or acid-base imbalance brought about by malnourished condition or self-induced vomiting]

Defining Characteristics ("evidenced by")

Decreased urine output
[Output greater than intake]
Increased urine concentration
Elevated hematocrit
Decreased blood pressure
Increased pulse rate
Increased body temperature
Dry skin
Decreased skin turgor
Weakness

Change in mental state
Dry mucous membranes

Goals/Objectives

Short-Term Goal

Client will drink 125 mL of fluid each hour during waking hours.

Long-Term Goal

By discharge from treatment, client will exhibit no signs or symptoms of dehydration (as evidenced by quantity of urinary output sufficient to individual client; normal specific gravity; vital signs within normal limits; moist, pink mucous membranes; good skin turgor; and immediate capillary refill).

Interventions with *Selected Rationales*

1. Keep strict record of intake and output. Teach client importance of daily fluid intake of 2000 to 3000 mL. ***This information is required to promote client safety and plan nursing care.***
2. Weigh client daily immediately on arising and following first voiding. Always use same scale, if possible. ***An accurate daily weight is needed to plan nursing care for the client.***
3. Assess and document condition of skin turgor and any changes in skin integrity. ***Condition of skin provides valuable data regarding client hydration.***
4. Discourage client from bathing every day if skin is very dry. ***Hot water and soap are drying to the skin.***
5. Monitor laboratory serum values, and notify physician of significant alterations. ***Laboratory data provide an objective measure for evaluating adequate hydration.***
6. Client should be observed for at least 1 hour following meals and may need to be accompanied to the bathroom if self-induced vomiting is suspected. ***Vomiting causes active loss of body fluids and can precipitate fluid volume deficit.***
7. Assess and document moistness and color of oral mucous membranes. ***Dry, pale mucous membranes may be indicative of malnutrition or dehydration.***
8. Encourage frequent oral care ***to moisten mucous membranes, reducing discomfort from dry mouth, and to decrease bacterial count, minimizing risk of tissue infection.***
9. Help client identify true feelings and fears that contribute to maladaptive eating behaviors. ***Emotional issues must be resolved if maladaptive behaviors are to be eliminated.***

Outcome Criteria

1. Client's vital signs, blood pressure, and laboratory serum studies are within normal limits.

2. No abnormalities of skin turgor and dryness of skin and oral mucous membranes are evident.
3. Client verbalizes knowledge regarding consequences of fluid loss due to self-induced vomiting and importance of adequate fluid intake.

INEFFECTIVE COPING

Definition: ***Inability to form a valid appraisal of the stressors, inadequate choices of practiced responses, and/or inability to use available resources.***

Possible Etiologies ("related to")

[Retarded ego development]
[Unfulfilled tasks of trust and autonomy]
[Dysfunctional family system]
[Unmet dependency needs]
[Feelings of helplessness and lack of control in life situation]
[Possible chemical imbalance caused by malfunction of hypothalamus]
[Unrealistic perceptions]

Defining Characteristics ("evidenced by")

[Preoccupation with extreme fear of obesity and distortion of own body image]
[Refusal to eat]
[Obsessed with talking about food]
[Compulsive behavior (e.g., excessive hand washing)]
[Excessive overeating, followed by self-induced vomiting and/or abuse of laxatives and diuretics]
[Poor self-esteem]
[Chronic fatigue]
[Chronic anxiety]
[Chronic depression]
Inability to problem-solve
Inability to meet role expectations
Destructive behavior toward self

Goals/Objectives

Short-Term Goal

Within 7 days, client will eat regular meals and attend activities without discussing food or physical appearance.

Long-Term Goal

Client will be able to verbalize adaptive coping mechanisms that can be realistically incorporated into his or her lifestyle, thereby eliminating the need for maladaptive eating behaviors.

Interventions with *Selected Rationales*

1. Establish a trusting relationship with client by being honest, accepting, and available and by keeping all promises. ***The therapeutic nurse-client relationship is built on trust.***
2. Acknowledge client's anger at feelings of loss of control brought about by established eating regimen (refer to interventions for Imbalanced Nutrition).
3. When nutritional status has improved, begin to explore with client the feelings associated with his or her extreme fear of gaining weight. ***Emotional issues must be resolved if maladaptive behaviors are to be eliminated.***
4. Explore family dynamics. Help client identify his or her role contributions and their appropriateness within the family system. Assist client to identify specific concerns within the family structure and ways to help relieve those concerns. Also, discuss importance of client's separation of self as individual within the family system and of identifying independent emotions and accepting them as his or her own. ***Client must recognize how maladaptive eating behaviors are related to emotional problems—often issues of control within the family structure.***
5. Initially, allow client to maintain dependent role. To deprive the individual of this role at this time could cause his or her anxiety to rise to an unmanageable level. As trust is developed and physical condition improves, encourage client to be as independent as possible in self-care activities. Offer positive reinforcement for independent behaviors and problem solving and decision making. ***Client must learn to function independently. Positive reinforcement increases self-esteem and encourages the client to use behaviors that are more acceptable.***
6. Explore with client ways in which he or she may feel in control within the environment, without resorting to maladaptive eating behaviors.

Outcome Criteria

1. Client is able to assess maladaptive coping behaviors accurately.
2. Client is able to verbalize adaptive coping strategies that can be used in the home environment.

ANXIETY (MODERATE TO SEVERE)

Definition: *Vague, uneasy feeling of discomfort or dread accompanied by an autonomic response (the source often nonspecific or unknown to the individual); a feeling of apprehension caused by anticipation of danger. It is an alerting signal that warns of impending danger and enables the individual to take measures to deal with threat.*

Possible Etiologies ("related to")

Situational and maturational crises
[Unmet dependency needs]
[Low self-esteem]
[Dysfunctional family system]
[Feelings of helplessness and lack of control in life situation]
[Unfulfilled tasks of trust and autonomy]

Defining Characteristics ("evidenced by")

[Increased tension]
Increased helplessness
Overexcited
Apprehensive; fearful
Restlessness
Poor eye contact
[Increased difficulty taking oral nourishment]
[Inability to learn]

Goals/Objectives

Short-Term Goal

Client will demonstrate use of relaxation techniques to maintain anxiety at manageable level within 7 days.

Long-Term Goal

By time of discharge from treatment, client will be able to recognize events that precipitate anxiety and intervene to prevent disabling behaviors.

Interventions with *Selected Rationales*

1. Be available to stay with client. Remain calm, and provide reassurance of safety. ***Client safety and security are a nursing priority.***
2. Help client identify the situation that precipitated onset of anxiety symptoms. ***Client may be unaware that emotional issues are related to symptoms of anxiety. Recognition may be the first step in elimination of this maladaptive response.***
3. Review client's methods of coping with similar situations in the past. ***In seeking to create change, it is helpful for client to identify past responses and determine whether they were successful and whether they could be employed again. Client strengths should be identified and used to his or her advantage.***
4. Provide quiet environment. Reduce stimuli: low lighting, few people. ***Anxiety level may be decreased in calm atmosphere with few stimuli.***
5. Administer antianxiety medications, as ordered by physician. Monitor for effectiveness of medication and for adverse side effects. ***Short-term use of antianxiety medications (e.g., diazepam,***

chlordiazepoxide, alprazolam) provides relief from the immobilizing effects of anxiety and facilitates client's cooperation with therapy.

6. Teach client to recognize signs of increasing anxiety and ways to intervene for maintaining the anxiety at a manageable level (e.g., exercise, walking, jogging, relaxation techniques). ***Anxiety and tension can be reduced safely and with benefit to the client through physical activities.***

Outcome Criteria

1. Client is able to verbalize events that precipitate anxiety and demonstrate techniques for its reduction.
2. Client is able to verbalize ways in which he or she may gain more control of the environment and thereby reduce feelings of helplessness.

DISTURBED BODY IMAGE/LOW SELF-ESTEEM

Definition: *Confusion in mental picture of one's physical self. Negative self-evaluation and feelings about self or self-capabilities.*

Possible Etiologies ("related to")

[Lack of positive feedback]
[Perceived failures]
[Unrealistic expectations (on the part of self and others)]
[Retarded ego development]
[Unmet dependency needs]
[Threat to security caused by dysfunctional family dynamics]
[Morbid fear of obesity]
[Perceived loss of control in some aspect of life]

Defining Characteristics ("evidenced by")

[Distorted body image; views self as fat, even in the presence of normal body weight or severe emaciation]
[Denial that problem with low body weight exists]
[Difficulty accepting positive reinforcement]
[Not taking responsibility for self-care (self-neglect)]
[Nonparticipation in therapy]
[Self-destructive behavior (self-induced vomiting, abuse of laxatives or diuretics, refusal to eat)]
Lack of eye contact
[Depressed mood and self-deprecating thoughts following episode of binging and purging]
[Preoccupation with appearance and how others perceive it]

Goals/Objectives

Short-Term Goal

Client will verbally acknowledge misperception of body image as "fat" within specified time (depending on severity and chronicity of condition).

Long-Term Goal

Client will demonstrate an increase in self-esteem as manifested by verbalizing positive aspects of self and exhibiting less preoccupation with own appearance as a more realistic body image is developed by time of discharge.

Interventions with *Selected Rationales*

1. Help client reexamine negative perceptions of self and recognize positive attributes. ***Client's own identification of strengths and positive attributes can increase sense of self-worth.***
2. Offer positive reinforcement for independently made decisions influencing client's life. ***Positive reinforcement enhances self-esteem and may encourage client to continue functioning more independently.***
3. Offer positive reinforcement when honest feelings related to autonomy and dependence issues remain separated from maladaptive eating behaviors.
4. Help client develop a realistic perception of body image and relationship with food. ***Client needs to recognize that his or her perception of body image is unhealthy and that maintaining control through maladaptive eating behaviors is dangerous, even life-threatening.***
5. Promote feelings of control within the environment through participation and independent decision making. Through positive feedback, help client learn to accept self as is, weaknesses as well as strengths. ***Client must come to understand that he or she is a capable, autonomous individual who can perform outside the family unit and who is not expected to be perfect. Control of his or her life must be achieved in ways other than dieting and weight loss.***
6. Help client realize that perfection is unrealistic, and explore this need with him or her. ***As client begins to feel better about self, identifies positive self-attributes, and develops the ability to accept certain personal inadequacies, the need for unrealistic achievements should diminish.***
7. Help client claim ownership of angry feelings and recognize that expressing them is acceptable if done so in an appropriate manner. Be an effective role model. ***Unexpressed anger is often turned inward on the self, resulting in a depreciation of self-esteem.***

Outcome Criteria

1. Client is able to verbalize positive aspects about self.

2. Client expresses interest in welfare of others and less preoccupation with own appearance.
3. Client verbalizes that image of body as "fat" was misperception and demonstrates ability to take control of own life without resorting to maladaptive eating behaviors.

Common Nursing Diagnoses and Interventions (for Obesity)

(Interventions are applicable to various health-care settings, such as inpatient and partial hospitalization, community outpatient clinic, home health, and private practice.)

IMBALANCED NUTRITION: MORE THAN BODY REQUIREMENTS

Definition: ***Intake of nutrients that exceeds metabolic needs.***

Possible Etiologies ("related to")

[Compulsive eating]
Excessive intake in relation to metabolic needs
[Sedentary lifestyle]
[Genetics]
[Unmet dependency needs—fixation in oral developmental stage]

Defining Characteristics ("evidenced by")

Weight 20 percent over ideal for height and frame
[BMI of 30 or more]

Goals/Objectives

Short-Term Goal

Client will verbalize understanding of what must be done to lose weight.

Long-Term Goal

Client will demonstrate change in eating patterns, resulting in a steady weight loss.

Interventions with *Selected Rationales*

1. Encourage the client to keep a diary of food intake. ***This provides the opportunity for the client to gain a realistic picture of the amount of food ingested and provides data on which to base the dietary program.***
2. Discuss feelings and emotions associated with eating. ***This helps to identify when client is eating to satisfy an emotional need rather than a physiological one.***

3. With input from the client, formulate an eating plan that includes food from the basic food pyramid, with emphasis on low-fat intake. It is helpful to keep the plan as similar to the client's usual eating pattern as possible. ***Diet must eliminate calories while maintaining adequate nutrition. Client is more likely to stay on the eating plan if he or she is able to participate in its creation and it deviates as little as possible from usual types of foods.***
4. Identify realistic increment goals for weekly weight loss. ***Reasonable weight loss (1 to 2 lb/wk) results in more lasting effects. Excessive, rapid weight loss may result in fatigue and irritability and may ultimately lead to failure in meeting goals for weight loss. Motivation is more easily sustained by meeting "stair-step" goals.***
5. Plan progressive exercise program tailored to individual goals and choice. ***Exercise may enhance weight loss by burning calories and reducing appetite, increasing energy, toning muscles, and enhancing sense of well-being and accomplishment. Walking is an excellent choice for overweight individuals.***
6. Discuss the probability of reaching plateaus when weight remains stable for extended periods. ***Client should know that this is likely to happen as changes in metabolism occur. Plateaus cause frustration, and client may need additional support during these times to remain on the weight loss program.***
7. Administer medications to assist with weight loss if ordered by the physician. ***Appetite-suppressant drugs (e.g., sibutramine and phentermine) may be helpful to someone who is obese. Drugs should be used for this purpose for only a short period while the individual attempts to adjust to the new pattern of eating.***

Outcome Criteria

1. Client has established a healthy pattern of eating for weight control, with weight loss progressing toward a desired goal.
2. Client verbalizes plans for future maintenance of weight control.

DISTURBED BODY IMAGE/LOW SELF-ESTEEM

Definition: *Confusion in mental picture of one's physical self. Negative self-evaluation and feelings about self or self-capabilities.*

Possible Etiologies ("related to")

[Dissatisfaction with appearance]
[Unmet dependency needs]
[Lack of adequate nurturing by maternal figure]

Defining Characteristics ("evidenced by")

Negative feelings about body (e.g., feelings of helplessness, hopelessness, or powerlessness)
[Verbalization of desire to lose weight]
[Failure to take responsibility for self-care (self-neglect)]
Lack of eye contact
[Expressions of low self-worth]

Goals/Objectives

Short-Term Goal

Client will begin to accept self based on self-attributes rather than on appearance.

Long-Term Goal

Client will pursue loss of weight as desired.

Interventions with *Selected Rationales*

1. Assess client's feelings and attitudes about being obese. ***Individuals who are overweight and who have compulsive eating behaviors may have deep-rooted psychological implications, such as compensation for lack of love and nurturing or a defense against intimacy.***
2. Ensure that client has privacy during self-care activities. ***The obese individual may be sensitive or self-conscious about his or her body.***
3. Have client recall coping patterns related to food in family of origin, and explore how these may affect current situation. ***Parents are role models for their children. Maladaptive eating behaviors are learned within the family system and are supported through positive reinforcement. Food may be substituted by the parent for affection and love, and eating is associated with a feeling of satisfaction, becoming the primary defense.***
4. Determine client's motivation for weight loss and set goals. ***The individual may harbor repressed feelings of hostility, which may be expressed inward on the self. Because of a poor self-concept, the person often has difficulty with relationships. When the motivation is to lose weight for someone else, successful weight loss is less likely to occur.***
5. Help client identify positive self-attributes. Focus on strengths and past accomplishments unrelated to physical appearance. ***It is important that self-esteem not be tied solely to size of the body. Client needs to recognize that obesity need not interfere with positive feelings regarding self-concept and self-worth.***
6. Refer client to support or therapy group. ***Support groups can provide companionship, increase motivation, decrease loneliness and social ostracism, and give practical solutions to common***

problems. Group therapy can be helpful in dealing with underlying psychological concerns.

Outcome Criteria

1. Client has established a healthy pattern of eating for weight control, with weight loss progressing toward a desired goal.
2. Client verbalizes plans for future maintenance of weight control.

■ INTERNET REFERENCES

Additional information about anorexia nervosa and bulimia nervosa may be located at the following websites:

- http://www.aabainc.org
- http://www.psych.org/public_info/eatingdisorders52201.cfm
- http://www.mentalhealth.com/dis/p20-et01.html
- http://www.anred.com/
- http://www.mentalhealth.com/dis/p20-et02.html
- http://www.nimh.nih.gov/publicat/eatingdisorder.cfm
- http://medlineplus.nlm.nih.gov/medlineplus/eatingdisorders.html

Additional information about obesity may be located at the following websites:

- http://www.shapeup.org/
- http://www.obesity.org/
- http://medlineplus.nlm.nih.gov/medlineplus/obesity.html
- http://www.asbp.org/
- http://www.niddk.nih.gov/health/nutrit/pubs/binge.htm

CHAPTER 12

*Adjustment Disorder**

BACKGROUND ASSESSMENT DATA

The essential feature of adjustment disorder is a maladaptive reaction to an identifiable psychosocial stressor that occurs within 3 months after the onset of the stressor and that has persisted for no longer than 6 months (APA, 2000). The response is considered maladaptive either because there is impairment in social or occupational functioning or because the behaviors are exaggerated beyond the usual, expected response to such a stressor. The impairment is corrected with the disappearance of or adaptation to the stressor. The following categories are defined:

1. **309.0 Adjustment Disorder with Depressed Mood.** This category is the most commonly diagnosed adjustment disorder. The major symptoms include depressed mood, tearfulness, and hopelessness. A differential diagnosis with the affective disorders must be considered.
2. **309.24 Adjustment Disorder with Anxiety.** The predominant manifestation of this adjustment disorder is anxiety. Major symptoms include nervousness, worry, and jitteriness. A differential diagnosis with the anxiety disorders must be considered.
3. **309.28 Adjustment Disorder with Mixed Anxiety and Depressed Mood.** The predominant manifestation of this adjustment disorder is a combination of depression and anxiety. A differential diagnosis must be made considering the affective and anxiety disorders.
4. **309.3 Adjustment Disorder with Disturbance of Conduct.** The major response involves conduct in which there is violation of the rights of others or of major age-appropriate societal norms and rules. A differential diagnosis with conduct disorder or antisocial personality disorder must be considered.

---

*Classification and criteria for all psychiatric diagnoses in this chapter are from the *Diagnostic and Statistical Manual of Mental Disorders, Fourth Edition, Text Revision, 2000.* Used with permission from the American Psychiatric Association.

5. **309.4 Adjustment Disorder with Mixed Disturbance of Emotions and Conduct.** The predominant manifestations are emotional symptoms (e.g., depression, anxiety) and disturbances in conduct.
6. **309.9 Adjustment Disorder Unspecified.** This diagnosis is used when the maladaptive reaction is not consistent with any of the other categories of adjustment disorder. Manifestations may include physical complaints, social withdrawal, or work or academic inhibition, without significant depressed or anxious mood.

Predisposing Factors

1. **Physiological**
   a. ***Developmental Impairment.*** The presence of chronic disorders, such as organic mental disorder or mental retardation, is thought to limit the general adaptive capacity of an individual. Yates (1994) suggests that genetic factors also may influence individual risks for maladaptive response to stress.
2. ***Psychosocial Theories***
   a. ***Psychoanalytical Theory.*** Some proponents of psychoanalytical theory view adjustment disorder as a maladaptive response to stress that is caused by early childhood trauma, increased dependency, and retarded ego development. Other psychoanalysts put considerable weight on constitutional factors, or birth characteristics, that contribute to the manner in which individuals respond to stress. In many instances, adjustment disorder is precipitated by a specific meaningful stressor having found a point of vulnerability in an individual of otherwise adequate ego strength.
   b. ***Developmental Model.*** Some studies relate a predisposition to adjustment disorder to factors such as developmental stage, timing of the stressor, and available support systems. When a stressor occurs and the individual does not have the developmental maturity, available support systems, or adequate coping strategies to adapt, normal functioning is disrupted, resulting in psychological or somatic symptoms. The disorder may also be related to a dysfunctional grieving process. The individual may remain in the denial or anger stage, with inadequate defense mechanisms to complete the grieving process.
   c. ***Stress-Adaptation Model.*** This model considers the type of stressor the individual experiences, the situational context in which it occurs, and intrapersonal factors in the predisposition to adjustment disorder. It has been found that continuous stressors (those to which an individual is exposed over an extended period) are more commonly cited than sudden-shock stressors (those that occur without warning) as precipitants to maladaptive functioning.

The situational context in which the stressor occurs may include factors such as personal and general economic conditions; occupational and recreational opportunities; availability of social supports, such as family, friends, and neighbors; and availability of cultural or religious support groups. Intrapersonal factors that have been implicated in the predisposition to adjustment disorder include birth temperament, learned social skills and coping strategies, the presence of psychiatric illness, extent of flexibility, and level of intelligence.

Symptomatology (Subjective and Objective Data)

1. Depressed mood
2. Tearfulness
3. Hopelessness
4. Nervousness
5. Worry
6. Jitteriness
7. Ambivalence
8. Anger, expressed inappropriately
9. Increased dependency
10. Violation of the rights of others
11. Violation of societal norms and rules, such as truancy, vandalism, reckless driving, fighting
12. Inability to function occupationally or academically
13. Manipulative behavior
14. Social isolation
15. Physical complaints, such as headache, backache, other aches and pains, fatigue

Common Nursing Diagnoses and Interventions

(Interventions are applicable to various health-care settings, such as inpatient and partial hospitalization, community outpatient clinic, home health, and private practice.)

RISK FOR SELF-DIRECTED OR OTHER-DIRECTED VIOLENCE

Definition: ***At risk for behaviors in which an individual demonstrates that he or she can be physically, emotionally, and/or sexually harmful either to self or to others.***

Related/Risk Factors ("related to")

[Fixation in earlier level of development]
[Negative role modeling]
[Dysfunctional family system]
[Low self-esteem]

[Unresolved grief]
[Psychic overload]
[Extended exposure to stressful situation]
[Lack of support systems]
[Biological factors, such as organic changes in the brain]
Body language—rigid posture, clenching of fists and jaw, hyperactivity, pacing, breathlessness, and threatening stances
[History or threats of violence toward self or others or of destruction to the property of others]
Impulsivity
Suicidal ideation, plan, available means
[Anger; rage]
[Increasing anxiety level]
[Depressed mood]

Goals/Objectives

Short-Term Goals

1. Client will seek out staff member when hostile or suicidal feelings occur.
2. Client will verbalize adaptive coping strategies for use when hostile or suicidal feelings occur.

Long-Term Goals

1. Client will demonstrate adaptive coping strategies for use when hostile or suicidal feelings occur.
2. Client will not harm self or others.

Interventions with *Selected Rationales*

1. Observe client's behavior frequently. Do this through routine activities and interactions; avoid appearing watchful and suspicious. ***Close observation is required so that intervention can occur if required to ensure client's (and others') safety.***
2. Observe for suicidal behaviors: verbal statements, such as "I'm going to kill myself." and "Very soon my mother won't have to worry herself about me any longer," and nonverbal behaviors, such as giving away cherished items and mood swings. ***Clients who are contemplating suicide often give clues regarding their potential behavior. The clues may be very subtle and require keen assessment skills by the nurse.***
3. Determine suicidal intent and available means. Ask direct questions, such as "Do you plan to kill yourself?" and "How do you plan to do it?" ***The risk of suicide is greatly increased if client has developed a plan and particularly if means exist for the client to execute the plan.***
4. Obtain verbal or written contract from client agreeing not to harm self and to seek out staff in the event that suicidal ideation occurs. ***Discussion of suicidal feelings with a trusted individual***

provides some relief to client. A contract gets the subject out in the open and places some of the responsibility for his or her safety with client. An attitude of acceptance of client as a worthwhile individual is conveyed.

5. Help client recognize when anger occurs and accept those feelings as his or her own. Have client keep an "anger notebook" in which feelings of anger experienced during a 24-hour period are recorded. Information regarding source of anger, behavioral response, and client's perception of the situation should also be noted. Discuss entries with client, and suggest alternative behavioral responses for those identified as maladaptive.
6. Act as a role model for appropriate expression of angry feelings, and give positive reinforcement to client for attempting to conform. ***It is vital that client express angry feelings, because suicide and other self-destructive behaviors are often viewed as the result of anger turned inward on the self.***
7. Remove all dangerous objects from client's environment (e.g., sharp items, belts, ties, straps, breakable items, smoking materials). ***Client safety is a nursing priority.***
8. Try to redirect violent behavior by means of physical outlets for client's anxiety (e.g., punching bag, jogging). ***Physical exercise is a safe and effective way of relieving pent-up tension.***
9. Be available to stay with client as anxiety level and tensions begin to rise. ***Presence of a trusted individual provides a feeling of security and may help to prevent rapid escalation of anxiety.***
10. Staff should maintain and convey a calm attitude to client. ***Anxiety is contagious and can be transmitted from staff members to client.***
11. Have sufficient staff available to indicate a show of strength to client if necessary. ***This conveys to the client evidence of control over the situation and provides some physical security for staff.***
12. Administer tranquilizing medications as ordered by physician, or obtain an order if necessary. Monitor client response for effectiveness of the medication and for adverse side effects. ***Short-term use of tranquilizing medications such as anxiolytics or antipsychotics can induce a calming effect on the client and may prevent aggressive behaviors.***
13. Use of mechanical restraints or isolation room may be required if less restrictive interventions are unsuccessful. Follow policy and procedure prescribed by the institution in executing this intervention. The Joint Commission on Accreditation of Healthcare Organizations (JCAHO) requires that the physician reevaluate and issue a new order for restraints every 4 hours for adults age 18 years and older. If client has previously refused medication, administer after restraints have been applied. Most states consider this intervention appropriate in emergency situations or in the event that a client would likely harm self or others.

14. Observe client in restraints every 15 minutes (or according to institutional policy). Ensure that circulation to extremities is not compromised (check temperature, color, pulses). Assist client with needs related to nutrition, hydration, and elimination. Position client so that comfort is facilitated and aspiration can be prevented. ***Client safety is a nursing priority.***
15. As agitation decreases, assess client's readiness for restraint removal or reduction. Remove one restraint at a time while assessing client's response. ***This minimizes risk of injury to the client and staff.***

Outcome Criteria

1. Anxiety is maintained at a level at which client feels no need for aggression.
2. Client denies any ideas of self-destruction.
3. Client demonstrates use of adaptive coping strategies when feelings of hostility or suicide occur.
4. Client verbalizes community support systems from which assistance may be requested when personal coping strategies are not successful.

ANXIETY (MODERATE TO SEVERE)

Definition: *Vague, uneasy feeling of discomfort or dread accompanied by an autonomic response (the source often nonspecific or unknown to the individual); a feeling of apprehension caused by anticipation of danger. It is an alerting signal that warns of impending danger and that enables the individual to take measures to deal with threat.*

Possible Etiologies ("related to")

Situational and maturational crises
[Low self-esteem]
[Dysfunctional family system]
[Feelings of powerlessness and lack of control in life situation]
[Retarded ego development]
[Fixation in earlier level of development]

Defining Characteristics ("evidenced by")

[Increased tension]
Increased helplessness
Overexcited
Apprehension; fear
Restlessness
Poor eye contact

Feelings of inadequacy
Insomnia
Focus on the self
Increased cardiac and respiratory rates
Diminished ability to problem-solve and learn

Goals/Objectives

Short-Term Goal

Client will demonstrate use of relaxation techniques to maintain anxiety at manageable level within 7 days.

Long-Term Goal

By time of discharge from treatment, client will be able to recognize events that precipitate anxiety and to intervene to prevent disabling behaviors.

Interventions with *Selected Rationales*

1. Be available to stay with client. Remain calm and provide reassurance of safety. ***Client safety and security is a nursing priority.***
2. Help client identify situation that precipitated onset of anxiety symptoms. ***Client may be unaware that emotional issues are related to symptoms of anxiety. Recognition may be the first step in elimination of this maladaptive response.***
3. Review client's methods of coping with similar situations in the past. Discuss ways in which client may assume control over these situations. ***In seeking to create change, it is helpful for client to identify past responses and to determine whether they were successful and if they could be employed again. A measure of control reduces feelings of powerlessness in a situation, ultimately decreasing anxiety. Client strengths should be identified and used to his or her advantage.***
4. Provide quiet environment. Reduce stimuli: low lighting, few people. ***Anxiety level may be decreased in calm atmosphere with few stimuli.***
5. Administer antianxiety medications as ordered by physician, or obtain order if necessary. Monitor client's response for effectiveness of the medication as well as for adverse side effects. ***Short-term use of antianxiety medications (e.g., diazepam, chlordiazepoxide, alprazolam) provides relief from the immobilizing effects of anxiety and facilitates client's cooperation with therapy.***
6. Discuss with client signs of increasing anxiety and ways of intervening to maintain the anxiety at a manageable level (e.g., exercise, walking, jogging, relaxation techniques). ***Anxiety and tension can be reduced safely and with benefit to the client through physical activities.***

Outcome Criteria

1. Client is able to verbalize events that precipitate anxiety and to demonstrate techniques for its reduction.
2. Client is able to verbalize ways in which he or she may gain more control of the environment and thereby reduce feelings of powerlessness.

INEFFECTIVE COPING

Definition: ***Inability to form a valid appraisal of the stressors, inadequate choices of practiced responses, and/or inability to use available resources.***

Possible Etiologies ("related to")

Situational crises
Maturational crises
[Inadequate support systems]
[Negative role modeling]
[Retarded ego development]
[Fixation in earlier level of development]
[Dysfunctional family system]
[Low self-esteem]
[Unresolved grief]

Defining Characteristics ("evidenced by")

Inability to meet role expectations
[Alteration in societal participation]
Inadequate problem solving
[Increased dependency]
[Manipulation of others in the environment for purposes of fulfilling own desires]
[Refusal to follow rules]

Goals/Objectives

Short-Term Goal

By the end of 1 week, client will comply with rules of therapy and refrain from manipulating others to fulfill own desires.

Long-Term Goal

By time of discharge from treatment, client will identify, develop, and use socially acceptable coping skills.

Interventions with *Selected Rationales*

1. Discuss with client the rules of therapy and consequences of noncompliance. Carry out the consequences matter-of-factly if rules

are broken. ***Negative consequences may work to decrease manipulative behaviors.***

2. Do not debate, argue, rationalize, or bargain with client regarding setting limit on manipulative behaviors. ***Ignoring these attempts may work to decrease manipulative behaviors. Consistency among all staff members is vital if this intervention is to be successful.***
3. Encourage discussion of angry feelings. Help client identify the true object of the hostility. Provide physical outlets for healthy release of the hostile feelings (e.g., punching bags, pounding boards). ***Verbalization of feelings with a trusted individual may help client work through unresolved issues. Physical exercise provides a safe and effective means of releasing pent-up tension.***
4. Take care not to reinforce dependent behaviors. Encourage client to perform as independently as possible, and provide positive feedback. ***Independent accomplishment and positive reinforcement enhance self-esteem and encourage repetition of desirable behaviors.***
5. Help client recognize some aspects of his or her life over which a measure of control is maintained. ***Recognition of personal control, however minimal, diminishes the feeling of powerlessness and decreases the need for manipulation of others.***
6. Identify the stressor that precipitated the maladaptive coping. If a major life change has occurred, encourage client to express fears and feelings associated with the change. Help client through the problem-solving process:
   a. Identify possible alternatives that indicate positive adaptation.
   b. Discuss benefits and consequences of each alternative.
   c. Select the most appropriate alternative.
   d. Implement the alternative.
   e. Evaluate the effectiveness of the alternative.
   f. Recognize areas of limitation, and make modifications. Request assistance with this process, if needed.
7. Provide positive reinforcement for application of adaptive coping skills and evidence of successful adjustment. ***Positive reinforcement enhances self-esteem and encourages repetition of desirable behaviors.***

Outcome Criteria

1. Client is able to verbalize alternative, socially acceptable, and lifestyle-appropriate coping skills he or she plans to use in response to stress.
2. Client is able to solve problems and fulfill activities of daily living (ADLs) independently.
3. Client does not manipulate others for own gratification.

IMPAIRED ADJUSTMENT†

Definition: ***Inability to modify lifestyle/behavior in a manner consistent with a change in health status.***

Possible Etiologies ("related to")

Low state of optimism
Intense emotional state
Negative attitudes toward health behavior
Absence of intent to change behavior
Multiple stressors
Absence of social support for changed beliefs and practices
Disability or health status change requiring change in lifestyle
Lack of motivation to change behaviors

Defining Characteristics ("evidenced by")

Denial of health status change
Failure to achieve optimal sense of control
Failure to take actions that would prevent further health problems
Demonstration of nonacceptance of health status change

Goals/Objectives

Short-Term Goals

1. Client will discuss with primary nurse the kinds of lifestyle changes that will occur because of the change in health status.
2. With the help of primary nurse, client will formulate a plan of action for incorporating those changes into his or her lifestyle.
3. Client will demonstrate movement toward independence, considering change in health status.

Long-Term Goal

Client will demonstrate competence to function independently to his or her optimal ability, considering change in health status, by time of discharge from treatment.

Interventions with *Selected Rationales*

1. Encourage client to talk about lifestyle prior to the change in health status. Discuss coping mechanisms that were used at stressful times in the past. ***It is important to identify client's strengths so that they may be used to facilitate adaptation to the change or loss that has occurred.***
2. Encourage client to discuss the change or loss and, particularly, to express anger associated with it. ***Some individuals may not real-***

† According to the North American Nursing Diagnosis Association definition, this diagnosis is appropriate for the person with adjustment disorder only if the precipitating stressor is a change in health status.

ize that anger is a normal stage in the grieving process. If anger is not released in an appropriate manner, it may be turned inward on the self, leading to pathological depression.

3. Encourage client to express fears associated with the change or loss or with the alteration in lifestyle that the change or loss has created. ***Change often creates a feeling of disequilibrium, and the individual may respond with fears that are irrational or unfounded. He or she may benefit from feedback that corrects misperceptions about how life will be with the change in health status.***
4. Provide assistance with ADLs as required, but encourage independence to the limit that client's ability will allow. Give positive feedback for activities accomplished independently. ***Independent accomplishments and positive feedback enhance self-esteem and encourage repetition of desired behaviors. Successes also provide hope that adaptive functioning is possible and decrease feelings of powerlessness.***
5. Help client with decision making regarding incorporation of change or loss into lifestyle. Identify problems that the change or loss is likely to create. Discuss alternative solutions, weighing potential benefits and consequences of each alternative. Support client's decision in the selection of an alternative. ***The great amount of anxiety that usually accompanies a major lifestyle change often interferes with an individual's ability to solve problems and to make appropriate decisions. Client may need assistance with this process in an effort to progress toward successful adaptation.***
6. Use role playing ***to decrease anxiety*** as client anticipates stressful situations that might occur in relation to the health status change. ***Role playing decreases anxiety and provides a feeling of security by giving client a plan of action to use in an appropriate manner when a stressful situation occurs.***
7. Ensure that client and family are fully knowledgeable regarding the physiology of the change in health status and its necessity for optimal wellness. Encourage them to ask questions, and provide printed material explaining the change to which they may refer following discharge.
8. Help client identify resources within the community from which he or she may seek assistance in adapting to the change in health status. Examples include self-help or support groups and public health nurse, counselor, or social worker. Encourage client to keep follow-up appointments with physician and to call physician's office before follow-up date if problems or concerns arise.

Outcome Criteria

1. Client is able to perform ADLs independently.
2. Client is able to make independent decisions regarding lifestyle, considering change in health status.

3. Client is able to express hope for the future with consideration of change in health status.

DYSFUNCTIONAL GRIEVING

Definition: ***Extended, unsuccessful use of intellectual and emotional responses by which individuals, families, and communities attempt to work through the process of modifying self-concept based on the perception of [actual or potential] loss.***

Possible Etiologies ("related to")

[Real or perceived loss of any concept of value to the individual]
[Bereavement overload (cumulative grief from multiple unresolved losses)]
[Thwarted grieving response to a loss]
[Absence of anticipatory grieving]
[Feelings of guilt generated by ambivalent relationship with lost concept]

Defining Characteristics ("evidenced by")

Verbal expression of distress at loss
Idealization of lost [concept]
Denial of loss
[Excessive anger, expressed inappropriately]
Developmental regression
Alterations in concentration or pursuit of tasks
Difficulty in expressing loss
Labile affect
Interference with life functioning
Repetitive use of ineffectual behaviors associated with attempts to reinvest in relationships
Reliving of past experiences with little or no reduction of intensity of the grief
Prolonged interference with life functioning
Onset or exacerbation of somatic or psychosomatic responses

Goals/Objectives

Short-Term Goal

By end of 1 week, client will express anger toward lost concept.

Long-Term Goal

Client will be able to verbalize behaviors associated with the normal stages of grief and identify own position in grief process while progressing at own pace toward resolution.

Interventions with *Selected Rationales*

1. Determine stage of grief in which client is fixed. Identify behaviors associated with this stage. ***Accurate baseline assessment data are necessary to plan effective care for the grieving client.***
2. Develop trusting relationship with client. Show empathy and caring. Be honest, and keep all promises. ***Trust is the basis for a therapeutic relationship.***
3. Convey an accepting attitude so that client is not afraid to express feelings openly. ***An accepting attitude conveys to client that you believe he or she is a worthwhile person. Trust is enhanced.***
4. Allow client to express anger. Do not become defensive if initial expression of anger is displaced on nurse or therapist. Help client explore angry feelings so that they may be directed toward the intended object or person. ***Verbalization of feelings in a nonthreatening environment may help client come to terms with unresolved issues.***
5. Help client discharge pent-up anger through participation in large-motor activities (e.g., brisk walks, jogging, physical exercises, volleyball, punching bag, exercise bike). ***Physical exercise provides a safe and effective method for discharging pent-up tension.***
6. Explain to client the normal stages of grief and the behaviors associated with each stage. Help client understand that feelings such as guilt and anger toward the lost concept are appropriate and acceptable during the grief process. ***Knowledge of the acceptability of the feelings associated with normal grieving may help to relieve some of the guilt that these responses generate.***
7. Encourage client to review relationship with lost concept. With support and sensitivity, point out reality of the situation in areas where misrepresentations are expressed. ***Client must give up idealized perception and be able to accept both positive and negative aspects about the lost concept before the grief process is complete.***
8. Communicate to client that crying is acceptable. Use of touch is therapeutic and appropriate with most clients. Knowledge of cultural influences specific to the client is important before employing this technique. ***Touch is considered inappropriate in some cultures.***
9. Help client solve problems as he or she attempts to determine methods for more adaptive coping with the experienced loss. Provide positive feedback for strategies identified and decisions made. ***Positive reinforcement enhances self-esteem and encourages repetition of desirable behaviors.***
10. Encourage client to reach out for spiritual support during this time in whatever form is desirable to him or her. Assess spiritual needs of client, and assist as necessary in the fulfillment of those

needs. ***Spiritual support can enhance successful adaptation to painful life experiences for some individuals.***

Outcome Criteria

1. Client is able to verbalize normal stages of grief process and behaviors associated with each stage.
2. Client is able to identify own position within the grief process and express honest feelings related to the lost concept.
3. Client is no longer manifesting exaggerated emotions and behaviors related to dysfunctional grieving and is able to carry out ADLs independently.

LOW SELF-ESTEEM

Definition: *Negative self-evaluation and feelings about self or self-capabilities.*

Possible Etiologies ("related to")

[Lack of positive feedback]
[Unmet dependency needs]
[Retarded ego development]
[Repeated negative feedback, resulting in diminished self-worth]
[Personal or situational factors such as dysfunctional family system or absence of social support]

Defining Characteristics ("evidenced by")

[Difficulty accepting positive reinforcement]
[Nonparticipation in therapy]
Self-negating verbalizations
Evaluation of self as unable to deal with events
Hesitant to try new things or situations [because of fear of failure]
[Projection of blame or responsibility for problems]
[Rationalization of personal failures]
[Hypersensitivity to slight or criticism]
[Grandiosity]
Lack of eye contact
[Manipulation of one staff member against another in an attempt to gain special privileges]
[Inability to form close, personal relationships]
[Degradation of others in an attempt to increase own feelings of self-worth]

Goals/Objectives

Short-Term Goal

1. Client will discuss fear of failure with nurse within (realistic period).

2. Client will verbalize things he or she likes about self within (realistic period).

Long-Term Goal

1. Client will exhibit increased feelings of self-worth as evidenced by verbal expression of positive aspects about self, past accomplishments, and future prospects.
2. Client will exhibit increased feelings of self-worth by setting realistic goals and trying to reach them, thereby demonstrating a decrease in fear of failure.

Interventions with *Selected Rationales*

1. Ensure that goals are realistic. It is important for client to achieve something, so plan for activities in which success is likely. ***Success enhances self-esteem.***
2. Convey unconditional positive regard for client. Promote understanding of your acceptance for him or her as a worthwhile human being.
3. Spend time with client, both on a one-to-one basis and in group activities. ***This conveys to client that you feel he or she is worth your time.***
4. Help client identify positive aspects of self and to develop plans for changing the characteristics he or she views as negative. ***Individuals with low self-esteem often have difficulty recognizing their positive attributes. They may also lack problem-solving ability and require assistance to formulate a plan for implementing the desired changes.***
5. Encourage and support client in confronting the fear of failure by attending therapy activities and undertaking new tasks. Offer recognition of successful endeavors and positive reinforcement for attempts made. ***Recognition and positive reinforcement enhance self-esteem.***
6. Do not allow client to ruminate about past failures. Withdraw attention if he or she persists. ***Lack of attention to these behaviors may discourage their repetition. Client must focus on positive attributes if self-esteem is to be enhanced.***
7. Minimize negative feedback to client. Enforce limit setting in matter-of-fact manner, imposing previously established consequences for violations. ***Negative feedback can be extremely threatening to a person with low self-esteem, possibly aggravating the problem. Consequences should convey unacceptability of the <u>behavior</u> but not of the <u>person.</u>***
8. Encourage independence in the performance of personal responsibilities as well as in decision making related to own self-care. Offer recognition and praise for accomplishments. ***The ability to perform self-care activities independently enhances self-esteem. Positive reinforcement encourages repetition of the desirable behavior.***

9. Help client increase level of self-awareness through critical examination of feelings, attitudes, and behaviors. Help him or her understand that it is perfectly acceptable for one's attitudes and behaviors to differ from those of others as long as they do not become intrusive. ***As the client achieves self-awareness and self-acceptance, the need for judging the behavior of others will diminish.***

Outcome Criteria

1. Client verbalizes positive perception of self.
2. Client demonstrates ability to manage own self-care, make independent decisions, and use problem-solving skills.
3. Client sets goals that are realistic and works to achieve those goals without evidence of fear of failure.

IMPAIRED SOCIAL INTERACTION

Definition: *Insufficient or excessive quantity or ineffective quality of social exchange.*

Possible Etiologies ("related to")

[Retarded ego development]
[Fixation in an earlier level of development]
[Negative role modeling]
[Low self-esteem]

Defining Characteristics ("evidenced by")

Verbalized or observed discomfort in social situations
Verbalized or observed inability to receive or communicate a satisfying sense of belonging, caring, interest, or shared history
Observed use of unsuccessful social interaction behaviors
Dysfunctional interaction with peers, family, or others
[Exhibiting behaviors unacceptable for age, as defined by dominant cultural group]

Goals/Objectives

Short-Term Goal

Client will develop trusting relationship with staff member within (realistic period), seeking out that staff member for one-to-one interaction.

Long-Term Goals

1. Client will be able to interact with others on a one-to-one basis with no indication of discomfort.

2. Client will voluntarily spend time with others in group activities, demonstrating acceptable, age-appropriate behavior.

Interventions with *Selected Rationales*

1. Develop trusting relationship with client. Be honest; keep all promises; convey acceptance of person, separate from unacceptable behaviors ("It is not *you*, but your *behavior*, that is unacceptable.") ***Unconditional acceptance of the client increases his or her feelings of self-worth.***
2. Offer to remain with client during initial interactions with others in the unit. ***Presence of a trusted individual provides a feeling of security.***
3. Provide constructive criticism and positive reinforcement for efforts. ***Positive reinforcement enhances self-esteem and encourages repetition of desirable behaviors.***
4. Confront client and withdraw attention when interactions with others are manipulative or exploitative. ***Attention to unacceptable behavior may reinforce it.***
5. Act as role model for client through appropriate interactions with him or her, other clients, and staff members.
6. Provide group situations for client. ***It is through these group interactions, with positive and negative feedback from his or her peers, that client will learn socially acceptable behavior.***

Outcome Criteria

1. Client seeks out staff member for social as well as therapeutic interaction.
2. Client has formed and satisfactorily maintained one interpersonal relationship with another client.
3. Client willingly and appropriately participates in group activities.
4. Client verbalizes reasons for inability to form close interpersonal relationships with others in the past.

RELOCATION STRESS SYNDROME†

Definition: *Physiological and/or psychosocial disturbance following transfer from one environment to another.*

Possible Etiologies ("related to")

[Change in environment or location]
Past, concurrent, and recent losses
[Losses involved with decision to move]

† This diagnosis would be appropriate for the individual with adjustment disorder if the precipitating stressor was relocation to a new environment.

Feeling of powerlessness
Lack of adequate support system
[Little or no preparation for the impending move]
[Moderate to high degree of environmental change]
[History and types of previous transfers]
Impaired psychosocial health status
Decreased physical health status

Defining Characteristics ("evidenced by")

Anxiety
Depression
Loneliness
[Verbalization of opposition to relocate]
Sleep disturbance
Increased physical symptoms
Dependency
Insecurity
Withdrawal
Anger, fear

Goals/Objectives

Short-Term Goal

Client will verbalize at least one positive aspect regarding relocation to new environment within (realistic period).

Long-Term Goal

Client will demonstrate positive adaptation to new environment, as evidenced by involvement in activities, expression of satisfaction with new acquaintances, and elimination of previously evident physical and psychological symptoms associated with the relocation (time dimension to be determined individually).

Interventions with *Selected Rationales*

1. Encourage individual to discuss feelings (concerns, fears, anger) regarding relocation. ***Exploration of feelings with a trusted individual may help the individual perceive the situation more realistically and come to terms with the inevitable change.***
2. Encourage individual to discuss how the change will affect his or her life. Ensure that the individual is involved in decision making and problem solving regarding the move. ***Taking responsibility for making choices regarding the relocation will increase feelings of control and decrease feelings of powerlessness.***
3. Help the individual identify positive aspects about the move. ***Anxiety associated with the opposed relocation may interfere with the individual's ability to recognize anything positive about it. Assistance may be required.***

4. Help the individual identify resources within the new community from which assistance with various types of services may be obtained. ***Because of anxiety and depression, the individual may not be able to identify these resources alone. Assistance with problem solving may be required.***
5. Identify groups within the community that specialize in helping individuals adapt to relocation. Examples include Newcomers' Club, Welcome Wagon Club, senior citizens' groups, and school and church organizations. ***These groups offer support from individuals who have often encountered similar experiences. Adaptation may be enhanced by the reassurance, encouragement, and support of peers who exhibit positive adaptation to relocation stress.***
6. Refer individual or family for professional counseling if deemed necessary. ***An individual who is experiencing dysfunctional grieving over loss of previous residence may require therapy to achieve resolution of the problem. It may be that other unresolved issues are interfering with successful adaptation to the relocation.***

Outcome Criteria

1. The individual no longer exhibits signs of anxiety, depression, or somatic symptoms.
2. The individual verbalizes satisfaction with new environment.
3. The individual willingly participates in social and vocational activities within his or her new environment.

■ INTERNET REFERENCES

Additional information about adjustment disorder may be located at the following websites:

- http://www.mentalhealth.com/rx/p23-aj01.html
- http://www.findarticles.com/cf_dls/g2601/0000/2601000025/p1/article.jhtml
- http://www.athealth.com/Consumer/disorders/Adjustment.html
- http://www.mentalhealth.com/dis/p20-aj01.html

CHAPTER 13

*Impulse Control Disorders**

■ BACKGROUND ASSESSMENT DATA

Impulse control disorders are characterized by a need or desire that must be satisfied immediately, regardless of the consequences. Many of the behaviors have adverse or even destructive consequences for the individuals affected, and seldom do these individuals know why they do what they do or why it is pleasurable.

The *Diagnostic and Statistical Manual of Mental Disorders, Fourth Edition, Text Revision, 2000 (DSM-IV-TR)* (APA, 2000) describes the essential features of impulse control disorders as follows:

1. Failure to resist an impulse, drive, or temptation to perform an act that is harmful to the person or others.
2. An increasing sense of tension or arousal before committing the act.
3. An experience of either pleasure, gratification, or relief at the time of committing the act. Following the act, there may or may not be regret, self-reproach, or guilt. The *DSM-IV-TR* (APA, 2000) describes the following categories of impulse control disorders:

312.34 Intermittent Explosive Disorder

This disorder is characterized by discrete episodes of failure to resist aggressive impulses, resulting in serious assaultive acts or destruction of property. Some clients report changes in sensorium, such as confusion during an episode or amnesia for events that occurred during an episode. Symptoms usually appear suddenly without apparent provocation and terminate abruptly, lasting only minutes to a few hours, followed by feelings of genuine remorse and self-reproach about the behavior.

---

*Classification and criteria for all psychiatric diagnoses in this chapter are from the *Diagnostic and Statistical Manual of Mental Disorders, Fourth Edition, Text Revision, 2000.* Used with permission from the American Psychiatric Association.

312.32 Kleptomania

Kleptomania is described as "the recurrent failure to resist impulses to steal items not needed for personal use or for their monetary value." Often the stolen items (for which the individual usually has enough money to pay) are given away, discarded, returned, or kept and hidden. The individual with kleptomania steals purely for the sake of stealing and for the sense of relief and gratification that follows an episode.

312.31 Pathological Gambling

Pathological gambling is defined as "persistent and recurrent maladaptive gambling behavior that disrupts personal, family, or vocational pursuits." The preoccupation with gambling and the impulse to gamble intensify when the individual is under stress. Many pathological gamblers exhibit characteristics associated with narcissism and grandiosity and often have difficulties with intimacy, empathy, and trust.

312.33 Pyromania

Pyromania is the inability to resist the impulse to set fires. The act itself is preceded by tension or affective arousal, and the individual experiences intense pleasure, gratification, or relief when setting the fires, witnessing their effects, or participating in their aftermath. Motivation for the behavior is self-gratification, and even though some individuals with pyromania may take precautions to avoid apprehension, many are totally indifferent to the consequences of their behavior.

312.39 Trichotillomania

This disorder is defined as "the recurrent pulling out of one's own hair that results in noticeable hair loss." The impulse is preceded by an increasing sense of tension, and the individual experiences a sense of release or gratification from pulling out the hair.

Predisposing Factors

1. **Physiological**
   a. ***Genetics.*** A familial tendency appears to be a factor in some cases of intermittent explosive disorder, pathological gambling, and trichotillomania.
   b. ***Physical Factors.*** Brain trauma or dysfunction and mental retardation have also been implicated in the predisposition to impulse control disorders (Kaplan & Sadock, 1998).
2. **Psychosocial**
   a. ***Family Dynamics.*** Various dysfunctional family patterns have been suggested as contributors in the predisposition to impulse control disorders. These include the following:

- Child abuse or neglect
- Parental rejection or abandonment
- Harsh or inconsistent discipline
- Emotional deprivation
- Parental substance abuse
- Parental unpredictability

Symptomatology (Subjective and Objective Data)

1. Sudden inability to control violent, aggressive impulses
2. Aggressive behavior accompanied by confusion or amnesia
3. Feelings of remorse following aggressive behavior
4. Inability to resist impulses to steal
5. Increasing tension before committing the theft, followed by pleasure or relief during and following the act
6. Sometimes discards, returns, or hides stolen items
7. Inability to resist impulses to gamble
8. Preoccupation with ways to obtain money with which to gamble
9. Increasing tension that is relieved only by placing a bet
10. The need to gamble or loss of money interferes with social and occupational functioning
11. Inability to resist the impulse to set fires
12. Increasing tension that is relieved only by starting a fire
13. Inability to resist impulses to pull out one's own hair
14. Increasing tension followed by a sense of release or gratification from pulling out the hair
15. Hair pulling may be accompanied by other types of self-mutilation (e.g., head banging, biting, scratching)

Common Nursing Diagnoses and Interventions

(Interventions are applicable to various health-care settings, such as inpatient and partial hospitalization, community outpatient clinic, home health, and private practice.)

RISK FOR OTHER-DIRECTED VIOLENCE

Definition: ***At risk for behaviors in which an individual demonstrates that he or she can be physically, emotionally, and/or sexually harmful to others.***

Related/Risk Factors ("related to")

[Possible familial tendency]
[Central nervous system trauma]
[Dysfunctional family system, resulting in behaviors such as the following:

Child abuse or neglect
Parental rejection or abandonment
Harsh or inconsistent discipline
Emotional deprivation
Parental substance abuse
Parental unpredictability]

Body language—rigid posture, clenching of fists and jaw, hyperactivity, pacing, breathlessness, and threatening stances

History of threats of violence [toward others or of destruction of the property of others]

Impulsivity

Goals/Objectives

Short-Term Goal

Client will recognize signs of increasing tension, anxiety, and agitation and will report to staff (or others) for assistance with intervention (time dimension to be individually determined).

Long-Term Goal

Client will not harm others or the property of others (time dimension to be individually determined).

Interventions with *Selected Rationales*

1. Convey an accepting attitude toward the client. Feelings of rejection are undoubtedly familiar to him or her. Work on the development of trust. Be honest, keep all promises, and convey the message that it is not the *person* but the *behavior* that is unacceptable. ***An attitude of acceptance promotes feelings of self-worth. Trust is the basis of a therapeutic relationship.***
2. Maintain low level of stimuli in client's environment (low lighting, few people, simple decor, low noise level). ***A stimulating environment may increase agitation and promote aggressive behavior. Make client's environment as safe as possible*** by removing all potentially dangerous objects.
3. Help client identify the true object of his or her hostility. ***Because of weak ego development, client may be unable to use ego defense mechanisms correctly. Helping him or her recognize this in a nonthreatening manner may help reveal unresolved issues so that they may be confronted.***
4. Staff should maintain and convey a calm attitude. ***Anxiety is contagious and can be transferred from staff to client. A calm attitude provides client with a feeling of safety and security.***
5. Help client recognize the signs that tension is increasing and ways in which violence can be averted. ***Activities that require physical exertion are helpful in relieving pent-up tension.***
6. Explain to client that should explosive behavior occur, staff will intervene in whatever way is required (e.g., tranquilizing medica-

tion, restraints, isolation) to protect client and others. ***This conveys to client evidence of control over the situation and provides a feeling of safety and security.***

Outcome Criteria

1. Anxiety is maintained at a level at which client feels no need for aggression.
2. The client is able to verbalize the symptoms of increasing tension and adaptive ways of coping with it.
3. The client is able to inhibit the impulse for violence and aggression.

RISK FOR SELF-MUTILATION

Definition: *At risk for deliberate self-injurious behavior causing tissue damage, with the intent of causing nonfatal injury to attain relief of tension.*

Related/Risk Factors ("related to")

[Possible familial tendency]
[Central nervous system trauma]
[Mental retardation]
[Early emotional deprivation]
[Parental rejection or abandonment]
[Child abuse or neglect]
[History of self-mutilative behaviors in response to increasing anxiety: hair pulling, biting, head banging, scratching]

Goals/Objectives

Short-Term Goals

1. Client will cooperate with plan of behavior modification in an effort to respond more adaptively to stress (time dimension ongoing).
2. Client will not harm self.

Long-Term Goal

Client will not harm self.

Interventions with *Selected Rationales*

1. Intervene to protect client when self-mutilative behaviors, such as head banging or hair pulling, become evident. ***The nurse is responsible for ensuring client safety.***
2. A helmet may be used to protect against head banging, hand mitts to prevent hair pulling, and appropriate padding to protect extremities from injury during hysterical movements.

3. Try to determine if self-mutilative behaviors occur in response to increasing anxiety, and, if so, to what the anxiety may be attributed. ***Self-mutilative behaviors may be averted if the cause can be determined.***
4. Work on one-to-one basis with client ***to establish trust.***
5. Assist with plan for behavior modification ***in an effort to teach the client more adaptive ways of responding to stress.***
6. Encourage client to discuss feelings, particularly anger, ***in an effort to confront unresolved issues and expose internalized rage that may be triggering self-mutilative behaviors.***
7. Offer self to client during times of increasing anxiety ***to provide feelings of security and decrease need for self-mutilative behaviors.***

Outcome Criteria

1. Anxiety is maintained at a level at which client feels no need for self-mutilation.
2. Client demonstrates ability to use adaptive coping strategies in the face of stressful situations.

INEFFECTIVE COPING

Definition: *Inability to form a valid appraisal of the stressors, inadequate choices of practiced responses, and/or inability to use available resources.*

Possible Etiologies ("related to")

[Possible hereditary factors]
[Brain trauma or dysfunction]
[Mental retardation]
[Dysfunctional family system, resulting in behaviors such as the following:
Child abuse or neglect
Parental rejection or abandonment
Harsh or inconsistent discipline
Emotional deprivation
Parental substance abuse
Parental unpredictability]

Defining Characteristics ("evidenced by")

[Inability to control impulse of violence or aggression]
[Inability to control impulse to steal]
[Inability to control impulse to gamble]
[Inability to control impulse to set fires]
[Inability to control impulse to pull out own hair]

[Feeling of intense anxiety and tension that precedes, and is relieved by, engaging in these impulsive behaviors]

Goals/Objectives

Short-Term Goal

Client will verbalize adaptive ways to cope with stress by means other than impulsive behaviors (time dimension to be individually determined).

Long-Term Goal

Client will be able to delay gratification and use adaptive coping strategies in response to stress (time dimension to be individually determined).

Interventions with *Selected Rationales*

1. Help client gain insight into his or her behaviors. Often these individuals rationalize to such an extent that they deny that what they have done is wrong. ***Client must come to understand that certain behaviors will not be tolerated within the society and that severe consequences will be imposed on those individuals who refuse to comply. Client must want to become a productive member of society before he or she can be helped.***
2. Talk about past behaviors with client. Discuss behaviors that are acceptable by societal norms and those that are not. Help client identify ways in which he or she has exploited others. Encourage client to explore how he or she would feel if the circumstances were reversed. ***An attempt may be made to enlighten client to the sensitivity of others by promoting self-awareness in an effort to help client gain insight into his or her own behavior.***
3. Throughout relationship with client, maintain attitude of "It is not *you*, but your *behavior*, that is unacceptable." ***An attitude of acceptance promotes feelings of dignity and self-worth.***
4. Work with client to increase the ability to delay gratification. Reward desirable behaviors, and provide immediate positive feedback. ***Rewards and positive feedback enhance self-esteem and encourage repetition of desirable behaviors.***
5. Help client identify and practice more adaptive strategies for coping with stressful life situations. ***The impulse to perform the maladaptive behavior may be so great that client is unable to see any other alternatives to relieve stress.***

Outcome Criteria

1. Client is able to demonstrate techniques that may be used in response to stress to prevent resorting to maladaptive impulsive behaviors.
2. Client verbalizes understanding that behavior is unacceptable and accepts responsibility for own behavior.

INTERNET REFERENCES

Additional information about impulse control disorders may be located at the following websites:

- http://www.ncpgambling.org/
- http://www.gamblersanonymous.org/
- http://www.crescentlife.com/disorders/pyromania.htm
- http://www.findarticles.com/cf_dls/m0UMR/9_21/65714216/p1/article.jhtml
- http://www.biopsychiatry.com/klepto.htm

CHAPTER 14

*Psychological Factors Affecting Medical Condition**

BACKGROUND ASSESSMENT DATA

The *Diagnostic and Statistical Manual of Mental Disorders, Fourth Edition, Text Revision, 2000 (DSM-IV-TR)* (APA, 2000) identifies psychological factors affecting medical condition as the presence of one or more specific psychological or behavioral factors that adversely affect a general medical condition. These factors can adversely affect the medical condition in several ways:

1. By influencing the course of the medical condition (i.e., contributing to the development or exacerbation of or delayed recovery from the medical condition).
2. By interfering with treatment of the medical condition.
3. By constituting an additional health risk for the individual (e.g., the individual who has peptic ulcers who continues to drink and smoke).

Several types of psychological factors are implicated by the *DSM-IV-TR* as those that can affect the general medical condition. They include:

1. Mental disorders (e.g., axis I disorders, such as major depression).
2. Psychological symptoms (e.g., depressed mood or anxiety).
3. Personality traits or coping style (e.g., denial of the need for medical care).
4. Maladaptive health behaviors (e.g., smoking or overeating).
5. Stress-related physiological responses (e.g., tension headaches).
6. Other or unspecified psychological factors (e.g., interpersonal or cultural factors).

---

*Classification and criteria for all psychiatric diagnoses in this chapter are from the *Diagnostic and Statistical Manual of Mental Disorders, Fourth Edition, Text Revision, 2000.* Used with permission from the American Psychiatric Association.

316 Psychological Factors Affecting Medical Condition

Defined

The *DSM-IV-TR* (APA, 2000) designates this diagnosis when there is evidence of a physical symptom or a physical disorder that is adversely affected by psychological factors. Common examples of medical conditions for which this category may be appropriate include, but are not limited to, tension headache, migraine headache, cardiospasm, pylorospasm, rheumatoid arthritis, asthma, ulcers, ulcerative colitis, regional enteritis, hypertension, nausea and vomiting, tachycardia, arrhythmia, acne, angina pectoris, painful menstruation, frequency of micturition, neurodermatitis, and sacroiliac pain. Kaplan and Sadock (1998) state "psychological or behavioral factors play a role in almost every medical condition." Virtually any organic disorder can be considered psychophysiological.

This category differs from somatoform disorders and conversion disorders in that there is evidence of either demonstrable organic pathology (such as the inflammation associated with rheumatoid arthritis) or a known pathophysiological process (such as the cerebral vasodilation of migraine headaches).

Predisposing Factors

1. **Physiological**
   a. ***Physical Factors.*** Selye (1956) believes that psychophysiological disorders occur when the body is exposed to prolonged stress, producing a number of physiological effects under direct control of the pituitary-adrenal axis. He also suggests that genetic predisposition influences which organ system will be affected and determines the type of psychophysiological disorder the individual will develop.
2. **Psychosocial**
   a. ***Emotional Response Pattern.*** It has been hypothesized that individuals exhibit specific physiological responses to certain emotions. For example, in response to the emotion of anger, one person may experience peripheral vasoconstriction, resulting in an increase in blood pressure. The same emotion in another individual may evoke the response of cerebral vasodilation, manifesting a migraine headache.
   b. ***Personality Traits.*** Various studies suggest that individuals with specific personality traits are predisposed to certain disease processes. Although personality cannot account totally for the development of psychophysiological disorders, the literature alludes to the following possible relationships:

Asthma	Dependent personality characteristics
Ulcers, hypertension	Repressed anger
Cancer	Depressive personality

Rheumatoid arthritis, ulcerative colitis	Self-sacrificing and inhibited
Migraine headaches	Compulsive and perfectionistic
Coronary heart disease	Aggressive and competitive

c. ***Learning Theory.*** A third psychosocial theory considers the role of learning in the psychophysiological response to stress. If a child grows up observing the attention, increased dependency, or other secondary gain an individual receives because of illness, such behaviors may be viewed as desirable and subsequently imitated by the child.

d. ***Theory of Family Dynamics.*** This theory relates to the predisposition of those individuals who are members of dysfunctional family systems to use psychophysiological problems to cover up interpersonal conflicts. The anxiety in a dysfunctional family situation is shifted from the conflict to the ailing individual. Anxiety decreases, the conflict is avoided, and the person receives positive reinforcement for his or her symptoms. The situation appears more comfortable, but the real problem remains unresolved.

Symptomatology (Subjective and Objective Data)

1. Complaints of physical illness that can be substantiated by objective evidence of physical pathology or known pathophysiological process.
2. Moderate to severe level of anxiety.
3. Denial of emotional problems; client unable to see a relationship between physical problems and response to stress.
4. Use of physical illness as excuse for noncompliance with psychiatric treatment plan.
5. Repressed anger or anger expressed inappropriately.
6. Verbal hostility.
7. Depressed mood.
8. Low self-esteem.
9. Dependent behaviors.
10. Attention-seeking behaviors.
11. Report (or other evidence) of numerous stressors occurring in person's life.

Common Nursing Diagnoses and Interventions†

(Interventions are applicable to various health-care settings, such as inpatient and partial hospitalization, community outpatient clinic, home health, and private practice.)

---

†A number of nursing diagnoses common to specific physical disorders or symptoms could be used (e.g., pain, activity intolerance, impaired tissue integrity, diarrhea). For purposes of this chapter, only nursing diagnoses common to the general category are presented.

INEFFECTIVE COPING

Definition: *Inability to form a valid appraisal of the stressors, inadequate choices of practiced responses, and/or inability to use available resources.*

Possible Etiologies ("related to")

[Repressed anxiety]
[Inadequate support systems]
[Inadequate coping methods]
[Low self-esteem]
[Unmet dependency needs]
[Negative role modeling]
[Dysfunctional family system]

Defining Characteristics ("evidenced by")

[Initiation or exacerbation of physical illness (specify)]
[Denial of relationship between physical symptoms and emotional problems]
[Use of sick role for secondary gains]
Inability to meet role expectations
Inadequate problem solving

Goals/Objectives

Short-Term Goal

Within 1 week, client will verbalize adaptive ways of coping with stressful situations.

Long-Term Goal

Client will achieve physical wellness and demonstrate the ability to prevent exacerbation of physical symptoms as a coping mechanism in response to stress.

Interventions with *Selected Rationales*

1. Perform thorough physical assessment ***in order to determine specific care required for client's physical condition.*** Monitor laboratory values, vital signs, intake and output, and other assessments necessary ***to maintain an accurate, ongoing appraisal.***
2. Together with client, identify goals of care and ways in which client believes he or she can best achieve those goals. Client may need assistance with problem solving. ***Personal involvement in his or her care provides a feeling of control and increases chances for positive outcomes.***
3. Encourage client to discuss current life situations that he or she perceives as stressful and the feelings associated with each. ***Verbalization of true feelings in a nonthreatening environment may help client come to terms with unresolved issues.***

4. During client's discussion, note times during which a sense of powerlessness or loss of control over life situation emerges. Focus on these times, and discuss ways in which client may maintain a feeling of control. ***A sense of self-worth develops and is maintained when an individual feels power over his or her own life situations.***
5. As client becomes able to discuss feelings more openly, help him or her in a nonthreatening manner to relate certain feelings to the appearance of physical symptoms. ***Client may be unaware of the relationship between physical symptoms and emotional problems.***
6. Discuss stressful times when physical symptoms did not appear and the adaptive coping strategies that were used during those situations. ***Therapy is facilitated by considering areas of strength and using them to client's benefit.***
7. Provide positive reinforcement for adaptive coping mechanisms identified or used. Suggest alternative coping strategies, but allow client to determine which can most appropriately be incorporated into his or her lifestyle. ***Positive reinforcement enhances self-esteem and encourages repetition of desirable behaviors. Client may require assistance with problem solving but must be allowed and encouraged to make decisions independently.***
8. Help client identify a resource within the community (friend, significant other, group) to use as a support system for the expression of feelings ***in an effort to prevent maladaptive coping through physical illness.***

Outcome Criteria

1. Client is able to demonstrate techniques that may be used in response to stress to prevent the occurrence or exacerbation of physical symptoms.
2. Client verbalizes an understanding of the relationship between emotional problems and physical symptoms.

LOW SELF-ESTEEM

Definition: *Negative self-evaluation and feelings about self or self-capabilities.*

Possible Etiologies ("related to")

[Lack of positive feedback]
[Unmet dependency needs]
[Retarded ego development]
[Repeated negative feedback, resulting in diminished self-worth]
[Dysfunctional family system]

Defining Characteristics ("evidenced by")

[Difficulty accepting positive reinforcement]
[Nonparticipation in therapy]
Self-negating verbalizations
Evaluation of self as unable to deal with events
Hesitant to try new things or situations [because of fear of failure]
[Hypersensitive to slight or criticism]
Lack of eye contact
[Inability to form close, personal relationships]
[Degradation of others in an attempt to increase own feelings of self-worth]

Goals/Objectives

Short-Term Goals

1. Client will discuss fear of failure with nurse within 3 days.
2. Client will verbalize aspects of self he or she likes within 5 days.

Long-Term Goals

1. Client will exhibit increased feelings of self-worth as evidenced by verbal expression of positive aspects about self, past accomplishments, and future prospects.
2. Client will exhibit increased feelings of self-worth by setting realistic goals and trying to reach them, thereby demonstrating a decrease of fear of failure.

Interventions with *Selected Rationales*

1. Ensure that goals are realistic. It is important for client to achieve something, so plan activities in which success is likely. ***Success increases self-esteem.***
2. Minimize amount of attention given to physical symptoms. Client must perceive self as a worthwhile person, separate and apart from the role of client. ***Lack of attention may discourage use of undesirable behaviors.***
3. Promote your acceptance of client as a worthwhile person by spending time with him or her. Develop trust through one-to-one interactions, then encourage client to participate in group activities. Support group attendance with your presence until client feels comfortable attending alone. ***The feeling of acceptance by others increases self-esteem.***
4. Ask client to make a written list of positive and negative aspects about self. Discuss each item on the list with client. Develop plans of change for the characteristics viewed as negative. Assist client in implementing the plans. Provide positive feedback for successful change. ***Individuals with low self-esteem often have difficulty recognizing their positive attributes. They may also lack problem-solving skills and require assistance to formulate a plan***

for implementing the desired changes. Positive feedback enhances self-esteem and encourages repetition of desired behaviors.

5. Avoid fostering dependence by "doing for" client. Allow client to perform as independently as physical condition will permit. Offer recognition and praise for accomplishments. ***The ability to perform self-care activities independently provides a feeling of self-control and enhances self-esteem. Positive reinforcement encourages repetition of desirable behavior.***
6. Allow client to be an active participant in his or her therapy. Promote feelings of control or power by encouraging input into decision making regarding treatment and for planning discharge from treatment. Provide positive feedback for adaptive responses. ***Control over own life experiences promotes feelings of self-worth.***

Outcome Criteria

1. Client verbalizes positive perception of self.
2. Client demonstrates ability to manage own self-care, make independent decisions, and use problem-solving skills.
3. Client sets goals that are realistic and works to achieve those goals without evidence of fear of failure.

INEFFECTIVE ROLE PERFORMANCE

Definition: *Patterns of behavior and self-expression that do not match the environmental context, norms, and expectations.*

Possible Etiologies ("related to")

[Physical illness accompanied by real or perceived disabling symptoms]
[Unmet dependency needs]
[Dysfunctional family system]

Defining Characteristics ("evidenced by")

Change in self-perception of role
Change in [physical] capacity to resume role
[Assumption of dependent role]
Changes in usual patterns of responsibility [because of conflict within dysfunctional family system]

Goals/Objectives

Short-Term Goal

Client will verbalize understanding that physical symptoms interfere with role performance in order to fill an unmet need.

Long-Term Goal

Client will be able to assume role-related responsibilities by time of discharge from treatment.

Interventions with *Selected Rationales*

1. Determine client's usual role within the family system. Identify roles of other family members. ***An accurate database is required in order to formulate appropriate plan of care for client.***
2. Assess specific disabilities related to role expectations. Assess relationship of disability to physical condition. ***It is important to determine the realism of client's role expectations.***
3. Encourage client to discuss conflicts evident within the family system. Identify ways in which client and other family members have responded to these conflicts. ***It is necessary to identify specific stressors as well as adaptive and maladaptive responses within the system before assistance can be provided in an effort to create change.***
4. Help client identify feelings associated with family conflict, the subsequent exacerbation of physical symptoms, and the accompanying disabilities. ***Client may be unaware of the relationship between physical symptoms and emotional problems. An awareness of the correlation is the first step toward creating change.***
5. Help client identify changes he or she would like to occur within the family system.
6. Encourage family participation in the development of plans to effect positive change, and work to resolve the conflict for which the client's sick role provides relief. ***Input from the individuals who will be directly involved in the change will increase the likelihood of a positive outcome.***
7. Allow input from all family members in the plan for change: knowledge of benefits and consequences for each alternative, selection of appropriate alternatives, methods for implementation of alternatives, alternate plan in the event initial change is unsuccessful. ***Family may require assistance with this problem-solving process.***
8. Ensure that client has accurate perception of role expectations within the family system. Use role playing to practice areas associated with his or her role that client perceives as painful. ***Repetition through practice may help to desensitize client to the anticipated distress.***
9. As client is able to understand the relationship between exacerbation of physical symptoms and existing conflict, discuss more adaptive coping strategies that may be used to prevent interference with role performance during times of stress.

Outcome Criteria

1. Client is able to verbalize realistic perception of role expectations.
2. Client is physically able to assume role-related responsibilities.
3. Client and family are able to verbalize plan for attempt at conflict resolution.

DEFICIENT KNOWLEDGE (Psychological Factors Affecting Medical Condition)

Definition: *Absence or deficiency of cognitive information related to specific topic.*

Possible Etiologies ("related to")

Lack of interest in learning
[Severe level of anxiety]
[Low self-esteem]
[Regression to earlier level of development]

Defining Characteristics ("evidenced by")

[Denial of emotional problems]
[Statements such as, "I don't know why the doctor put me in the psychiatric unit. I have a physical problem."]
[History of numerous exacerbations of physical illness]
[Noncompliance with psychiatric treatment]
Inappropriate or exaggerated behaviors (e.g., hysterical, hostile, agitated, apathetic)

Goals/Objectives

Short-Term Goal

Client will cooperate with plan for teaching provided by primary nurse.

Long-Term Goal

By time of discharge from treatment, client will be able to verbalize psychological factors affecting his or her medical condition.

Interventions with *Selected Rationales*

1. Assess client's level of knowledge regarding effects of psychological problems on the body. ***An adequate database is necessary for the development of an effective teaching plan.***
2. Assess client's level of anxiety and readiness to learn. ***Learning does not occur beyond the moderate level of anxiety.***
3. Discuss physical examinations and laboratory tests that have been conducted. Explain purpose and results of each. ***Fear of the unknown may contribute to elevated level of anxiety. Client has the right to know about and accept or refuse any medical treatment.***
4. Explore client's feelings and fears. Go slowly. These feelings may have been suppressed or repressed for so long that their disclosure may be very painful. Be supportive. ***Verbalizing feelings in a nonthreatening environment and with a trusting individual may help client come to terms with unresolved issues.***

5. Have client keep a diary of appearance, duration, and intensity of physical symptoms. A separate record of situations that client finds especially stressful should also be kept. ***Comparison of these records may provide objective data from which to observe the relationship between physical symptoms and stress.***
6. Help client identify needs that are met through the sick role. Together, formulate more adaptive means for fulfilling these needs. Practice by role playing. ***Repetition through practice serves to reduce discomfort in the actual situation.***
7. Provide instruction in assertiveness techniques, especially the ability to recognize the differences among passive, assertive, and aggressive behaviors and the importance of respecting the human rights of others while protecting one's own basic human rights. ***These skills will preserve client's self-esteem while also improving his or her ability to form satisfactory interpersonal relationships.***
8. Discuss adaptive methods of stress management such as relaxation techniques, physical exercise, meditation, breathing exercises, and autogenics. ***Use of these adaptive techniques may decrease appearance of physical symptoms in response to stress.***

Outcome Criteria

1. Client verbalizes an understanding of the relationship between psychological stress and exacerbation of physical illness.
2. Client demonstrates the ability to use adaptive coping strategies in the management of stress.

■ INTERNET REFERENCES

Additional information about psychophysiological disorders discussed in this chapter may be located at the following websites:

- http://www.nci.nih.gov
- http://www.cancer.org
- http://www.americanheart.org/
- http://www.headaches.org/
- http://www.pslgroup.com/ASTHMA.HTM
- http://www.gastro.org/
- http://www.pslgroup.com/HYPERTENSION.HTM
- http://content.health.msn.com/condition_center/rha
- http://www.niddk.nih.gov/health/digest/pubs/colitis/colitis.htm

CHAPTER 15

*Personality Disorders**

BACKGROUND ASSESSMENT DATA

The *Diagnostic and Statistical Manual of Mental Disorders, Fourth Edition, Text Revision, 2000 (DSM-IV-TR)* (APA, 2000) describes personality *traits* as "enduring patterns of perceiving, relating to, and thinking about the environment and oneself that are exhibited in a wide range of social and personal contexts." A personality *disorder* is said to exist only when these traits become inflexible and maladaptive and cause either significant functional impairment or subjective distress.

The *DSM-IV-TR* groups the personality disorders into three clusters. They are coded on axis II in the *DMS-IV-TR* Classification. These clusters, and the disorders classified under each, are as follows:

1. **Cluster A:** Behaviors described as odd or eccentric
   a. 301.0 Paranoid personality disorder
   b. 301.20 Schizoid personality disorder
   c. 301.22 Schizotypal personality disorder
2. **Cluster B:** Behaviors described as dramatic, emotional, or erratic
   a. 301.7 Antisocial personality disorder
   b. 301.83 Borderline personality disorder
   c. 301.50 Histrionic personality disorder
   d. 301.81 Narcissistic personality disorder
3. **Cluster C:** Behaviors described as anxious or fearful
   a. 301.82 Avoidant personality disorder
   b. 301.6 Dependent personality disorder
   c. 301.4 Obsessive-compulsive personality disorder
   d. Passive-aggressive personality disorder

NOTE: The third edition of the *DSM* included passive-aggressive personality disorder in cluster C. In the *DSM-IV-TR*, this disorder is included in the section on *Criteria Provided for Further Study*. For

---

*Classification and criteria for all psychiatric diagnoses in this chapter are from the *Diagnostic and Statistical Manual of Mental Disorders, Fourth Edition, Text Revision, 2000.* Used with permission from the American Psychiatric Association.

purposes of this text, passive-aggressive personality disorder is described with the cluster C disorders.

Categories of personality disorders described by the *DSM-IV-TR* include the following:

1. **Cluster A**
   a. ***Paranoid Personality Disorder.*** The essential feature is a pervasive and unwarranted suspiciousness and mistrust of people. There is a general expectation of being exploited or harmed by others in some way. Symptoms include guardedness in relationships with others, pathological jealousy, hypersensitivity, inability to relax, unemotionality, and lack of a sense of humor. These individuals are very critical of others but have much difficulty accepting criticism themselves.
   b. ***Schizoid Personality Disorder.*** This disorder is characterized by an inability to form close, personal relationships. Symptoms include social isolation; absence of warm, tender feelings for others; indifference to praise, criticism, or the feelings of others; and flat, dull affect (appears cold and aloof).
   c. ***Schizotypal Personality Disorder.*** This disorder is characterized by peculiarities of ideation, appearance, behavior, and deficits in interpersonal relatedness that are not severe enough to meet the criteria for schizophrenia. Symptoms include magical thinking; ideas of reference; social isolation; illusions; odd speech patterns; aloof, cold, suspicious behavior; and undue social anxiety.
2. **Cluster B**
   a. ***Antisocial Personality Disorder.*** This disorder is characterized by a pattern of socially irresponsible, exploitative, and guiltless behavior, as evidenced by the tendency to fail to conform to the law or to sustain consistent employment; to exploit and manipulate others for personal gain; to deceive; and to fail to develop stable relationships. The individual must be at least 18 years of age and have a history of conduct disorder before the age of 15. (Symptoms of this disorder are identified later in this chapter, along with predisposing factors and nursing care.)
   b. ***Borderline Personality Disorder.*** The features of this disorder are described as marked instability in interpersonal relationships, mood, and self-image. The instability is significant to the extent that the individual seems to hover on the border between neurosis and psychosis. (Symptoms of this disorder are identified later in this chapter, along with predisposing factors and nursing care.)
   c. ***Histrionic Personality Disorder.*** The essential feature of this disorder is described as a pervasive pattern of excessive emotionality and attention-seeking behavior. Symptoms include exaggerated expression of emotions, incessant drawing of attention to oneself, overreaction to minor events, constantly

seeking approval from others, egocentricity, vain and demanding behavior, extreme concern with physical appearance, and inappropriately sexually seductive appearance or behavior.

d. ***Narcissistic Personality Disorder.*** This disorder is characterized by a grandiose sense of self-importance; preoccupation with fantasies of success, power, brilliance, beauty, or ideal love; a constant need for admiration and attention; exploitation of others for fulfillment of own desires; lack of empathy; response to criticism or failure with indifference or humiliation and rage; and preoccupation with feelings of envy.

3. **Cluster C**

a. ***Avoidant Personality Disorder.*** This disorder is characterized by social withdrawal brought about by extreme sensitivity to rejection. Symptoms include unwillingness to enter into relationships unless given unusually strong guarantees of uncritical acceptance; low self-esteem; and social withdrawal in spite of a desire for affection and acceptance. Depression and anxiety are common. Social phobia may be a complication of this disorder.

b. ***Dependent Personality Disorder.*** Individuals with this disorder passively allow others to assume responsibility for major areas of life because of their inability to function independently. They lack self-confidence, are unable to make decisions, perceive themselves as helpless and stupid, possess fear of being alone or abandoned, and seek constant reassurance and approval from others.

c. ***Obsessive-Compulsive Personality Disorder.*** This disorder is characterized by a pervasive pattern of perfectionism and inflexibility. Interpersonal relationships have a formal and serious quality, and others often perceive these individuals as stilted or "stiff." Other symptoms include difficulty expressing tender feelings, insistence that others submit to his or her way of doing things, excessive devotion to work and productivity to the exclusion of pleasure, indecisiveness, perfectionism, preoccupation with details, depressed mood, and being judgmental of self and others.

d. ***Passive-Aggressive Personality Disorder.*** Characteristic of this disorder is a passive resistance to demands for adequate performance in both occupational and social functioning. Symptoms include obstructionism, procrastination, stubbornness, intentional inefficiency, dawdling, "forgetfulness," criticism of persons in authority, dependency, and low self-esteem. Oppositional defiant disorder in childhood or adolescence is a predisposing factor.

Many of the behaviors associated with the personality disorders may be manifested by clients with other psychiatric diagnoses as well as by individuals described as "healthy." It is only when personality traits or styles repetitively interfere with an individual's ability to function within age-appropriate cultural and developmental expectations, disrupt interpersonal relationships, or distort a person's pattern of perception and thinking about the environment that a diagnosis of personality disorder is assigned.

Individuals with personality disorders may be encountered in all types of treatment settings. They are not often treated in acute care settings, but because of the instability of the borderline client, hospitalization is necessary from time to time. The individual with antisocial personality disorder also may be hospitalized as an alternative to imprisonment when a legal determination is made that psychiatric intervention may be helpful. Because of these reasons, suggestions for inpatient care are included in this chapter; however, these interventions may also be used in other types of treatment settings. Undoubtedly, these clients represent the ultimate challenge for the psychiatric nurse.

Borderline Personality Disorder

Defined

This personality disorder is characterized by instability of affect, behavior, object relationships, and self-image. The term "borderline" came into being because the emotionally unstable behavior seems to fall *on the border* between neurotic and psychotic. Transient psychotic symptoms appear during periods of extreme stress. The disorder is more commonly diagnosed in women than in men.

Predisposing Factors

1. **Theory of Object Relations.** This theory suggests that the basis for borderline personality lies in the ways the child relates to the mother and does not separate from her. Mahler and associates (1975) define this process in a series of phases described as follows:
    a. **Phase 1 (Birth to 1 month), Autistic Phase.** Most of the infant's time is spent in a half-waking, half-sleeping state.
    b. **Phase 2 (1 to 5 months), Symbiotic Phase.** A type of psychic fusion of mother and child. Child views self as extension of mother.
    c. **Phase 3 (5 to 10 months), Differentiation Phase.** Child begins to become aware of separateness between self and mother.
    d. **Phase 4 (10 to 16 months), Practicing Phase.** The child displays increased independence in terms of ability to ambulate and explore on his or her own.
    e. **Phase 5 (16 to 24 months), Rapprochement Phase.** Awareness of separateness from mother increases. This is frightening to the child, who wants to regain some lost closeness but not return to symbiosis. The child just wants mother there as needed for "emotional refueling."

f. **Phase 6 (24 to 36 months), On the Way to Object Constancy Phase.** The child completes the individuation process and learns to relate to objects in an effective, constant manner.

The theory of object relations suggests that the individual with borderline personality is fixed in the rapprochement phase of development. This fixation occurs when the mother begins to feel threatened by the increasing autonomy of her child and so withdraws her emotional support during those times *or* she may reward clinging, dependent behaviors. In this way, the child comes to believe that

"To grow up and be independent = a 'bad' child."
"To stay immature and dependent = a 'good' child."
"Mom withholds nurturing from 'bad' child."

Consequently, the child develops a deep fear of abandonment that persists into adulthood. In addition, because object constancy is never achieved, the child continues to view objects (people) as parts—either good or bad. This is called splitting, the primary defense mechanism of borderline personality.

Symptomatology (Subjective and Objective Data)

At least five of the following criteria are required by the *DSM-IV-TR* (APA, 2000) for a diagnosis of borderline personality disorder:

1. Frantic efforts to avoid real or imagined abandonment (not to include suicidal or self-mutilating behavior covered in criterion 5).
2. A pattern of unstable and intense interpersonal relationships characterized by alternating between extremes of idealization and devaluation.
3. Identity disturbance: markedly and persistently unstable self-image or sense of self.
4. Impulsivity in at least two areas, which is potentially self-damaging, such as spending, sex, substance abuse, reckless driving, binge eating (not to include behavior covered in criterion 5).
5. Recurrent suicidal behavior, gestures, or threats or self-mutilating behavior.
6. Affective instability caused by marked reactivity of mood (e.g., intense episodic dysphoria, irritability, or anxiety, usually lasting a few hours and only rarely more than a few days).
7. Chronic feelings of emptiness.
8. Inappropriate, intense anger or difficulty controlling anger (e.g., frequent displays of temper, constant anger, recurrent physical fights).
9. Transient, stress-related paranoid ideation or severe dissociative symptoms.

Other symptoms include the following:

10. Alternating clinging and distancing behaviors.
11. Projection—seeing in others attitudes they fail to see in themselves.

12. Poor reality testing—misinterpretations of the environment and relationships, resulting from poor ego development.

Common Nursing Diagnoses and Interventions

(Interventions are applicable to various health-care settings, such as inpatient and partial hospitalization, community outpatient clinic, home health, and private practice.)

RISK FOR SELF-MUTILATION/RISK FOR SELF-DIRECTED OR OTHER-DIRECTED VIOLENCE

Definition: ***At risk for deliberate self-injurious behavior causing tissue damage with the intent of causing nonfatal injury to attain relief of tension. At risk for behaviors in which an individual demonstrates that he/she can be physically, emotionally, and/or sexually harmful either to self or to others.***

Related/Risk Factors ("related to")

[Extreme fears of abandonment]
[Feelings of unreality]
[Depressed mood]
[Use of suicidal gestures for manipulation of others]
[Unmet dependency needs]
[Low self-esteem]
[Unresolved grief]
[Rage reactions]
[Physically self-damaging acts (cutting, burning, drug overdose, etc.)]
Body language—rigid posture, clenching of fists and jaw, hyperactivity, pacing, breathlessness, and threatening stances
History or threats of violence toward self or others or of destruction to the property of others
Impulsivity
Suicidal ideation, plan, available means
[History of suicide attempts]

Goals/Objectives

Short-Term Goal

1. Client will seek out staff member if feelings of harming self or others emerge.
2. Client will not harm self or others.

Long-Term Goal

Client will not harm self or others.

Interventions with *Selected Rationales*

1. Observe client's behavior frequently. Do this through routine activities and interactions; avoid appearing watchful and suspicious. ***Close observation is required so that intervention can occur if required to ensure client's (and others') safety.***
2. Secure a verbal contract from client that he or she will seek a staff member when the urge for self-mutilation is experienced. ***Discussing feelings of self-harm with a trusted individual provides some relief to client. A contract gets the subject out in the open and places some of the responsibility for his or her safety with the client. An attitude of acceptance of client as a worthwhile individual is conveyed.***
3. If self-mutilation occurs, care for client's wounds in a matter-of-fact manner. Do not give positive reinforcement to this behavior by offering sympathy or additional attention. ***Lack of attention to the maladaptive behavior may decrease repetition of its use.***
4. Encourage client to talk about feelings he or she was having just before this behavior. ***To problem-solve the situation with client, knowledge of the precipitating factors is important.***
5. Act as a role model for appropriate expression of angry feelings, and give positive reinforcement to client when attempts to conform are made. ***It is vital that client express angry feelings, because suicide and other self-destructive behaviors are often viewed as a result of anger turned inward on the self.***
6. Remove all dangerous objects from client's environment. ***Client safety is a nursing priority.***
7. Try to redirect violent behavior by means of physical outlets for client's anxiety (e.g., punching bag, jogging). ***Physical exercise is a safe and effective way of relieving pent-up tension.***
8. Have sufficient staff available to indicate a show of strength to client if necessary. ***This conveys to client evidence of control over the situation and provides some physical security for staff.***
9. Administer tranquilizing medications as ordered by physician or obtain an order if necessary. Monitor client for effectiveness of the medication and for the appearance of adverse side effects. ***Tranquilizing medications such as anxiolytics or antipsychotics may have a calming effect on client and may prevent aggressive behaviors.***
10. Use of mechanical restraints or isolation room may be required if less restrictive interventions are unsuccessful. Follow policy and procedure prescribed by the institution in executing this intervention. The Joint Commission on Accreditation of Healthcare Organizations (JCAHO) requires that the physician reevaluate and issue a new order for restraints every 4 hours for adults age 18 years and older. If client has previously refused medication, administer after restraints have been applied. Most states con-

sider this intervention appropriate in emergency situations or in the event that a client would likely harm self or others.

11. Observe client in restraints every 15 minutes (or according to institutional policy). Ensure that circulation to extremities is not compromised (check temperature, color, pulses). Assist client with needs related to nutrition, hydration, and elimination. Position client so that comfort is facilitated and aspiration can be prevented. ***Client safety is a nursing priority.***
12. May need to assign staff on a one-to-one basis if warranted by acuity of the situation. ***Clients with borderline personality disorder have extreme fear of abandonment; leaving them alone at such a time may cause an acute rise in level of anxiety and agitation.***

Outcome Criteria

1. Client has not harmed self or others.
2. Anxiety is maintained at a level in which client feels no need for aggression.
3. Client denies any ideas of self-harm.
4. Client verbalizes community support systems from which assistance may be requested when personal coping strategies are unsuccessful.

ANXIETY (Severe to Panic)

Definition: *A vague uneasy feeling of discomfort or dread accompanied by an autonomic response (the source often nonspecific or unknown to the individual); a feeling of apprehension caused by anticipation of danger. It is an alerting signal that warns of impending danger and enables the individual to take measures to deal with threat.*

Possible Etiologies ("related to")

Threat to self-concept
Unmet needs
[Extreme fear of abandonment]
Unconscious conflicts [associated with fixation in earlier level of development]

Defining Characteristics ("evidenced by")

[Transient psychotic symptoms in response to severe stress, manifested by disorganized thinking, confusion, altered communication patterns, disorientation, misinterpretation of the environment]
[Excessive use of projection (attributing own thoughts and feelings to others)]

[Depersonalization (feelings of unreality)]
[Derealization (a feeling that the environment is unreal)]
[Acts of self-mutilation in an effort to find relief from feelings of unreality]

Goals/Objectives

Short-Term Goal

Client will demonstrate use of relaxation techniques to maintain anxiety at manageable level.

Long-Term Goal

Client will be able to recognize events that precipitate anxiety and intervene to prevent disabling behaviors.

Interventions with *Selected Rationales*

1. Symptoms of depersonalization often occur at the panic level of anxiety. Clients with borderline personality disorder often resort to cutting or other self-mutilating acts in an effort to relieve the anxiety. Being able to feel pain or see blood is a reassurance of existence to the person. If injury occurs, care for the wounds in a matter-of-fact manner without providing reinforcement for this behavior. ***Lack of reinforcement may discourage repetition of the maladaptive behavior.***
2. During periods of panic anxiety, stay with client and provide reassurance of safety and security. Orient client to the reality of the situation. ***Client comfort and safety are nursing priorities.***
3. Administer tranquilizing medications as ordered by physician, or obtain order if necessary. Monitor client for effectiveness of the medication as well as for adverse side effects. ***Antianxiety medications (e.g., diazepam, chlordiazepoxide, alprazolam) provide relief from the immobilizing effects of anxiety and facilitate client's cooperation with therapy.***
4. Correct misinterpretations of the environment as expressed by client. ***Confronting misinterpretations honestly, with a caring and accepting attitude, provides a therapeutic orientation to reality and preserves client's feelings of dignity and self-worth.***
5. Encourage client to talk about true feelings. Help him or her recognize ownership of these feelings rather than projecting them onto others in the environment. ***Exploration of feelings with a trusted individual may help client perceive the situation more realistically and come to terms with unresolved issues.***
6. Help client work toward achievement of object constancy. Client may feel totally abandoned when nurse or therapist leaves at shift change or at end of therapy session. There may even be feelings that the therapist ceases to exist. Leaving a signed note or card with client for reassurance may help. It is extremely important for more

than one nurse to develop a therapeutic relationship with the borderline client. It is also necessary that staff maintain open communication and consistency in the provision of care for these individuals. ***Individuals with borderline personality disorder have a tendency to cling to one staff member, if allowed, transferring their maladaptive dependency to that individual. This dependency can be avoided if client is able to establish therapeutic relationships with two or more staff members who encourage independent self-care activities.***

Outcome Criteria

1. Client is able to verbalize events that precipitate anxiety and demonstrate techniques for its reduction.
2. Client manifests no symptoms of depersonalization.
3. Client interprets the environment realistically.

DYSFUNCTIONAL GRIEVING

Definition: *Extended, unsuccessful use of intellectual and emotional responses by which individuals, families, and communities attempt to work through the process of modifying self-concept based upon the perception of loss.*

Possible Etiologies ("related to")

[Maternal deprivation during rapprochement phase of development (internalized as a loss, with fixation in the anger stage of the grieving process)]

Defining Characteristics ("evidenced by")

Anger
[Internalized rage]
[Depressed mood]
Labile affect
[Extreme fear of being alone (fear of abandonment)]
[Acting-out behaviors, such as sexual promiscuity, suicidal gestures, temper tantrums, substance abuse]
[Difficulty expressing feelings]
Alterations in eating habits, sleep patterns, dream patterns, activity level, libido
Repetitive use of ineffectual behaviors associated with attempts to reinvest in relationships
Reliving of past experiences with little or no reduction of intensity of the grief
Prolonged interference with life functioning

Goals/Objectives

Short-Term Goal

Client will discuss with nurse or therapist maladaptive patterns of expressing anger.

Long-Term Goal

Client will be able to identify the true source of angry feelings, accept ownership of these feelings, and express them in a socially acceptable manner, in an effort to satisfactorily progress through the grieving process.

Interventions with *Selected Rationales*

1. Convey an accepting attitude—one that creates a nonthreatening environment for client to express feelings. Be honest, and keep all promises. ***An accepting attitude conveys to client that you believe he or she is a worthwhile person. Trust is enhanced.***
2. Identify the function that anger, frustration, and rage serve for client. Allow client to express these feelings within reason. ***Verbalization of feelings in a nonthreatening environment may help client come to terms with unresolved issues.***
3. Encourage client to discharge pent-up anger through participation in large-motor activities (e.g., brisk walks, jogging, physical exercises, volleyball, punching bag, exercise bike). ***Physical exercise provides a safe and effective method for discharging pent-up tension.***
4. Explore with client the true source of the anger. This is painful therapy that often leads to regression as client deals with the feelings of early abandonment. It seems that sometimes client must "get worse before he or she can get better." ***Reconciliation of the feelings associated with this stage is necessary before progression through the grieving process can continue.***
5. As anger is displaced onto the nurse or therapist, caution must be taken to guard against the negative effects of countertransference. These are very difficult clients who have the capacity for eliciting a whole array of negative feelings from the therapist. These feelings must be acknowledged but not allowed to interfere with the therapeutic process.
6. Explain the behaviors associated with the normal grieving process. Help client to recognize his or her position in this process. ***Knowledge of the acceptability of the feelings associated with normal grieving may help to relieve some of the guilt that these responses generate.***
7. Help client understand appropriate ways of expressing anger. Give positive reinforcement for behaviors used to express anger appropriately. Act as a role model. ***Positive reinforcement enhances self-esteem and encourages repetition of desirable behaviors. It is appropriate to let client know when he or she has done something

that has generated angry feelings in you. Role modeling ways to express anger in an appropriate manner is a powerful learning tool.

8. Set limits on acting-out behaviors, and explain consequences of violation of those limits. Be supportive, yet consistent and firm, in caring for this client. ***Client lacks sufficient self-control to limit maladaptive behaviors, so assistance is required from staff. Without consistency on the part of all staff members working with this client, a positive outcome will not be achieved.***

Outcome Criteria

1. Client is able to verbalize how anger and acting-out behaviors are associated with maladaptive grieving.
2. Client is able to discuss the original source of the anger and demonstrates socially acceptable ways of expressing the emotion.

IMPAIRED SOCIAL INTERACTION

Definition: *Insufficient or excessive quantity or ineffective quality of social exchange.*

Possible Etiologies ("related to")

[Fixation in rapprochement phase of development]
[Extreme fears of abandonment and engulfment]
[Lack of personal identity]

Defining Characteristics ("evidenced by")

[Alternating clinging and distancing behaviors]
[Inability to form satisfactory intimate relationship with another person]
Observed use of unsuccessful social interaction behaviors
[Use of primitive dissociation (splitting) in their relationships (viewing others as all good or all bad)]

Goals/Objectives

Short-Term Goal

Client will discuss with nurse or therapist behaviors that impede the development of satisfactory interpersonal relationships.

Long-Term Goals

1. Client will interact with others in the therapy setting in both social and therapeutic activities without difficulty by time of discharge from treatment.
2. Client will display no evidence of splitting or clinging and distancing behaviors in relationships by time of discharge from treatment.

Interventions with *Selected Rationales*

1. Encourage client to examine these behaviors (to recognize that they are occurring). ***Client may be unaware of splitting or of clinging and distancing pattern of interaction with others.***
2. Help client realize that you will be available, without reinforcing dependent behaviors. ***Knowledge of your availability may provide needed security for client.***
3. Give positive reinforcement for independent behaviors. ***Positive reinforcement enhances self-esteem and encourages repetition of desirable behaviors.***
4. Rotate staff who work with client in order to avoid client's developing dependence on particular staff members. ***Client must learn to relate to more than one staff member in an effort to decrease use of splitting and to diminish fears of abandonment.***
5. Explore with client feelings that relate to fears of abandonment and engulfment. Help client understand that clinging and distancing behaviors are engendered by these fears. ***Exploration of feelings with a trusted individual may help client come to terms with unresolved issues.***
6. Help client understand how these behaviors interfere with satisfactory relationships. ***Client may be unaware of others' perception of him or her and why these behaviors are not acceptable to others.***
7. Help client work toward achievement of object constancy. Be available, without promoting dependency, ***so that client may resolve fears of abandonment and develop the ability to establish satisfactory intimate relationships.***

Outcome Criteria

1. Client is able to interact with others in both social and therapeutic activities in a socially acceptable manner.
2. Client does not use splitting or clinging and distancing behaviors in relationships and is able to relate the use of these behaviors to failure of past relationships.

DISTURBED PERSONAL IDENTITY

Definition: *Inability to distinguish between self and nonself.*

Possible Etiologies ("related to")

[Failure to complete tasks of separation/individuation stage of development]

[Underdeveloped ego]

[Unmet dependency needs]

[Absence of, or rejection by, parental sex-role model]

Defining Characteristics ("evidenced by")

[Excessive use of projection]
[Uncertainties regarding gender identity]
[Uncertainties about long-term goals or career choice]
[Ambiguous value system]
[Vague self-image]
[Unable to tolerate being alone]
[Feelings of depersonalization and derealization]
[Self-mutilation (cutting, burning) to validate existence of self]

Goals/Objectives

Short-Term Goal

Client will describe characteristics that make him or her a unique individual.

Long-Term Goal

Client will be able to distinguish own thoughts, feelings, behaviors, and image from those of others, as the initial step in the development of a healthy personal identity.

Interventions with *Selected Rationales*

1. Help client recognize the reality of his or her separateness. Do not attempt to translate client's thoughts and feelings into words. ***Because of the blurred ego boundaries, client may believe you can read his or her mind.*** For this reason, caution should be taken in the use of empathetic understanding. For example, avoid statements such as "I know how you must feel about that."
2. Help client recognize separateness from nurse by clarifying which behaviors and feelings belong to whom. If deemed appropriate, allow client to touch your hand or arm. ***Touch and physical presence provide reality for client and serve to strengthen weak ego boundaries.***
3. Encourage client to discuss thoughts and feelings. Help client recognize ownership of these feelings rather than projecting them onto others in the environment. ***Verbalization of feelings in a nonthreatening environment may help client come to terms with unresolved issues.***
4. Confront statements that project client's feelings onto others. Ask client to validate that others possess those feelings. The expression of *reasonable doubt* as a therapeutic technique may be helpful ("I find that hard to believe").
5. If the problem is with gender identity, ask client to describe his or her perception of appropriate male and female behaviors. Provide information about role behaviors and sex education, if necessary. Client may require clarification of distorted ideas or misinformation. Convey acceptance of the person regardless of preferred identity. ***An attitude of acceptance reinforces client's feelings of self-worth.***

6. Always call client by his or her name. If client experiences feelings of depersonalization or derealization, orientation to the environment and correction of misperceptions may be helpful. ***These interventions help to preserve client's feelings of dignity and self-worth.***
7. Help client understand that there are more adaptive ways of validating his or her existence than self-mutilation. Contract with client to seek out staff member when these feelings occur. ***A contract gets the subject out in the open and places some of the responsibility for his or her safety with client. Client safety is a nursing priority.***
8. Work with client to clarify values. Discuss beliefs, attitudes, and feelings underlying his or her behaviors. Help client identify those values that have been (or are intended to be) incorporated as his or her own. Care must be taken by the nurse to avoid imposing his or her own value system on the client. ***Because of underdeveloped ego and fixation in early developmental level, client may not have established own value system. In order to accomplish this, ownership of beliefs and attitudes must be identified and clarified.***
9. Use of photographs of client may help establish or clarify ego boundaries. ***Photographs may help to increase client's awareness of self as separate from others.***
10. Alleviate anxiety by assuring client that he or she will not be left alone. ***Early childhood traumas may predispose borderline clients to extreme fears of abandonment.***
11. Touch is sometimes therapeutic in identity confirmation. Before this technique is used, however, assess cultural influences and degree of trust. ***Touch and physical presence provide reality for client and serve to strengthen weak ego boundaries.***

Outcome Criteria

1. Client is able to distinguish between own thoughts and feelings and those of others.
2. Client claims ownership of those thoughts and feelings and does not use projection in relationships with others.
3. Client has clarified own feelings regarding sexual identity.

LOW SELF-ESTEEM

Definition: *Negative self-evaluation and feelings about self or self-capabilities.*

Possible Etiologies ("related to")

[Lack of positive feedback]
[Unmet dependency needs]

[Retarded ego development]
[Repeated negative feedback, resulting in diminished self-worth]
[Dysfunctional family system]
[Fixation in earlier level of development]

Defining Characteristics ("evidenced by")

[Difficulty accepting positive reinforcement]
[Self-destructive behavior]
[Frequent use of derogatory and critical remarks against the self]
Lack of eye contact
[Manipulation of one staff member against another in an attempt to gain special privileges]
[Inability to form close, personal relationships]
[Inability to tolerate being alone]
[Degradation of others in an attempt to increase own feelings of self-worth]
Hesitancy to try new things or situations [because of fear of failure]

Goals/Objectives

Short-Term Goals

1. Client will discuss fear of failure with nurse or therapist.
2. Client will verbalize things he or she likes about self.

Long-Term Goals

1. Client will exhibit increased feelings of self-worth as evidenced by verbal expression of positive aspects about self, past accomplishments, and future prospects.
2. Client will exhibit increased feelings of self-worth by setting realistic goals and trying to reach them, thereby demonstrating a decrease in fear of failure.

Interventions with *Selected Rationales*

1. Ensure that goals are realistic. It is important for client to achieve something, so plan for activities in which success is likely. ***Success increases self-esteem.***
2. Convey unconditional positive regard for client. Promote understanding of your acceptance for him or her as a worthwhile human being. ***Acceptance by others increases feelings of self-worth.***
3. Set limits on manipulative behavior. Identify the consequences for violation of those limits. Minimize negative feedback to client. Enforce the limits, and impose the consequences for violations in a matter-of-fact manner. Consistency among all staff members is essential. ***Negative feedback can be extremely threatening to a person with low self-esteem and possibly aggravate the problem. Consequences should convey unacceptability of the behavior, not the person.***

4. Recognize when client is playing one staff member against another. Remember that splitting is the primary defense mechanism of these individuals, and the impressions they have of others as either "good" or "bad" are a manifestation of this defense. Do not listen as client tries to degrade other staff members. Suggest that client discuss the problem directly with staff person involved. ***Lack of reinforcement for these maladaptive behaviors may discourage their repetition.***
5. Encourage independence in the performance of personal responsibilities as well as in decision making related to client's self-care. Offer recognition and praise for accomplishments. ***Positive reinforcement enhances self-esteem and encourages repetition of desirable behaviors.***
6. Help client increase level of self-awareness through critical examination of feelings, attitudes, and behaviors. ***Self-exploration in the presence of a trusted individual may help client come to terms with unresolved issues.***
7. Help client identify positive self-attributes as well as those aspects of the self he or she finds undesirable. Discuss ways to effect change in these areas. ***Individuals with low self-esteem often have difficulty recognizing their positive attributes. They may also lack problem-solving ability and require assistance to formulate a plan for implementing the desired changes.***
8. Discuss client's future. Help client establish short-term and long-term goals. What are his or her strengths? How can he or she best use those strengths to achieve those goals? Encourage client to perform at a level realistic to his or her ability. Offer positive reinforcement for decisions made.

Outcome Criteria

1. Client verbalizes positive aspects about self.
2. Client demonstrates ability to make independent decisions regarding management of own self-care.
3. Client expresses some optimism and hope for the future.
4. Client sets realistic goals for self and demonstrates willingness to reach them.

ANTISOCIAL PERSONALITY DISORDER

Defined

This personality disorder is characterized by a pattern of antisocial behavior that begins before the age of 15 years. These behaviors violate the rights of others, and individuals with this disorder display no evidence of guilt feelings at having done so. There is often a long history of involvement with law-enforcement agencies. Substance abuse is not uncommon. The disorder is more frequently diagnosed in men than in women. Individuals with antisocial personalities are often labeled *sociopathic* or *psychopathic* in the lay literature.

Predisposing Factors

1. **Physiological**
   a. ***Genetics.*** The *DSM-IV-TR* reports that antisocial personality is more common among first-degree biological relatives of those with the disorder than among the general population (APA, 2000). Cadoret (1994) reports on studies that implicate the role of genetics. These studies of families of individuals with antisocial personality show higher numbers of relatives with antisocial personality or alcoholism than are found in the general population. Additional studies have shown that children of parents with antisocial behavior are more likely to be diagnosed as antisocial personality, even when they are separated at birth from their biological parents and reared by individuals without the disorder.
   b. ***Temperament.*** Characteristics associated with temperament in the newborn may be significant in the predisposition to antisocial personality. Parents who bring their children with behavior disorders to clinics often report that the child displayed temper tantrums from infancy and would become furious when awaiting a bottle or a diaper change. As these children mature, they commonly develop a bullying attitude toward other children. Parents report that they are undaunted by punishment and are generally quite unmanageable. They are daring and foolhardy in their willingness to chance physical harm, and they seem unaffected by pain.
2. **Psychosocial**
   a. ***Theories of Family Dynamics.*** Antisocial personality disorder frequently arises from a chaotic home environment (Cadoret, 1994). Parental deprivation during the first 5 years of life appears to be a critical predisposing factor. Separation due to parental delinquency appears to be more highly correlated with the disorder than is parental loss from other causes. The presence or intermittent appearance of inconsistent, impulsive parents, not the loss of a consistent parent, is environmentally *most* damaging.

Studies have shown that individuals with antisocial personality disorder often have been severely physically abused in childhood. The abuse contributes to the development of antisocial behavior in several ways. First, it provides a model for behavior. Second, it may result in injury to the child's central nervous system, thereby impairing the child's ability to function appropriately. Finally, it engenders rage in the victimized child, which is then displaced onto others in the environment.

Disordered family functioning has been implicated as an important factor (Cadoret, 1994; Phillips, Yen, & Gunderson, 2003). The following circumstances may be influential in the predisposition to the disorder:

- Absence of parental discipline
- Extreme poverty
- Removal from the home
- Growing up without parental figures of both sexes
- Erratic and inconsistent methods of discipline
- Being "rescued" each time they are in trouble (never having to suffer the consequences of their own behavior)
- Maternal deprivation

Symptomatology (Subjective and Objective Data)

1. Extremely low-self esteem (abuses other people in an attempt to validate his or her own superiority).
2. Inability to sustain satisfactory job performance.
3. Inability to function as a responsible parent.
4. Failure to follow social and legal norms; repeated performance of antisocial acts that are grounds for arrest (whether arrested or not).
5. Inability to develop satisfactory, enduring, intimate relationship with a sexual partner.
6. Aggressive behaviors; repeated physical fights; spouse or child abuse.
7. Extreme impulsivity.
8. Repeated lying for personal benefit.
9. Reckless driving; driving while intoxicated.
10. Inability to learn from punishment.
11. Lack of guilt or remorse felt in response to exploitation of others.
12. Difficulty with interpersonal relationships.
13. Social extroversion; stimulation through interaction with and abuse of others.
14. Repeated failure to honor financial obligations.

Common Nursing Diagnoses and Interventions

(Interventions are applicable to various health-care settings, such as inpatient and partial hospitalization, community outpatient clinic, home health, and private practice.)

RISK FOR OTHER-DIRECTED VIOLENCE

Definition: *At risk for behaviors in which an individual demonstrates that he/she can be physically, emotionally, and/or sexually harmful to others.*

Related/Risk Factors ("related to")

[Rage reactions]
History of witnessing family violence
Neurological impairment (e.g., positive EEG)
[Suspiciousness of others]
[Interruption of client's attempt to fulfill own desires]
[Inability to tolerate frustration]
[Learned behavior within client's subculture]
[Vulnerable self-esteem]
Body language—rigid posture, clenching of fists and jaw, hyperactivity, pacing, breathlessness, and threatening stances
History or threats of violence toward self or others or of destruction to the property of others
Impulsivity
Availability and/or possession of weapon(s)
[Substance abuse or withdrawal]
[Provocative behavior: argumentative, dissatisfied, overreactive, hypersensitive]
History of violence against others
History of childhood abuse

Goals/Objectives

Short-Term Goals

1. Client will discuss angry feelings and situations that precipitate hostility.
2. Client will not harm others.

Long-Term Goal

Client will not harm others.

Interventions with *Selected Rationales*

1. Convey an accepting attitude toward this client. Feelings of rejection are undoubtedly familiar to him or her. Work on development of trust. Be honest, keep all promises, and convey the message to client that it is not *him* or *her*, but the *behavior,* that is unacceptable. ***An attitude of acceptance promotes feelings of self-worth. Trust is the basis of a therapeutic relationship.***
2. Maintain low level of stimuli in client's environment (low lighting, few people, simple decor, low noise level). ***A stimulating environment may increase agitation and promote aggressive behavior.***
3. Observe client's behavior frequently. Do this through routine activities and interactions; avoid appearing watchful and suspicious. ***Close observation is required so that intervention can occur if needed to ensure client's (and others') safety.***
4. Remove all dangerous objects from client's environment. ***Client safety is a nursing priority.***

5. Help client identify the true object of his or her hostility (e.g., "You seem to be upset with . . ."). ***Because of weak ego development, client may be misusing the defense mechanism of displacement. Helping him or her recognize this in a nonthreatening manner may help reveal unresolved issues so that they may be confronted.***
6. Encourage client to gradually verbalize hostile feelings. ***Verbalization of feelings in a nonthreatening environment may help client come to terms with unresolved issues.***
7. Explore with client alternative ways of handling frustration (e.g., large-motor skills that channel hostile energy into socially acceptable behavior). ***Physically demanding activities help to relieve pent-up tension.***
8. Staff should maintain and convey a calm attitude toward client. ***Anxiety is contagious and can be transferred from staff to client. A calm attitude provides client with a feeling of safety and security.***
9. Have sufficient staff available to present a show of strength to client if necessary. ***This conveys to client evidence of control over the situation and provides some physical security for staff.***
10. Administer tranquilizing medications as ordered by physician or obtain an order if necessary. Monitor client for effectiveness of the medication as well as for appearance of adverse side effects. ***Antianxiety agents (e.g., diazepam, chlordiazepoxide, oxazepam) produce a calming effect and may help to allay hostile behaviors.*** (NOTE: Medications are often not prescribed for clients with antisocial personality disorder because of these individuals' strong susceptibility to addictions.)
11. If client is not calmed by "talking down" or by medication, use of mechanical restraints may be necessary. Be sure to have sufficient staff available to assist. Follow protocol established by the institution in executing this intervention. JCAHO requires that the physician reevaluate and issue a new order for restraints every 4 hours for adults age 18 years and older. If client has refused medication, administer after restraints have been applied. Most states consider this intervention appropriate in emergency situations or in the event that a client would likely harm self or others. Never use restraints as a punitive measure but rather as a protective measure for a client who is out of control.
12. Observe client in restraints every 15 minutes (or according to institutional policy). Ensure that circulation to extremities is not compromised (check temperature, color, pulses). Assist client with needs related to nutrition, hydration, and elimination. Position client so that comfort is facilitated and aspiration can be prevented. ***Client safety is a nursing priority.***

Outcome Criteria

1. Client is able to rechannel hostility into socially acceptable behaviors.
2. Client is able to discuss angry feelings and verbalize ways to tolerate frustration appropriately.

INEFFECTIVE COPING

Definition: *Inability to form a valid appraisal of the stressors, inadequate choices of practiced responses, and/or inability to use available resources.*

Possible Etiologies ("related to")

[Inadequate support systems]
[Inadequate coping method]
[Underdeveloped ego]
[Underdeveloped superego]
[Dysfunctional family system]
[Negative role modeling]
[Absent, erratic, or inconsistent methods of discipline]
[Extreme poverty]

Defining Characteristics ("evidenced by")

[Disregard for societal norms and laws]
[Absence of guilt feelings]
[Inability to delay gratification]
[Extreme impulsivity]
[Inability to learn from punishment]

Goals/Objectives

Short-Term Goal

Within 24 hours after admission, client will verbalize understanding of unit rules and regulations and the consequences for violation of them.

Long-Term Goal

Client will be able to cope more adaptively by delaying gratification of own desires and following rules and regulations of the unit by time of discharge from treatment.

Interventions with *Selected Rationales*

1. From the onset, client should be made aware of which behaviors will not be accepted in the unit. Explain consequences of violation of the limits. Consequences must involve something of value to the client. All staff must be consistent in enforcing these limits.

Consequences should be administered in a matter-of-fact manner immediately after the infraction. ***Because client cannot (or will not) impose own limits on maladaptive behaviors, these behaviors must be delineated and enforced by staff. Undesirable consequences may help to decrease repetition of these behaviors.***

2. Do not attempt to coax or convince client to do the "right thing." Do not use the words "You should (or shouldn't) . . ."; instead, use "You will be expected to . . . ." The ideal would be for this client to eventually internalize societal norms, beginning with this step-by-step "either/or" approach in the unit (*either* you do [don't do] this, *or* this will occur). ***Explanations must be concise, concrete, and clear, with little or no capacity for misinterpretation.***
3. Provide positive feedback or reward for acceptable behaviors. ***Positive reinforcement enhances self-esteem and encourages repetition of desirable behaviors.***
4. ***In an attempt to assist client to delay gratification,*** begin to increase the length of time requirement for acceptable behavior in order to achieve the reward. For example, 2 hours of acceptable behavior may be exchanged for a phone call; 4 hours of acceptable behavior for 2 hours of television; 1 day of acceptable behavior for a recreational therapy bowling activity; 5 days of acceptable behavior for a weekend pass.
5. A milieu unit provides the appropriate environment for the client with antisocial personality. ***The democratic approach, with specific rules and regulations, community meetings, and group therapy sessions, emulates the type of societal situation in which the client must learn to live. Feedback from peers is often more effective than confrontation from an authority figure. Client learns to follow the rules of the group as a positive step in the progression toward internalizing the rules of society.***
6. Help client gain insight into own behavior. Often, these individuals rationalize to such an extent that they deny that their behavior is inappropriate. (For example, "The owner of this store has so much money, he'll never miss the little bit I take. He has everything, and I have nothing. It's not fair! I deserve to have some of what he has.") ***Client must come to understand that certain behaviors will not be tolerated within the society and that severe consequences will be imposed on those individuals who refuse to comply. Client must want to become a productive member of society before he or she can be helped.***
7. Talk about past behaviors with client. Discuss which behaviors are acceptable by societal norms and which are not. Help client identify ways in which he or she has exploited others. Encourage client to explore how he or she would feel if the circumstances were reversed. ***An attempt may be made to enlighten client to the sensi-***

tivity of others by promoting self-awareness in an effort to help client gain insight into his or her own behavior.

8. Throughout relationship with client, maintain attitude of "It is not *you*, but your *behavior*, that is unacceptable." ***An attitude of acceptance promotes feelings of dignity and self-worth.***

Outcome Criteria

1. Client follows rules and regulations of the milieu environment.
2. Client is able to verbalize which of his or her behaviors are not acceptable.
3. Client shows regard for the rights of others by delaying gratification of own desires when appropriate.

DEFENSIVE COPING

Definition: *Repeated projection of falsely positive self-evaluation based on a self-protective pattern that defends against underlying perceived threats to positive self-regard.*

Possible Etiologies ("related to")

[Low self-esteem]
[Retarded ego development]
[Underdeveloped superego]
[Negative role models]
[Lack of positive feedback]
[Absent, erratic, or inconsistent methods of discipline]
[Dysfunctional family system]

Defining Characteristics ("evidenced by")

Denial of obvious problems or weaknesses
Projection of blame or responsibility
Rationalization of failures
Hypersensitivity to criticism
Grandiosity
Superior attitude toward others
Difficulty establishing or maintaining relationships
Hostile laughter at or ridicule of others
Difficulty in perception of reality
Lack of follow-through or participation in treatment or therapy

Goals/Objectives

Short-Term Goal

Client will verbalize personal responsibility for difficulties experienced in interpersonal relationships within (period reasonable for client).

Long-Term Goal

Client will demonstrate ability to interact with others without becoming defensive, rationalizing behaviors, or expressing grandiose ideas.

Interventions with *Selected Rationales*

1. Recognize and support basic ego strengths. ***Focusing on positive aspects of the personality may help to improve self-concept.***
2. Encourage client to recognize and verbalize feelings of inadequacy and need for acceptance from others and how these feelings provoke defensive behaviors, such as blaming others for own behaviors. ***Recognition of the problem is the first step in the change process toward resolution.***
3. Provide immediate, matter-of-fact, nonthreatening feedback for unacceptable behaviors. ***Client may lack knowledge about how he or she is being perceived by others. Providing this information in a nonthreatening manner may help to eliminate these undesirable behaviors.***
4. Help client identify situations that provoke defensiveness, and practice through role playing more appropriate responses. ***Role playing provides confidence to deal with difficult situations when they actually occur.***
5. Provide immediate positive feedback for acceptable behaviors. ***Positive feedback enhances self-esteem and encourages repetition of desirable behaviors.***
6. Help client set realistic, concrete goals, and determine appropriate actions to meet those goals. ***Success increases self-esteem.***
7. Evaluate with client the effectiveness of the new behaviors, and discuss any modifications for improvement. ***Because of limited problem-solving ability, assistance may be required to reassess and develop new strategies in the event that certain of the new coping methods prove ineffective.***

Outcome Criteria

1. Client verbalizes and accepts responsibility for own behavior.
2. Client verbalizes correlation between feelings of inadequacy and the need to defend the ego through rationalization and grandiosity.
3. Client does not ridicule or criticize others.
4. Client interacts with others in group situations without taking a defensive stance.

LOW SELF-ESTEEM

Definition: *Negative self-evaluation and feelings about self or self-capabilities.*

Possible Etiologies ("related to")

[Lack of positive feedback]
[Unmet dependency needs]
[Retarded ego development]
[Repeated negative feedback, resulting in diminished self-worth]
[Dysfunctional family system]
[Absent, erratic, or inconsistent parental discipline]
[Extreme poverty]
[History of childhood abuse]

Defining Characteristics ("evidenced by")

[Denial of problems obvious to others]
[Projection of blame or responsibility for problems]
[Grandiosity]
[Aggressive behavior]
[Frequent use of derogatory and critical remarks against others]
[Manipulation of one staff member against another in an attempt to gain special privileges]
[Inability to form close, personal relationships]

Goals/Objectives

Short-Term Goal

Client will verbalize an understanding that derogatory and critical remarks against others reflect feelings of self-contempt.

Long-Term Goal

Client will experience an increase in self-esteem, as evidenced by verbalizations of positive aspects of self and the lack of manipulative behaviors toward others.

Interventions with *Selected Rationales*

1. Ensure that goals are realistic. It is important for client to achieve something, so plan for activities in which success is likely. ***Success increases self-esteem.***
2. Identify ways in which client is manipulating others. Set limits on manipulative behavior. ***Because client is unable (or unwilling) to limit own maladaptive behaviors, assistance is required from staff.***
3. Explain consequences of manipulative behavior. All staff must be consistent and follow through with consequences in a matter-of-fact manner. ***From the onset, client must be aware of the outcomes his or her maladaptive behaviors will effect. Without consistency of follow-through from all staff, a positive outcome cannot be achieved.***
4. Encourage client to talk about his or her behavior, the limits, and consequences for violation of those limits. ***Discussion of feelings regarding these circumstances may help the client achieve some insight into his or her situation.***

5. Discuss how manipulative behavior interferes with formation of close, personal relationships. ***Client may be unaware of others' perception of him or her and of why these behaviors are not acceptable to others.***
6. Help client identify more adaptive interpersonal strategies. Provide positive feedback for nonmanipulative behaviors. ***Client may require assistance with solving problems. Positive reinforcement enhances self-esteem and encourages repetition of desirable behaviors.***
7. Encourage client to confront the fear of failure by attending therapy activities and undertaking new tasks. Offer recognition of successful endeavors.
8. Help client identify positive aspects of the self and develop ways to change the characteristics that are socially unacceptable. ***Individuals with low self-esteem often have difficulty recognizing their positive attributes. They may also lack problem-solving ability and require assistance to formulate a plan for implementing the desired changes.***
9. Minimize negative feedback to client. Enforce limit setting in a matter-of-fact manner, imposing previously established consequences for violations. ***Negative feedback can be extremely threatening to a person with low self-esteem, possibly aggravating the problem. Consequences should convey unacceptability of the behavior but not of the person.***
10. Encourage independence in the performance of personal responsibilities and in decision making related to own self-care. Offer recognition and praise for accomplishments. ***Positive reinforcement enhances self-esteem and encourages repetition of desirable behaviors.***
11. Help client increase level of self-awareness through critical examination of feelings, attitudes, and behaviors. Help client understand that it is perfectly acceptable for attitudes and behaviors to differ from those of others as long as they do not become intrusive. ***As client becomes more aware and accepting of himself or herself, the need for judging the behavior of others will diminish.***
12. Teach client assertiveness techniques, especially the ability to recognize the differences among passive, assertive, and aggressive behaviors and the importance of respecting the human rights of others while protecting one's own basic human rights. ***These techniques increase self-esteem while enhancing the ability to form satisfactory interpersonal relationships.***

Outcome Criteria

1. Client verbalizes positive aspects about self.
2. Client does not manipulate others in an attempt to increase feelings of self-worth.
3. Client considers the rights of others in interpersonal interactions.

IMPAIRED SOCIAL INTERACTION

Definition: *Insufficient or excessive quantity or ineffective quality of social exchange.*

Possible Etiologies ("related to")

[Low self-esteem]
[Unmet dependency needs]
[Retarded ego development]
[Retarded superego development]
[Negative role modeling]
Knowledge deficit about ways to enhance mutuality

Defining Characteristics ("evidenced by")

Verbalized or observed discomfort in social situations
Verbalized or observed inability to receive or communicate a satisfying sense of belonging, caring, interest, or shared history
Observed use of unsuccessful social interaction behaviors
Dysfunctional interaction with peers, family, or others
[Exploitation of others for the fulfillment of own desires]
[Inability to develop satisfactory, enduring, intimate relationship with a sexual partner]
[Physical and verbal hostility toward others when fulfillment of own desires is thwarted]

Goals/Objectives

Short-Term Goal

Client will develop satisfactory relationship (no evidence of manipulation or exploitation) with nurse or therapist within 1 week.

Long-Term Goal

Client will interact appropriately with others, demonstrating concern for the needs of others as well as for his or her own needs, by time of discharge from treatment.

Interventions with *Selected Rationales*

1. Develop therapeutic rapport with client. Establish trust by always being honest; keep all promises; convey acceptance of person, separate from unacceptable behaviors ("It is not *you*, but your *behavior*, that is unacceptable"). ***An attitude of acceptance promotes feelings of self-worth. Trust is the basis of a therapeutic relationship.***
2. Offer to remain with client during initial interactions with others in the unit. ***Presence of a trusted individual increases feelings of security during uncomfortable situations.***

3. Provide constructive criticism and positive reinforcement for efforts. ***Positive feedback enhances self-esteem and encourages repetition of desirable behaviors.***
4. Confront client as soon as possible when interactions with others are manipulative or exploitative. Establish consequences for unacceptable behavior, and always follow through. ***Because of the strong id influence on client's behavior, client should receive immediate feedback when behavior is unacceptable. Consistency in enforcing the consequences is essential if positive outcomes are to be achieved. Inconsistency creates confusion and encourages testing of limits.***
5. Act as a role model for client through appropriate interactions with him or her and with others. ***Role modeling is a powerful and effective form of learning.***
6. Provide group situations for client. ***It is through these group interactions, with positive and negative feedback from peers, that client will learn socially acceptable behavior.***

Outcome Criteria

1. Client willingly and appropriately participates in group activities.
2. Client has satisfactorily established and maintained one interpersonal relationship with nurse or therapist, without evidence of manipulation or exploitation.
3. Client demonstrates ability to interact appropriately with others, showing respect for self and others.
4. Client is able to verbalize reasons for inability to form close interpersonal relationships with others in the past.

DEFICIENT KNOWLEDGE (Self-Care Activities to Achieve and Maintain Optimal Wellness)

Definition: *Absence or deficiency of cognitive information related to a specific topic.*

Possible Etiologies ("related to")

Lack of interest in learning
[Low self-esteem]
[Denial of need for information]
[Denial of risks involved with maladaptive lifestyle]
Unfamiliarity with information sources

Defining Characteristics ("evidenced by")

[History of substance abuse]
[Statement of lack of knowledge]
[Statement of misconception]

[Request for information]
[Demonstrated lack of knowledge regarding basic health practices]
[Reported or observed inability to take the responsibility for meeting basic health practices in any or all functional pattern areas]
[History of lack of health-seeking behavior]
Inappropriate or exaggerated behaviors (e.g., hysterical, hostile, agitated, apathetic)

Goals/Objectives

Short-Term Goal

Client will verbalize understanding of knowledge required to fulfill basic health needs following implementation of teaching plan.

Long-Term Goal

Client will be able to demonstrate skills learned for fulfillment of basic health needs by time of discharge from therapy.

Interventions with *Selected Rationales*

1. Assess client's level of knowledge regarding positive self-care practices. ***An adequate database is necessary for the development of an effective teaching plan.***
2. Assess client's level of anxiety and readiness to learn. ***Learning does not occur beyond the moderate level of anxiety.***
3. Determine method of learning most appropriate for client (e.g., discussion, question and answer, use of audio or visual aids, oral, written). Be sure to consider level of education and development. ***Teaching will be ineffective if presented at a level or by a method inappropriate to the client's ability to learn.***
4. Develop teaching plan, including measurable objectives for the learner. Provide information regarding healthful strategies for activities of daily living as well as about harmful effects of substance abuse on the body. Include suggestions for community resources to assist client when adaptability is impaired.
5. Include significant others in the learning activity, if possible. ***Input from individuals who are directly involved in the potential change increases the likelihood of a positive outcome.***
6. Implement teaching plan at a time that facilitates, and in a place that is conducive to, optimal learning (e.g., in the evening when family members visit; in an empty, quiet classroom or group therapy room). ***Learning is enhanced by an environment with few distractions.***
7. Begin with simple concepts, and progress to the more complex. ***Retention is increased if introductory material is easy to understand.***
8. Provide activities for client and significant others in which to actively participate during the learning exercise. ***Active participation increases retention.***

9. Ask client and significant others to demonstrate knowledge gained by verbalizing information regarding positive self-care practices. ***Verbalization of knowledge gained is a measurable method of evaluating the teaching experience.***
10. Provide positive feedback for participation as well as for accurate demonstration of knowledge gained. ***Positive feedback enhances self-esteem and encourages repetition of desirable behaviors.***
11. Evaluate the teaching plan. Identify strengths and weaknesses and any changes that may enhance the effectiveness of the plan.

Outcome Criteria

1. Client is able to verbalize information regarding positive self-care practices.
2. Client is able to verbalize community resources for obtaining knowledge about and help with deficits related to health care.

■ INTERNET REFERENCES

Additional information about personality disorders may be located at the following websites:

- http://www.mentalhealth.com/dis/p20-pe04.html
- http://www.mentalhealth.com/dis/p20-pe08.html
- http://www.mentalhealth.com/dis/p20-pe05.html
- http://www.mentalhealth.com/dis/p20-pe09.html
- http://www.mentalhealth.com/dis/p20-pe06.html
- http://www.mentalhealth.com/dis/p20-pe07.html
- http://www.mentalhealth.com/dis/p20-pe10.html
- http://www.mentalhealth.com/dis/p20-pe01.html
- http://www.mentalhealth.com/dis/p20-pe02.html
- http://www.mentalhealth.com/dis/p20-pe03.html
- http://www.mentalhealth.com/p13.html#Per

UNIT THREE

SPECIAL TOPICS IN PSYCHIATRIC/MENTAL HEALTH NURSING

CHAPTER 16

Problems Related to Abuse or Neglect

BACKGROUND ASSESSMENT DATA

The *DSM-IV-TR* (APA, 2000) lists the following categories for this classification:

1. **V61.21 Physical Abuse of Child.** Physical injury to a child includes any *nonaccidental* physical injury caused by the parent or caretaker. The most obvious way to detect it is by outward physical signs. However, behavioral indicators may also be evident (Townsend, 2003).
2. **V61.21 Sexual Abuse of Child.** This category is defined as "employment, use, persuasion, inducement, enticement, or coercion of any child to engage in, or assist any other person to engage in, any sexually explicit conduct or any simulation of such conduct for the purpose of producing any visual depiction of such conduct; or the rape, and in cases of caretaker or inter-familial relationships, statutory rape, molestation, prostitution, or other form of sexual exploitation of children, or incest with children"

(National Clearinghouse on Child Abuse and Neglect [NCCAN], 2002). **Incest** is the occurrence of sexual contacts or interaction between, or sexual exploitation of, close relatives or between participants who are related to each other by a kinship bond that is regarded as a prohibition to sexual relations (e.g., caretakers, stepparents, stepsiblings) (Kaplan & Sadock, 1998).

3. **V61.21 Neglect of Child.** Physical neglect of a child includes refusal of or delay in seeking health care, abandonment, expulsion from the home or refusal to allow a runaway to return home, and inadequate supervision (NCCAN, 2002). Emotional neglect refers to a chronic failure by the parent or caretaker to provide the child with the hope, love, and support necessary for the development of a sound, healthy personality (Kansas Child Abuse Prevention Council, 1992).
4. **Physical Abuse of Adult:**
   •**V61.12** (if by partner)
   •**V62.83** (if by person other than partner)

Physical abuse of an adult may be defined as behavior used with the intent to cause harm and to establish power and control over another person. It may include slaps, punches, biting, hair-pulling, choking, kicking, stabbing, shooting, or forcible restraint.

5. **Sexual Abuse of Adult:**
   •**V61.12**(if by partner)
   •**V62.83**(if by person other than partner)

Sexual abuse of an adult may be defined as the expression of power and dominance by means of sexual violence, most commonly by men over women, although men may also be victims of sexual assault. Sexual assault is identified by the use of force and executed against the person's will.

Predisposing Factors (Contributing to Patterns of Abuse)

1. **Physiological**
   a. *Neurophysiological Influences.* Components of the neurological system in humans and animals have been implicated in the facilitation and inhibition of aggressive impulses. Areas of the brain that may be involved include the temporal lobe, the limbic system, and the amygdaloid nucleus (Tardiff, 1994).
   b. *Biochemical Influences.* Studies show that various neurotransmitters—in particular, norepinephrine, dopamine, and serotonin—may play a role in the facilitation and inhibition of aggressive impulses (Silver & Yudofsky, 1992).
   c. *Genetic Influences.* Some studies have implicated heredity as a component in the predisposition to aggressive behavior. Direct genetic links and the genetic karyotype XYY have been investigated as possibilities. Evidence remains inconclusive.
   d. *Disorders of the Brain.* Tumors, trauma, and certain diseases

(e.g., encephalitis and epilepsy) have been implicated in the predisposition to aggressive behavior (Silver & Yudofsky, 1992).

2. **Psychosocial**
   a. ***Psychodynamic Theory.*** The psychodynamic theorists imply that unmet needs for satisfaction and security result in an underdeveloped ego and a weak superego. It is thought that when frustration occurs, aggression and violence supply this individual with a dose of power and prestige that boosts the self-mage and validates a significance to his or her life that is lacking. The immature ego cannot prevent dominant id behaviors from occurring, and the weak superego is unable to produce feelings of guilt.
   b. ***Learning Theory.*** This theory postulates that aggressive and violent behaviors are learned from prestigious and influential role models. Individuals who were abused as children or whose parents disciplined with physical punishment are more likely to behave in a violent manner as adults (Tardiff, 1994).
   c. ***Societal Influences.*** Social scientists believe that aggressive behavior is primarily a product of one's culture and social structure. Societal influences may contribute to violence when individuals believe their needs and desires cannot be met through conventional means, and they resort to delinquent behaviors in an effort to obtain desired ends.

Symptomatology (Subjective and Objective Data)

1. Signs of physical abuse may include the following:
   a. Bruises over various areas of the body. Bruises may present with different colors of bluish-purple to yellowish-green (indicating various stages of healing).
   b. Bite marks, skin welts, burns.
   c. Fractures, scars, serious internal injuries, brain damage.
   d. Lacerations, abrasions, or unusual bleeding.
   e. Bald spots indicative of severe hair pulling.
   f. In a child, regressive behaviors (such as thumb sucking and enuresis) are common.
   g. Extreme anxiety and mistrust of others.
2. Signs of neglect of a child may include the following:
   a. Soiled clothing that does not fit and that may be inappropriate for the weather.
   b. Poor hygiene.
   c. Always hungry, with possible signs of malnutrition (e.g., emaciated with swollen belly).
   d. Listless and tired much of the time.
   e. Unattended medical problems.
   f. Social isolation; unsatisfactory peer relationships.
   g. Poor school performance and attendance record.

3. Signs of sexual abuse of a child include the following:
   a. Frequent urinary infections.
   b. Difficulty or pain in walking or sitting.
   c. Rashes or itching in the genital area; scratching the area a great deal or fidgeting when seated.
   d. Frequent vomiting.
   e. Seductive behavior, compulsive masturbation, precocious sex play.
   f. Excessive anxiety and mistrust of others.
   g. Sexually abusing another child.
4. Signs of sexual abuse of an adult include the following (Burgess, 1984):
   a. Contusions and abrasions in various parts of the body.
   b. Headaches, fatigue, sleep-pattern disturbances.
   c. Stomach pains, nausea, and vomiting.
   d. Vaginal discharge and itching, burning on urination, rectal bleeding and pain.
   e. Rage, humiliation, embarrassment, desire for revenge, self-blame.
   f. Fear of physical violence and death.
   g. Overwhelming sense of helplessness and personal violation.

Common Nursing Diagnoses and Interventions

(Interventions are applicable to various health-care settings, such as inpatient and partial hospitalization, community outpatient clinic, home health, and private practice.)

RAPE-TRAUMA SYNDROME

Definition: ***Sustained maladaptive response to a forced, violent sexual penetration against the victim's will and consent.***

Possible Etiologies ("related to")

[Having been the victim of sexual violence executed with the use of force and against one's personal will and consent]

Defining Characteristics ("evidenced by")

Disorganization
Change in relationships
Confusion
Physical trauma (e.g., bruising, tissue irritation)
Suicide attempts
Denial; guilt
Paranoia; humiliation, embarrassment

Aggression; muscle tension and/or spasms
Mood swings
Dependence
Powerlessness; helplessness
Nightmares and sleep disturbances
Sexual dysfunction
Revenge; phobias
Loss of self-esteem
Inability to make decisions
Substance abuse; depression
Anger; anxiety; agitation
Shame; shock; fear

Goals/Objectives

Short-Term Goal

The client's physical wounds will heal without complication.

Long-Term Goal

The client will begin a healthy grief resolution, initiating the process of psychological healing (time to be individually determined).

Interventions with *Selected Rationales*

1. Smith (1987a) relates the importance of communicating the following four phrases to the rape victim:
   a. I am very sorry this happened to you.
   b. You are safe here.
   c. I am very glad you are alive.
   d. You are not to blame. You are a victim. It was not your fault. Whatever decisions you made at the time of the victimization were the right ones because you are alive.

   The woman who has been sexually assaulted fears for her life and must be reassured of her safety. She may also be overwhelmed with self-doubt and self-blame, and these statements instill trust and validate self-worth.
2. Explain every assessment procedure that will be conducted and why. Ensure that data collection is conducted in a caring, nonjudgmental manner ***to decrease fear and anxiety and increase trust.***
3. Ensure that client has adequate privacy for all immediate postcrisis interventions. Try to have as few people as possible providing the immediate care or collecting immediate evidence. ***The post-trauma client is extremely vulnerable. Additional people in the environment increase this feeling of vulnerability and escalate anxiety.***
4. Encourage client to give an account of the assault. Listen, but do not probe. ***Nonjudgmental listening provides an avenue for catharsis that client needs to begin healing. A detailed account***

may be required for legal follow-up, and a caring nurse, as client advocate, may help to lessen the trauma of evidence collection.

5. Discuss with client whom to call for support or assistance. Provide information about referrals for aftercare. ***Because of severe anxiety and fear, client may need assistance from others during this immediate postcrisis period. Provide referral information in writing for later reference (e.g., psychotherapist, mental health clinic, community advocacy group).***

Outcome Criteria

1. Client is no longer experiencing panic anxiety.
2. Client demonstrates some trust in the primary nurse.
3. Client has received immediate attention to physical injuries.
4. Client has initiated behaviors consistent with the grief response.

POWERLESSNESS

Definition: *Perception that one's own action will not significantly affect an outcome; a perceived lack of control over a current situation or immediate happening.*

Possible Etiologies ("related to")

Lifestyle of helplessness
[Low self-esteem]
[Living with, or in a long-term relationship with, an individual who victimizes by inflicting physical pain or injury with the intent to cause harm and continues to do so over a long period of time]
[Lack of support network of caring others]
[Lack of financial independence]

Defining Characteristics ("evidenced by")

Verbal expressions of having no control or influence over situation or outcome
Reluctance to express true feelings
Passivity
[Verbalizations of abuse]
[Lacerations over areas of body]
[Fear for personal and children's safety]
[Verbalizations of no way to get out of relationship]

Goals/Objectives

Short-Term Goal

Client will recognize and verbalize choices that are available, thereby perceiving some control over life situation (time to be individually determined).

Long-Term Goal

Client will exhibit control over life situation by making decision about what to do regarding living with cycle of abuse (time to be individually determined).

Interventions with Selected Rationales

1. In collaboration with physician, ensure that all physical wounds, fractures, and burns receive immediate attention. Take photographs, if the victim will permit. ***Client safety is a nursing priority. Photographs may be called in as evidence if charges are filed.***
2. Take the woman to a private area to do the interview. ***If client is accompanied by the man who did the battering, she is not likely to be truthful about her injuries.***
3. If woman has come alone or with her children, assure her of her safety. Encourage her to discuss the battering incident. Ask questions about whether this has happened before; whether the abuser takes drugs; whether the woman has a safe place to go; and whether she is interested in pressing charges. ***Some women will attempt to keep secret how their injuries occurred in an effort to protect the partner or because they are fearful that the partner will kill them if they tell.***
4. Ensure that "rescue" efforts are not attempted by the nurse. Offer support, but remember that the final decision must be made by client. ***Making her own decision will give client a sense of control over her life situation. Imposing judgments and giving advice are nontherapeutic.***
5. Stress the importance of safety. Smith (1987b) suggests a statement such as, "Yes, it has happened. Now where do you want to go from here?" Burgess (1990) states, "The victim needs to be made aware of the variety of resources that are available to her. These may include crisis hotlines, community groups for women who have been abused, shelters, a variety of counseling opportunities (i.e., couples, individual, or group), and information regarding the victim's rights in the civil and criminal justice system." After a discussion of these available resources, the woman may choose for herself. If her decision is to return to the marriage and home, this choice, too, must be respected. ***Knowledge of available choices can serve to decrease the victim's sense of powerlessness, but true empowerment comes only when she chooses to use that knowledge for her own benefit.***

Outcome Criteria

1. Client has received immediate attention to physical injuries.
2. Client verbalizes assurance of her immediate safety.
3. Client discusses life situation with primary nurse.

4. Client is able to verbalize choices available to her from which she may receive assistance.

DELAYED GROWTH AND DEVELOPMENT

Definition: *Deviations from age-group norms.*

Possible Etiologies ("related to")

Inadequate caretaking
[The infliction by caretakers of physical or sexual abuse, usually occurring over an extended period of time]
[Ignoring the child's basic physiological needs]
[Indifference to the child]
[Ignoring the child's presence]
[Ignoring the child's social, educational, recreational, and developmental needs]

Defining Characteristics ("evidenced by")

Delay or difficulty in performing skills (motor, social, or expressive) typical of age group
Altered physical growth
Inability to perform self-care or self-control activities appropriate for age
Flat affect
Listlessness
Decreased responses
[Evidence of bruises, burns, lacerations, or other types of physical injury not consistent with performance of everyday activities]
[Expression of fear of parent or caretaker]
[Social isolation]
[Regressive behaviors (e.g., rocking, thumb sucking, enuresis)]
[Wearing clothing inappropriate to weather in order to cover up the injuries]
[Seductive behavior, precocious sex play, sexually abusing another child]

Goals/Objectives

Short-Term Goal

Client will develop trusting relationship with nurse and report how evident injuries were sustained (time to be individually determined).

Long-Term Goal

Client will demonstrate behaviors consistent with age-appropriate growth and development.

Interventions with *Selected Rationales*

1. Perform complete physical assessment of the child. Take particular note of bruises (in various stages of healing), lacerations, and client complaints of pain in specific areas. Do not overlook or discount the possibility of sexual abuse. Assess for nonverbal signs of abuse: aggressive conduct, excessive fears, extreme hyperactivity, apathy, withdrawal, age-inappropriate behaviors. ***An accurate and thorough physical assessment is required in order to provide appropriate care for client.***
2. Conduct an in-depth interview with the parent or adult who accompanies the child. Consider: If the injury is being reported as an accident, is the explanation reasonable? Is the injury consistent with the explanation? Is the injury consistent with the child's developmental capabilities? ***Fear of imprisonment or loss of child custody may place the abusive parent on the defensive. Discrepancies may be evident in the description of the incident, and lying to cover up involvement is a common defense that may be detectable in an in-depth interview.***
3. Use games or play therapy to gain child's trust. Use these techniques to assist in describing his or her side of the story. ***Establishing a trusting relationship with an abused child is extremely difficult. The child may not want to be touched. Play activities can provide a nonthreatening environment that may enhance the child's attempt to discuss these painful issues (Celano, 1990).***
4. Determine whether nature of the injuries warrants reporting to authorities. Specific state statutes must enter into the decision whether to report suspected child abuse. ***A report is commonly made if there is reason to suspect that a child has been injured as a result of physical, mental, emotional, or sexual abuse. "Reason to suspect" exists when there is evidence of a discrepancy or inconsistency in explaining a child's injury. Most states require that the following individuals report cases of suspected child abuse: all health-care workers, all mental health therapists, teachers, child-care providers, firefighters, emergency medical personnel, and law enforcement personnel. Reports are made to the Department of Health and Human Services or to a law enforcement agency.***

Outcome Criteria

1. Client has received immediate attention to physical injuries.
2. Client demonstrates trust in primary nurse by discussing abuse through the use of play therapy.
3. Client is demonstrating a decrease in regressive behaviors.

■ INTERNET REFERENCES

Additional information related to child abuse may be located at the following websites:

- http://www.calib.com/nccanch
- http://www.childabuse.org/
- http://www.fvpf.org
- http://www.child-abuse.com

Additional information related to sexual assault may be located at the following websites:

- http://www.vaw.umn.edu/Vawnet/mrape.htm
- http://www.ncweb.com/org/rapecrisis

Additional information related to domestic violence may be located at the following websites:

- http://www.ndvh.org/
- http://www.cpsdv.org/
- http://home.cybergrrl.com/dv/book/toc.html
- http://crisis-support.org/
- http://www.ama-assn.org/ama/pub/category/3242.html

CHAPTER 17

*Premenstrual Dysphoric Disorder**

BACKGROUND ASSESSMENT DATA

Defined

Premenstrual dysphoric disorder (PMDD)[†] is identified by a variety of physical and emotional symptoms that occur during the last week of the luteal phase of the menstrual cycle and that remit within a few days after the onset of the follicular phase. In most women, these symptoms occur in the week before, and remit within a few days after, the onset of menses. The disorder has also been reported in nonmenstruating women who have had a hysterectomy but who retain ovarian function. The diagnosis is given only when the symptoms are sufficiently severe to cause marked impairment in social or occupational functioning and have occurred during a majority of menstrual cycles in the past year (APA, 2000).

Predisposing Factors

1. **Physiological**
   a. ***Biochemical.*** An imbalance of the hormones estrogen and progesterone has been implicated in the predisposition to PMDD. It is postulated that excess estrogen or a high estrogen-to-progesterone ratio during the luteal phase causes water retention and that this hormonal imbalance has other effects as well, resulting in the symptoms associated with premenstrual syndrome (Kaplan & Sadock, 1998).

*Classification and criteria for all psychiatric diagnoses in this chapter are from the *Diagnostic and Statistical Manual of Mental Disorders, Fourth Edition, Text Revision, 2000 (DSM-IV-TR)*. Used with permission from the American Psychiatric Association.

†Text and criteria are provided in the *DSM-IV-TR* to facilitate systematic clinical research (APA, 2000).

b. ***Nutritional.*** A number of nutritional alterations have been implicated in the cause of PMDD. They include deficiencies in the B vitamins, calcium, magnesium, manganese, vitamin E, and linolenic acid (Frackiewicz & Shiovitz, 2001). Glucose tolerance fluctuations, abnormal fatty acid metabolism, and sensitivity to caffeine and alcohol may also play a role in bringing about the symptoms associated with this disorder.

Symptomatology (Subjective and Objective Data)

The American Psychiatric Association (2000) has identified the following symptoms as diagnostic for PMDD:

1. Markedly depressed mood, feelings of hopelessness, or self-deprecating thoughts
2. Marked anxiety, tension, feelings of being "keyed up" or "on edge"
3. Marked affective lability (e.g., feeling suddenly sad or tearful or increased sensitivity to rejection)
4. Persistent and marked anger or irritability or increased interpersonal conflicts
5. Decreased interest in usual activities (e.g., work, school, friends, hobbies)
6. Subjective sense of difficulty in concentrating
7. Lethargy, easy fatigability, or marked lack of energy
8. Marked change in appetite, overeating, or specific food cravings
9. Hypersomnia or insomnia
10. A subjective sense of being overwhelmed or out of control
11. Other physical symptoms, such as breast tenderness or swelling, headaches, joint or muscle pain, a sensation of "bloating," weight gain

Other subjective symptoms that have been reported include (Doenges, Townsend & Moorhouse, 1998):

12. Cramps
13. Alcohol intolerance
14. Acne
15. Cystitis
16. Oliguria
17. Altered sexual drive
18. Forgetfulness
19. Suicidal ideations or attempts

Common Nursing Diagnoses and Interventions

(Interventions are applicable to various health-care settings, such as inpatient and partial hospitalization, community outpatient clinic, home health, and private practice.)

ACUTE PAIN

Definition: *Sudden or slow onset of any intensity from mild to severe, with an anticipated or predictable end and a duration of less than 6 months*

Possible Etiologies ("related to")

[Imbalance in estrogen and progesterone levels]
[Possible nutritional alterations, including the following:
- Vitamin B deficiencies
- Glucose tolerance fluctuations
- Abnormal fatty acid metabolism, which may contribute to alteations in prostaglandin synthesis
- Magnesium deficiency
- Vitamin E deficiency
- Caffeine sensitivity
- Alcohol intolerance]

[Fluid retention]

Defining Characteristics ("evidenced by")

[Subjective communication of:
- Headache
- Backache
- Joint or muscle pain
- A sensation of "bloating"
- Abdominal cramping
- Breast tenderness and swelling]

Facial mask [of pain]
Sleep disturbance
Self-focus
Changes in appetite and eating

Goals/Objectives

Short-Term Goal

Client cooperates with efforts to manage symptoms of premenstrual syndrome (PMS) and minimize feelings of discomfort.

Long-Term Goal

Client verbalizes relief from discomfort associated with symptoms of PMS.

Interventions with *Selected Rationales*

1. Assess and record location, duration, and intensity of pain. ***Background assessment data are necessary to formulate an accurate plan of care for client.***

2. Provide nursing comfort measures with a matter-of-fact approach that does not give positive reinforcement to the pain behavior (e.g., backrub, warm bath, heating pad). Give additional attention at times when client is not focusing on physical symptoms. ***These measures may serve to provide some temporary relief from pain. Absence of secondary gains in the form of positive reinforcement may discourage client's use of the pain as attention-seeking behavior.***
3. Encourage client to get adequate rest and sleep, and avoid stressful activity during the premenstrual period. ***Fatigue exaggerates symptoms associated with PMS. Stress elicits heightened symptoms of anxiety, which may contribute to exacerbation of symptoms and altered perception of pain.***
4. Assist client with activities that distract from focus on self and pain. Demonstrate techniques such as visual or auditory distractions, guided imagery, breathing exercises, massage, application of heat or cold, and relaxation techniques that may provide symptomatic relief. ***These techniques may help to maintain anxiety at a manageable level and prevent the discomfort from becoming disabling.***
5. ***In an effort to correct the possible nutritional alterations that may be contributing to PMS,*** the following guidelines may be suggested (Doenges, Townsend & Moorhouse, 1998):
   a. Reduce intake of fats in the diet, particularly saturated fats.
   b. Limit intake of dairy products to two servings a day (excessive dairy products block the absorption of magnesium).
   c. Increase intake of complex carbohydrates (vegetables, legumes, cereals, and whole grains) and *cis*-linoleic acid–containing foods (e.g., safflower oil). Decrease refined and simple sugars. (Excess sugar is thought to cause nervous tension, palpitations, headache, dizziness, drowsiness, and excretion of magnesium in the urine.)
   e. Decrease salt intake to 3 g per day but not less than 0.5 g per day. (Salt restriction prevents edema; too little salt stimulates norepinephrine and causes sleep disturbances.)
   f. Limit intake of caffeine (coffee, tea, colas, and chocolate) and alcohol (one to two drinks a week). Caffeine increases breast tenderness and pain. Alcohol can cause reactive hypoglycemia and fluid retention.
   g. Because some women crave junk food during the premenstrual period, it is important that they take a multiple vitamin or mineral tablet daily to ensure that adequate nutrients are consumed.
6. Administer medications as prescribed. Monitor client response for effectiveness of the medication as well as for appearance of adverse side effects. ***When other measures are insufficient to bring***

about relief, physician may prescribe symptomatic drug therapy. Provide client with information about the medication to be administered. ***Client has the right to know about the treatment she is receiving.*** Some medications commonly used for symptomatic treatment of PMS are presented in Table 17–1. Some women have experienced relief from the symptoms of PMS and PMDD with herbal medications. Some of these medications are listed in Table 17–2.

Outcome Criteria

1. Client demonstrates ability to manage premenstrual symptoms with minimal discomfort.
2. Client verbalizes relief of painful symptoms.

TABLE 17–1 **Medications for Symptomatic Relief of PMS**

Medication	*Indication*
Fluoxetine (Sarafem), sertraline (Zoloft)	These medications have been approved by the FDA for treatment of PMS/PMDD. (All of the selective serotonin reuptake inhibitors have been used with positive results.)
Hydrochlorothiazide (Esidrix, HydroDiuril), furosemide (Lasix)	Diuretics may provide relief from edema when diet and sodium restriction are not sufficient.
Ibuprofen (Advil, Motrin, Nuprin), naproxen (Naprosyn)	Nonsteroidal anti-inflammatory agents may provide relief from joint, muscle, and lower abdominal pain related to increased prostaglandins.
Propranolol (Inderal), verapamil (Isoptin)	β-Blockers and calcium channel blockers are often given for prophylactic treatment of migraine headaches.
Sumatriptan (Imitrex), naratriptan (Amerge), rizatriptan (Maxalt), zolmitriptan (Zomig), frovatriptan (Frova), almotriptan (Axert)	These serotonin 5-HT_1 receptor agonists are highly effective in the treatment of acute migraine attack.
Bromocriptine (Parlodel)	This drug may be prescribed to relieve breast pain and other symptoms of PMS that may be caused by elevated prolactin.

TABLE 17–2 **Herbals Used for Symptoms of PMS**

Herbal	***Precautions/ Adverse Effects***	***Contraindications***
Black cohosh (*Cimicifuga racemosa*)	May potentiate the effects of antihypertensive medications. Some individuals may experience nausea or headache.	Pregnancy
Bugleweed (*Lycopus virginicus*)	No side effects known. Should not be taken concomitantly with thyroid preparations.	Thyroid disease
Chaste tree (*Vitex agnus castus*)	Occasional rashes may occur. Should not be taken concomitantly with dopamine-receptor antagonists.	Pregnancy and lactation
Evening primrose (*Oenothera biennis*)	May lower the seizure threshold. Should not be taken concomitantly with other drugs that lower the seizure threshold.	
Potentilla (*Potentilla anserina*)	May cause stomach irritation.	
Shepherd's purse (*Capsella bursa pastoris*)	No side effects known.	Pregnancy
Valerian (*Valeriana officinalis*)	With long-term use: headache, restless states, sleeplessness, mydriasis, disorders of cardiac function. Should not be taken concomitantly with CNS depressants.	Pregnancy and lactation

Source: PDR for Herbal Medicines, 2nd ed., 2000.

INEFFECTIVE COPING

Definition: *Inability to form a valid appraisal of the stressors, inadequate choices of practiced responses, and/or inability to use available resources.*

Possible Etiologies ("related to")

[Imbalance in estrogen and progesterone levels]
[Possible nutritional alterations, including the following:
Vitamin B deficiencies
Glucose tolerance fluctuations

Abnormal fatty acid metabolism, which may contribute to alterations in prostaglandin synthesis
Magnesium deficiency
Vitamin E deficiency
Caffeine sensitivity
Alcohol intolerance]

Defining Characteristics ("evidenced by")

[Affective liability (sad one minute, angry the next)]
[Marked anger or irritability]
[Feelings of elevated anxiety, tension, being "keyed up" or "on edge"]
[Depressed mood, feelings of hopelessness, or self-deprecating thoughts]
[Decreased interest in usual activities]
[Easy fatigability or marked lack of energy]
[Difficulty concentrating; forgetfulness]
[Changes in appetite]
[Hypersomnia or insomnia]
[Altered sexual drive]
[Suicidal ideations or attempts]
Inability to problem-solve
Inability to meet role expectations

Goals/Objectives

Short-Term Goals

1. Client will seek out support person if thoughts of suicide emerge.
2. Client will verbalize ways to express anger in an appropriate manner and maintain anxiety at a manageable level.

Long-Term Goals

1. Client will not harm self while experiencing symptoms associated with PMS.
2. Client will demonstrate adaptive coping strategies to use in an effort to minimize disabling behaviors during the premenstrual and perimenstrual periods.

Interventions with *Selected Rationales*

1. Assess client's potential for suicide. Has she expressed feelings of not wanting to live? Does she have a plan? A means? ***Depression is the most prevalent disorder that precedes suicide. The risk of suicide is greatly increased if client has developed a plan and particularly if means exist for client to execute the plan.***
2. Formulate a short-term verbal contract with client that she will not harm herself during specific period of time. When that contract expires, make another, and so forth. ***Discussion of suicidal feelings with a trusted individual provides some relief to client. A contract gets the subject out in the open and places some of the***

responsibility for client's safety with client. An attitude of acceptance of client as a worthwhile individual is conveyed.

3. Secure a promise from client that she will seek out a staff member if thoughts of suicide emerge. ***Suicidal clients are often very ambivalent about their feelings. Discussion of feelings with a trusted individual may provide assistance before client experiences a crisis situation.***
4. Encourage client to express angry feelings within appropriate limits. Provide safe method of hostility release. Help client identify source of anger, if possible. Work on adaptive coping skills for use outside the health-care system. ***Depression and suicidal behaviors are sometimes viewed as anger turned inward on the self. If this anger can be verbalized in a nonthreatening environment, client may be able to resolve these feelings, regardless of the discomfort involved.***
5. Encourage client to discharge pent-up anger through participation in large-motor activities (e.g., brisk walks, jogging, physical exercises, volleyball, punching bag, exercise bike). ***Physical exercise provides a safe and effective method for discharging pent-up tension.***
6. Help client identify stressors that precipitate anxiety and irritability and develop new methods of coping with these situations (e.g., stress reduction techniques, relaxation, and visualization skills). ***Knowing stress factors and ways of handling them reduces anxiety and allows client to feel a greater measure of control over the situation.***
7. Identify extent of feelings and situations when loss of control occurs. Assist with problem solving to identify behaviors for protection of self and others (e.g., call support person, remove self from situation). ***Recognition of potential for harm to self or others and development of a plan enable client to take effective actions to meet safety needs.***
8. Encourage client to reduce or shift workload and social activities during the premenstrual period as part of a total stress management program. ***Stress may play a role in the exacerbation of stress.***
9. At each visit, evaluate symptoms, discuss those that may be most troublesome, and continue to persist well after initiation of therapy. ***If traditional measures are inadequate, pharmacological intervention may be required to enhance coping abilities. For example, antidepressants may be administered for depression that remains unresolved after other symptoms have been relieved.***
10. Encourage participation in support group, psychotherapy, marital counseling, or other type of therapy as deemed necessary. ***Professional assistance may be required to help client and fam-***

ily members learn effective coping strategies and support lifestyle changes that may be needed.

Outcome Criteria

1. Client participates willingly in treatment regimen and initiates necessary lifestyle changes.
2. Client demonstrates adaptive coping strategies to deal with episodes of depression and anxiety.
3. Client verbalizes that she has no suicidal thoughts or intentions.

■ INTERNET REFERENCES

- http://www.aafp.org/afp/980700ap/daughert.html
- http://www.pmsinst.com
- http://www.obgyn.net/women/articles/coffee_talk/ct007.htm
- http://www.usdoctor.com/pms.htm

CHAPTER 18

HIV Disease

BACKGROUND ASSESSMENT DATA

The Immune Response to HIV

The cells responsible for nonspecific immune reactions include neutrophils, monocytes, and macrophages. In the normal immune response, they work to destroy an invasive organism and initiate and facilitate repair to damaged tissue. If these cells are not effective in accomplishing a satisfactory healing response, specific immune mechanisms take over.

The elements of the cellular response include the T4 lymphocytes (also called helper T cells). When the body is invaded by a foreign antigen, these T4 cells divide many times, producing antigen-specific T4 cells with other functions. One of these is the T4 killer cell, which helps to destroy the antigen.

The most conspicuous immunologic abnormality associated with HIV infection is a striking depletion of T4 lymphocytes. The HIV infects the T4 lymphocyte, thereby destroying the cell the body needs to direct an attack on the virus. An individual with a healthy immune system may present with a T4 count between 600 and 1200 mm^3.

Stages and Symptoms of HIV Disease

1. **Early Stage (T4 Cells 1000–500 mm^3)**
   a. ***Acute HIV Infection.*** The acute HIV infection is identified by a characteristic syndrome of symptoms that occurs from 6 days to 6 weeks after exposure to the virus. The symptoms have an abrupt onset, are somewhat vague, and are similar to those sometimes seen in mononucleosis. Symptoms of acute HIV infection include fever, myalgia, malaise, lymphadenopathy, sore throat, anorexia, nausea and vomiting, headaches, skin rash, and diarrhea. Most symptoms resolve in 1 to 3 weeks, with the exception of fever, myalgia, lymphadenopathy, and malaise, which may continue for several months.
   b. ***Seroconversion.*** Seroconversion, the detectability of HIV antibodies in the blood, is most often detected between 6 and 12 weeks. More than 95 percent of people test positive for

HIV by 3 months after infection, and more than 99 percent test positive by 6 months (Bartlett & Finkbeiner, 1996). The time between infection and seroconversion is called the *window period.*

   c. ***Asymptomatic Infection.*** During this stage, there are no manifestations of illness. Blood tests may reveal immunologic and hematologic abnormalities, such as leukopenia, anemia, or thrombocytopenia. This period may last 5 to 10 years or longer. The progression of the illness is faster in infants and children than in adults.

2. **Middle Stage (T4 Cells 500–200 mm^3)**
   a. ***Persistent Generalized Lymphadenopathy.*** Lymph nodes in at least two different locations in the body (usually the neck, armpit, and groin) swell and remain swollen for months, with no other signs of a related infectious disease.
   b. ***Systemic Complaints.*** Fever, night sweats, chronic diarrhea, fatigue, minor oral infections, headaches, weight loss.
3. **Late Stage (T4 Cells ≤200 mm^3)**
   a. ***HIV Wasting Syndrome.*** Severe weight loss, large-volume diarrhea, fever, and weakness.
   b. ***Opportunistic Infections.*** Opportunistic infections are those that occur because of the altered immune state of the host. These infections, which are protozoan, fungal, viral, and bacterial, have long been a defining characteristic of AIDS. The most common, life-threatening opportunistic infection seen in clients with AIDS is *pneumocystis* pneumonia.
   c. ***AIDS-Related Malignancies.*** HIV-positive individuals are at risk for developing certain types of malignancies. These include Kaposi's sarcoma, non-Hodgkin's lymphoma, Hodgkin's disease, malignant melanoma, testicular cancers, primary hepatocellular carcinoma, and invasive cervical cancer.
   d. ***Altered Mental States.*** The most common alterations in mental states observed in AIDS clients include delirium (fluctuating consciousness, abnormal vital signs, and psychotic phenomena) and dementia (called HIV-associated dementia [HAD]. Symptoms of HAD include cognitive, motor, and behavioral changes similar to those in individuals with other cognitive disorders [see Chapter 3]). NOTE: Depression is common in HIV disease and can occur at any time during the disease process.

Predisposing Factors

1. **Sexual Transmission**
   a. ***Heterosexual Transmission.*** Because the virus is found in greater concentration in semen than in vaginal secretions, it is more readily transmitted from men to women than from

women to men. However, female-to-male transmission is possible, as HIV has been isolated in vaginal secretions.

b. ***Homosexual Transmission.*** The most significant risk factors for homosexual transmission of HIV are receptive anal intercourse and the number of male sexual partners. The lining of the anal canal is delicate and prone to tearing and bleeding, making anal intercourse an easy way for infections to be passed from one person to another.

2. **Bloodborne Transmission**
   a. ***Transfusion with Blood Products.*** Although laboratory tests are more than 99 percent sensitive, screening problems may occur when donations are received from individuals recently infected with HIV who have not yet developed antibodies or from persistently antibody-negative donors who are infected with HIV.
   b. ***Transmission by Needles Infected with HIV.*** The highest number of this type of infection comes from intravenous drug users who share needles and other equipment contaminated with HIV-infected blood. Other bloodborne modes of transmission of HIV are by health-care workers who experience accidental needle sticks with contaminated needles and who may become infected from other contaminated equipment used for therapeutic purposes.
3. **Perinatal Transmission**
   a. Modes of transmission include transplacental, exposure to maternal blood and vaginal secretions during delivery, and breast milk. The risk of perinatal transmission has been significantly reduced in recent years with the advent of free or low-cost prenatal care, provision of access to anti-HIV medication during pregnancy, and education about the dangers of breast-feeding.
4. **Other Possible Modes of Transmission**
   a. To date, HIV has been isolated from blood, semen, vaginal secretions, saliva, tears, breast milk, cerebrospinal fluid, and amniotic fluid. However, only blood, semen, vaginal secretions, and breast milk have been epidemiologically linked to transmission of the virus.

Common Nursing Diagnoses and Interventions*

(Interventions are applicable to various health-care settings, such as inpatient and partial hospitalization, community outpatient clinic, home health, and private practice.)

---

*The interventions for this care plan have been adapted from "Nursing Care Plan for the AIDS Patient," written by the nursing staff of Hospice, Inc., Wichita, KS.

INEFFECTIVE PROTECTION

Definition: *Decrease in the ability to guard self from internal or external threats such as illness or injury.*

Possible Etiologies ("related to")

[Compromised immune status secondary to diagnosis of HIV disease]

Defining Characteristics ("evidenced by")

[Laboratory values indicating decreased numbers of T4 cells]
[Presence of opportunistic infections]
[Manifestations of:
Fever, night sweats, diarrhea
Anorexia, weight loss
Fatigue, malaise
Swollen lymph glands
Cough, dyspnea
Rash, skin lesions, white patches in mouth
Headache
Ataxia
Bleeding, bruising
Neurological defects]

Goals/Objectives

Short-Term Goal

Client will exhibit no new signs or symptoms of infection.

Long-Term Goal

Client safety and comfort will be maximized.

Interventions with *Selected Rationales*

1. ***To prevent infection in an immunocompromised individual:***
   a. Implement universal blood and body fluid precautions.
   b. Wash hands with antibacterial soap before entering and after leaving client's room.
   c. Monitor vital signs at regular intervals.
   d. Monitor complete blood counts (CBCs) for leukopenia/neutropenia.
   e. Monitor for signs and symptoms of specific opportunistic infections.
   f. Protect client from individuals with infections.
   g. Maintain meticulous sterile technique for dressing changes and any invasive procedure.
   h. Administer antibiotics as ordered.

2. ***To restore nutritional status and decrease nausea, vomiting, and diarrhea:***
   a. Provide low-residue, high-protein, high-calorie, soft, bland diet. Maintain hydration with adequate fluid intake.
   b. Obtain daily weight, and record intake and output.
   c. Monitor serum electrolytes and CBCs.
   d. If client is unable to eat, provide isotonic tube feedings as tolerated. Check for gastric residual frequently.
   e. If client is unable to tolerate oral intake or tube feedings, consult physician regarding possibility of parenteral hyperalimentation. Observe hyperalimentation administration site for signs of infection.
   f. Administer antidiarrheals and antiemetics as ordered.
   g. Perform frequent oral care. Promote prevention and healing of lesions in the mouth.
   h. Have client eat small, frequent meals with high-calorie snacks rather than three large meals per day.
3. ***To promote improvement of skin and mucous membrane integrity:***
   a. Monitor skin condition for signs of redness and breakdown.
   b. Reposition client every 1 to 2 hours.
   c. Encourage ambulation and chair activity as tolerated.
   d. Use "egg crate" mattress or air mattress on bed.
   e. Wash skin daily with soap, and rinse well with water.
   f. Apply lotion to skin to maintain skin softness.
   g. Provide wound care as ordered for existing pressure sores or lesions.
   h. Cleanse skin exposed to diarrhea thoroughly, and protect rectal area with ointment.
   i. Apply artificial tears to eyes as appropriate.
   j. Perform frequent oral care; apply ointment to lips.
4. ***To maximize oxygen consumption and minimize respiratory distress:***
   a. Assess respiratory status frequently:
      - Monitor depth, rate, and rhythm of respirations.
      - Auscultate lung fields every 2 hours and as needed.
      - Monitor arterial blood gases.
      - Check color of skin, nail beds, and sclerae.
      - Assess sputum for color, odor, and viscosity.
   b. Encourage coughing and deep-breathing exercises.
   c. Provide humidified oxygen as ordered.
   d. Suction as needed, using sterile technique.
   e. Time nursing care to allow client adequate rest between procedures.
   f. Administer analgesics or sedatives judiciously to prevent respiratory depression.
   g. Administer bronchodilators and antibiotics as ordered.

5. ***To minimize the potential for easy bleeding caused by HIV-induced thrombocytopenia:***
   a. Follow protocol for maintenance of skin integrity.
   b. Provide safe environment to minimize falling or bumping into objects.
   c. Provide soft toothbrush or "toothette" swabs for cleaning teeth and gums.
   d. Ensure that client does not take aspirin or other medications that increase the potential for bleeding.
   e. Clean areas contaminated by client's blood with household bleach (5.25% sodium hypochlorite) diluted 1:10 with water (Bartlett & Finkbeiner, 1996).
6. ***To maintain near-normal body temperature:***
   a. Provide frequent tepid-water sponge baths.
   b. Provide antipyretic as ordered by physician (avoid aspirin).
   c. Place client in cool room, with minimal clothing and bed covers.
   d. Encourage intake of cool liquids (if not contraindicated).

Outcome Criteria

1. Client does not experience respiratory distress.
2. Client maintains optimal nutrition and hydration.
3. Client has experienced no further weight loss.
4. Client maintains integrity of skin and mucous membranes.
5. Client shows no new signs or symptoms of infection.

INTERRUPTED FAMILY PROCESSES

Definition: *Change in family relationships and/or functioning.*

Possible Etiologies ("related to")

[Crisis associated with having a family member diagnosed with HIV disease]

Defining Characteristics ("evidenced by")

Changes in availability for affective responsiveness and intimacy
Changes in participation in problem solving and decision making
Changes in communication patterns
Changes in availability for emotional support
Changes in satisfaction with family
Changes in expressions of conflict within family

Goals/Objectives

Short-Term Goal

Family members will express feelings regarding loved one's diagnosis and prognosis.

Long-Term Goal

Family will verbalize areas of dysfunction and demonstrate ability to cope more effectively.

Interventions with *Selected Rationales*

1. Create an environment that is comfortable, supportive, private, and trusting. ***Basic needs of the family must be met before crisis resolution can be attempted.***
2. Encourage each member to express feelings regarding loved one's diagnosis and prognosis. ***Every individual is unique and must feel that his or her private needs can be met within the family constellation.***
3. If client is homosexual, and this is the family's first awareness, help family members deal with guilt and shame they may experience. Help parents understand they are not responsible, and their child is still the same individual they have always loved. ***Resolving guilt and shame enables family members to respond adaptively to the crisis. Their response can affect the client's remaining future and the family's future.***
4. Serve as facilitator between client's family and homosexual partner. The family may have difficulty accepting the partner as a person who is as significant as a spouse. Clarify roles and responsibilities of family and partner. Do this by bringing both parties together to define and distribute the tasks involved in the client's care. ***By minimizing the lack of legally defined roles and by focusing on the need for making realistic decisions about client's care, communication and resolution of conflict are enhanced.***
5. Encourage use of stress management techniques (e.g., relaxation exercises, guided imagery, attendance at support group meetings for significant others of AIDS clients). ***Reduction of stress and support from others who share similar experiences enable individuals to begin to think more clearly and develop new behaviors to cope with this situational crisis.***
6. Provide educational information about AIDS and opportunities to ask questions and express concerns. ***Many misconceptions about the disease abound within the public domain. Clarification may calm some of the family's fears and facilitate interaction with client.***
7. Make family referrals to community organizations that provide supportive help or financial assistance to AIDS clients. ***Extended care can place a financial burden on client and family members. Respite care may provide family members with occasional much-needed relief from the stress of physical and emotional caregiving responsibilities.***

Outcome Criteria

1. Family members are able to discuss feelings regarding client's diagnosis and prognosis.

2. Family members are able to make rational decisions regarding care of their loved one and the effect on family functioning.

DEFICIENT KNOWLEDGE (PREVENTION OF TRANSMISSION AND PROTECTION OF THE CLIENT)

Definition: *Absence or deficiency of cognitive information related to a specific topic.*

Possible Etiologies ("related to")

Cognitive limitation
Information misinterpretation
Lack of exposure [to accurate information]

Defining Characteristics ("evidenced by")

Verbalization of the problem
Inappropriate or exaggerated behaviors
Inaccurate follow-through of instruction
[Inaccurate statements by client and family]

Goals/Objectives

Short-Term Goal

Client and family verbalize understanding about disease process, modes of transmission, and prevention of infection.

Long-Term Goals

1. Client and family demonstrate ability to execute precautions for preventing transmission of HIV and infection of the client.
2. Transmission of HIV and infection of the client are prevented.

Interventions with *Selected Rationales*

1. Present the following information ***in an effort to clarify misconceptions, calm fears, and support an environment of appropriate interventions for care of the client with AIDS.*** Teach that HIV cannot be contracted from:
   a. Casual or household contact with an individual with HIV infection.
   b. Shaking hands, hugging, social (dry) kissing, holding hands, or other nonsexual physical contact.
   c. Touching unsoiled linens or clothing, money, furniture, or other inanimate objects.
   d. Being near someone with HIV infection at work, school, or restaurants or in elevators.
   e. Toilet seats, bathtubs, towels, showers, or swimming pools.

   f. Dishes, silverware, or food handled by a person with HIV infection.
   g. Animals (pets may transmit opportunistic organisms).
   h. (Very unlikely spread by) coughing, sneezing, spitting, kissing, tears, or saliva.
2. HIV dies quickly outside the body because it requires living tissue to survive. It is readily killed by soap, cleansers, hot water, and disinfectants.
3. Teach client to protect self from infections by taking the following precautions:
   a. Avoid unpasteurized milk or milk products.
   b. Cook all raw vegetables and fruits before eating. ***Raw or improperly washed foods may transmit microbes.***
   c. Cook all meals well before eating.
   d. Avoid direct contact with persons with known contagious illnesses.
   e. Consult physician before getting a pet. ***Pets require extra infection control precautions because of the opportunistic organisms carried by animals.***
   f. Avoid touching animal feces, urine, emesis, litter boxes, aquariums, or bird cages.
   g. Always wear mask and gloves when cleaning up after a pet.
   h. Avoid traveling in countries with poor sanitation.
   i. Avoid vaccines or vaccinations that contain live organisms. ***Vaccination with live organisms may be fatal to severely immunosuppressed persons.***
   j. Exercise regularly.
   k. Control stress factors. A counselor or support group may be helpful.
   l. Stop smoking. ***Smoking predisposes to respiratory infections.***
   m. Maintain good personal hygiene.
4. Teach client/significant others about prevention of transmission:
   a. Do not donate blood, plasma, body organs, tissues, or semen.
   b. Inform physician, dentist, and anyone providing care that you have HIV infection.
   c. Do not share needles or syringes.
   d. Do not share personal items such as toothbrushes, razors, or other implements that may be contaminated with blood or body fluids.
   e. Do not eat or drink from the same dinnerware and utensils without washing them between use.
   f. Avoid becoming pregnant if at risk for HIV infection.
   g. Engage in only "safer" sexual practices (those ***not*** involving exchange of body fluids).
   h. Avoid sexual practices medically classified as "unsafe," such as anal or vaginal intercourse and oral sex.

i. Avoid the use of recreational drugs because of their immunosuppressive effects.

5. Teach the home caregiver(s) to protect self from HIV infection by taking the following precautions:
   a. Wash hands thoroughly with liquid antibiotic soap before and after each client contact. Use moisturizing lotion afterward to prevent dry, cracking skin.
   b. Wear gloves when in contact with blood or body fluids (e.g., open wounds, suctioning, and feces). Gown or aprons may be worn if soiling is likely.
   c. Wear a mask:
      - When client has a productive cough and tuberculosis has not been ruled out.
      - To protect client if caregiver has a cold.
      - During suctioning.
   d. Bag disposable gloves and masks with client's trash.
   e. Dispose of the following in the toilet:
      - Organic material on clothes or linen before laundering.
      - Blood or body fluids.
      - Soiled tissue or toilet paper.
      - Cleaners or disinfectants used to clean contaminated articles.
      - Solutions contaminated with blood or body fluids.
   f. Double-bag client's trash and soiled dressings in an impenetrable plastic bag. *Tie* the bag shut, and discard it with household trash.
   g. Do not recap needles, syringes, and other sharp items. Use puncture-proof covered containers for disposal (e.g., coffee cans and jars are appropriate for home use).
   h. Place soiled linen and clothing in a plastic bag and tie shut until washed. Launder these separately from other laundry. Use bleach or other disinfectant in hot water.
   i. When house-cleaning, all equipment used in care of the client as well as bathroom and kitchen surfaces should be cleaned with a 1:10 dilute bleach solution.
   j. Mops, sponges, and other items used for cleaning should be reserved specifically for that purpose.

Outcome Criteria

1. Client, family, and significant other(s) are able to verbalize information presented regarding ways in which HIV can and cannot be transmitted, ways to protect client from infections, and ways to prevent transmission to caregivers and others.
2. Transmission to others and infection of the client have been avoided.

INTERNET REFERENCES

Additional information about HIV/AIDS may be located at the following websites:

- http://www.avert.org/
- http://www.kc-reach.org/
- http:/www.infoweb.org/
- http://www.aegis.com/main/
- http://www.aidsnews/
- http://www.critpath.org/
- http://www.HIVpositive.com/index.html
- http://www.guides4living.com/links.html
- http://research.med.umkc.edu/teams/cml/AIDS.html
- http://www.cdc.gov/hiv

CHAPTER 19

Homelessness

BACKGROUND ASSESSMENT DATA

It is difficult to determine how many individuals are homeless in the United States. Estimates have been made at somewhere between 250,000 and 4 million.

Who Are the Homeless?

1. **Age.** Studies have produced a variety of statistics related to age of the homeless: 25% are younger than 18 years of age; 51 percent are between 31 and 50 years, and an estimated 2.5 to 19.4 percent are 55 to 60 years.
2. **Gender.** More men than women are homeless. The U.S. Conference of Mayors (2001) study found that single men comprised 45 percent of the urban homeless population and single women 14 percent.
3. **Families.** Families with children are among the fastest growing segments of the homeless population. Families comprise 40 percent of the urban homeless population, but research indicates that this number is likely higher in rural areas, where families, single mothers, and children make up the largest group of homeless people.
4. **Ethnicity.** The study by the U.S. Conference of Mayors found that the homeless population was 50 percent African-American, 35 percent Caucasian, 12 percent Hispanic, 2 percent Native American, and 1 percent Asian. The ethnic makeup of homeless populations varies according to geographic location.

Mental Illness and Homelessness

It is thought that approximately 22 percent of the homeless population suffers from some form of mental illness (U.S. Conference of Mayors, 2001). Schizophrenia is frequently described as the most common diagnosis. Other prevalent disorders include bipolar affective disorder, substance abuse and dependence, depression, personality disorders, and organic mental disorders.

Predisposing Factors to Homelessness Among Mentally Ill People

1. **Deinstitutionalization.** Deinstitutionalization is frequently implicated as a contributing factor to homelessness among persons with mental illness. Deinstitutionalization began out of expressed concern by mental health professionals and others who described the "deplorable conditions" in which mentally ill individuals were housed. Some believed that institutionalization deprived mentally ill people of their civil rights. Not the least of the motivating factors for deinstitutionalization was the financial burden these clients placed on state governments.
2. **Poverty.** Cuts in government entitlement programs have depleted the allotments available for chronically mentally ill individuals living in the community. The job market is prohibitive for individuals whose behavior is incomprehensible or even frightening to many. The stigma and discrimination associated with mental illness may be diminishing slowly, but they are still highly evident to those who suffer from mental illness.
3. **A Scarcity of Affordable Housing.** Wallsten (1992) states:

> Economic policies and issues have contributed to the growing numbers and different profiles of the homeless. Urban redevelopment projects eliminated a considerable amount of low-cost housing options for poor people. A growing number of impoverished families have been doubling and tripling up in single housing units as affordable housing becomes more scarce. A sizable proportion of residents in these renewal areas were poor elderly renting rooms in houses, residential hotels, and missions. (p. 21)

In addition, the number of single-room-occupancy (SRO) hotels has diminished drastically. These SRO hotels provided a means of relatively inexpensive housing for chronic psychiatric clients. Although some people believe that these facilities nurtured isolation, they provided adequate shelter from the elements for their occupants. So many individuals currently frequent the shelters of our cities that there is concern that the shelters are becoming mini-institutions for the chronically mentally ill.

4. **Lack of Affordable Health Care.** For families barely able to scrape together enough money to pay for day-to-day living, a catastrophic illness can create the level of poverty that starts the downward spiral to homelessness.
5. **Domestic Violence.** A study by the U.S. Conference of Mayors (1998) revealed that 46 percent of cities surveyed identified domestic violence as a primary cause of homelessness. Battered women are often forced to choose between an abusive relationship and homelessness.
6. **Addiction Disorders.** For individuals with alcohol or drug addictions, in the absence of appropriate treatment the chances increase for being forced into life on the street. The following have been

cited as obstacles to addiction treatment for homeless persons: lack of health insurance, lack of documentation, waiting lists, scheduling difficulties, daily contact requirements, lack of transportation, ineffective treatment methods, lack of supportive services, and cultural insensitivity.

Symptomatology (Commonly Associated with Homelessness)

1. Mobility and migration (the penchant for frequent movement to various geographic locations).
2. Substance abuse
3. Nutritional deficiencies
4. Difficulty with thermoregulation
5. Increased incidence of tuberculosis
6. Increased incidence of sexually transmitted diseases
7. Increased incidence of gastrointestinal (GI) and respiratory disorders
8. Among homeless children (compared with control samples), increased incidence of:
   a. Ear disorders
   b. GI disorders
   c. Infestational ailments
   d. Developmental delays
   e. Psychological problems

Common Nursing Diagnoses and Interventions

(Interventions are applicable to various health-care settings, such as inpatient and partial hospitalization, community health clinic, "street clinic," and homeless shelters.)

INEFFECTIVE HEALTH MAINTENANCE

Definition: ***Inability to identify, manage, and/or seek out help to maintain health.***

Possible Etiologies ("related to")

Perceptual/cognitive impairment
Lack of, or significant alteration in, communication skills
Unachieved developmental tasks
Lack of material resources
Lack of ability to make deliberate and thoughtful judgments
Ineffective individual coping

Defining Characteristics ("evidenced by")

History of lack of health-seeking behavior
Reported or observed lack of equipment, financial, and/or other resources

Reported or observed impairment of personal support systems
Demonstrated lack of knowledge regarding basic health practices
Demonstrated lack of adaptive behaviors to internal/external environmental changes
Reported or observed inability to take responsibility for meeting basic health practices in any or all functional pattern areas

Goals/Objectives

Short-Term Goal

Client will seek and receive assistance with current health matters.

Long-Term Goals

1. Client will assume responsibility for own health-care needs within level of ability.
2. Client will adopt lifestyle changes that support individual health-care needs.

Interventions with *Selected Rationales*

1. The triage nurse in the emergency department, street clinic, or shelter will begin the biopsychosocial assessment of the homeless client. ***An adequate assessment is required to ensure appropriate nursing care is provided.***
2. Assess developmental level of functioning and ability to communicate. Use language that the client can comprehend. ***This information is essential to ensure that client achieves an accurate understanding of information presented and that the nurse correctly interprets what client is attempting to convey.***
3. Assess client's use of substances, including use of tobacco. Discuss eating and sleeping habits. ***These actions may be contributing to current health problems.***
4. Assess sexual practices ***to determine level of personal risk.***
5. Assess oral hygiene practices ***to determine specific self-care needs.***
6. Assess client's ability to make decisions. ***Client may need assistance in determining the type of care that is required and how to determine the most appropriate time to seek that care.***
7. Hunter (1992) suggests three basic questions that must be asked of the homeless client:
   a. Do you understand what your problem is?
   b. How will you get your prescriptions filled?
   c. Where are you going when you leave here, or where will you sleep tonight?

   Answers to these questions at admission will initiate discharge planning for client.
8. Teach client the basics of self-care (e.g., proper hygiene; facts about nutrition). ***Client must have this type of knowledge if he or she is to become more self-sufficient.***
9. Teach client about safe sex practices ***in an effort to avoid sexually transmitted diseases.***

10. Identify immediate problems, and assist with crisis intervention. ***Emergency departments, "store-front" clinics, or shelters may be the homeless client's only resource in a crisis situation.***
11. Tend to physical needs immediately. Ensure that client has thorough physical examination. ***Client cannot deal with psychosocial issues until physical problems have been addressed.***
12. Assess mental health status. ***Many homeless individuals have some form of mental illness.*** Ensure that appropriate psychiatric care is provided. If possible, inquire about possible long-acting medication injections for client. ***Client may be less likely to discontinue the medication if he or she does not have to take pills every day.***
13. Refer client to others who can provide assistance (e.g., case manager; social worker). ***If client is to be discharged to a shelter, a case manager or social worker may be the best link between client and the health-care system to ensure that he or she obtains appropriate follow-up care.***

Outcome Criteria

1. Client verbalizes understanding of information presented regarding optimal health maintenance.
2. Client is able to verbalize signs and symptoms that should be reported to a health-care professional.
3. Client verbalizes knowledge of available resources from which he or she may seek assistance as required.

POWERLESSNESS

Definition: *Perception that one's own action will not significantly affect an outcome; a perceived lack of control over a current situation or immediate happening.*

Possible Etiologies ("related to")

Lifestyle of helplessness
[Homelessness]

Defining Characteristics ("evidenced by")

Verbal expressions of having no control over self-care
Verbal expressions of having no control or influence over situation
Verbal expressions of having no control or influence over outcome
Apathy

Goals/Objectives

Short-Term Goal

Client will identify areas over which he or she has control.

Long-Term Goal

Client will make decisions that reflect control over present situation and future outcome.

Interventions with *Selected Rationales*

1. Provide opportunities for client to make choices about his or her present situation. ***Providing client with choices will increase his or her feeling of control.***
2. Avoid arguing or using logic with client who feels powerless. ***Client will not believe it can make a difference.***
3. Accept expressions of feelings, including anger and hopelessness. ***An attitude of acceptance enhances feelings of trust and self-worth.***
4. Help client identify personal strengths and establish realistic life goals. ***Unrealistic goals set client up for failure and reinforce feelings of powerlessness.***
5. Help client identify areas of life situation that he or she can control. ***Client's emotional condition interferes with his or her ability to solve problems. Assistance is required to perceive accurately the benefits and consequences of available alternatives.***
6. Help client identify areas of life situation that are not within his or her ability to control. Encourage verbalization of feelings related to this inability ***in an effort to deal with unresolved issues and accept what cannot be changed.***
7. Encourage client to seek out support group or shelter resources. ***Social isolation promotes feelings of powerlessness and hopelessness.***

Outcome Criteria

1. Client verbalizes choices made in a plan to maintain control over his or her life situation.
2. Client verbalizes honest feelings about life situations over which he or she has no control.
3. Client is able to verbalize system for problem solving as required to maintain hope for the future.

■ INTERNET REFERENCES

- http://earthsystems.org/ways/
- http://www.chn.org/homeless/
- http://www.qvctc.commnet.edu/student/GaryOKeefe/homeless/frame.html
- http://www.nationalhomeless.org/

CHAPTER 20

Psychiatric Home Nursing Care

■ BACKGROUND ASSESSMENT DATA

Dramatic changes in the health-care delivery system and skyrocketing costs have created a need to find a way to provide quality, cost-effective care to psychiatric clients. Home care has become one of the fastest growing areas in the health-care system and is now recognized by many reimbursement agencies as a preferred method of community-based service. Just what is home health care? The National Association for Home Care (NAHC) (1996) contributes the following definition: "Home care is a simple phrase that encompasses a wide range of health and social services. These services are delivered at home to recovering, disabled, chronically or terminally ill persons in need of medical, nursing, social, or therapeutic treatment and/or assistance with essential activities of daily living."

Duffey and Miller (1996) expound on the role of *psychiatric* home care in the delivery of mental health services to clients in their home setting:

> Psychiatric home care nurses must have physical and psychosocial nursing skills to meet the demands of the patient population they serve. Inpatient psychiatric nurses are likely to have some familiarity with physical nursing skills. Psychiatric nurses in home care must adapt their skills to fit within the home care nursing arena. (p. 104)

Predisposing Factors

In 1998, 3.2 percent of all clients receiving home care services had a primary psychiatric diagnosis (NAHC, 2001). The increase in psychiatric home care may be related to a number of factors:

1. Earlier hospital discharges
2. Increased demand for home care as an alternative to institutional care
3. Broader third party payment coverage
4. Greater physician acceptance of home care
5. The increasing need to contain health-care costs and the growth of managed care

Psychiatric home nursing care is provided through private home health agencies, private hospitals, public hospitals, government institutions such as the Veterans Administration, and community mental health centers. Most often, home care is viewed as follow-up care to inpatient, partial, or outpatient hospitalization.

The majority of home health care is paid by Medicare. Other sources include Medicaid, private insurance, and self-pay. Medicare requires the following criteria for psychiatric home care:

1. A physician certifies that the client is homebound.
2. The client has a primary psychiatric diagnosis.
3. The client requires the knowledge and skills of a psychiatric nurse.

Case (1993) reports:

> Medicare's interpretation of "homebound" status for psychiatric clients diverges from the medical application with which most have been familiar in the past. Patients don't have to be physically homebound; they can be mentally homebound. In other words, they can be patients physically able to leave their homes but mentally unwilling. It deals more with not wanting to leave the home because of factors such as anxiety, cognitive impairment, and vegetative depression. Agency nurses must be able to document that patients truly are homebound by such factors. (p. 61)

Although Medicare and Medicaid are the largest reimbursement providers, a growing number of health maintenance organizations and preferred provider organizations are beginning to recognize the cost-effectiveness of psychiatric home nursing care and are including it as part of their benefit packages. Most managed care agencies require that treatment, or even a specific number of visits, be preauthorized for psychiatric home nursing care. The plan of treatment and subsequent charting must explain why the client's psychiatric disorder keeps him or her at home and justify the need for services.

Symptomatology (Subjective and Objective Data)

Homebound clients most often have diagnoses of depression, dementia, anxiety disorders, bipolar affective disorder, and schizophrenia (Duffey & Miller, 1996). Many elderly clients are homebound because of medical conditions that impair mobility and necessitate home care. Finkelman (1997) states:

> Psychiatric home care is provided to patients with psychiatric diagnoses who may or may not have been hospitalized in the past, to medical patients who do not have a formal psychiatric diagnosis but do have major psychiatric symptoms, and to medical patients with psychological responses to their medical illnesses. (p. xv)

Client populations that benefit from psychiatric home health nursing include:

1. **Elderly Clients.** These individuals may not have a psychiatric diagnosis, but they may be experiencing emotional difficulties that

have arisen from medical, sociocultural, or developmental factors. Depressed mood and social isolation are common.

2. **Persons with Chronic Mental Illness.** These individuals have a history of psychiatric illness and hospitalization. They require long-term medications and continual supportive care. Common diagnoses include recurrent major depression, schizophrenia, and borderline personality disorder.
3. **Individuals in Acute Crisis Situations.** These individuals are in need of crisis intervention and/or short-term psychotherapy.

The following components should be included in the comprehensive assessment of the homebound client (Wheeler, 1998):

1. Client's perception of the problem and need for assistance
2. Information regarding client's strengths and personal habits
3. Health history
4. Recent changes
5. Support systems
6. Vital signs
7. Current medications
8. Client's understanding of and compliance with medications
9. Nutritional and elimination assessment
10. Activities of daily living (ADLs) assessment
11. Substance use assessment
12. Neurological assessment
13. Mental status examination (See Appendix H)
14. Comprehension of proverbs
15. Global Assessment of Functioning scale rating

Other important assessments include information about acute or chronic medical conditions, patterns of sleep and rest, solitude and social interaction, use of leisure time, education and work history, issues related to religion or spirituality, and adequacy of the home environment.

Nursing Diagnoses and Interventions Common to Psychiatric Homebound Clients

INEFFECTIVE THERAPEUTIC REGIMEN MANAGEMENT

Definition: *Pattern of regulating and integrating into daily living a program for treatment of illness and the sequelae of illness that is unsatisfactory for meeting specific health goals.*

Possible Etiologies ("related to")

Perceived barriers
Social support deficits

Powerlessness
Perceived benefits
Mistrust of regimen and/or health-care personnel
Knowledge deficit
Complexity of therapeutic regimen

Defining Characteristics ("evidenced by")

Choices of daily living ineffective for meeting the goals of a treatment or prevention program
Verbalizes that did not take action to reduce risk factors for progression of illness and sequelae
Verbalizes difficulty with regulation/integration of one or more prescribed regimens for prevention of complications and the treatment or illness or its effects
[Acceleration of illness symptoms]
Verbalizes that did not take action to include treatment regimens in daily routines

Goals/Objectives

Short-Term Goals

1. Client will verbalize understanding of barriers to management of therapeutic regimen.
2. Client will participate in problem-solving efforts toward adequate management of therapeutic regimen.

Long-Term Goal

Client will incorporate changes in lifestyle necessary to maintain therapeutic regimen.

Interventions with *Selected Rationales*

1. Assess client's knowledge of condition and treatment needs. ***Client may lack full comprehension of need for treatment regimen.***
2. Identify client's perception of treatment regimen. ***Client may be mistrustful of treatment regimen or of health-care system in general.***
3. ***Promote a trusting relationship with client*** by being honest, encouraging client to participate in decision making, and conveying genuine positive regard.
4. Assist client in recognizing strengths and past successes. ***Recognition of strengths and past successes increases self-esteem and indicates to client that he or she can be successful in managing therapeutic regimen.***
5. Provide positive reinforcement for efforts. ***Positive reinforcement increases self-esteem and encourages repetition of desirable behaviors.***

6. Emphasize importance of need for treatment/medication. ***Client must understand that the consequence of lack of follow-through is possible decompensation.***
7. ***In an effort to incorporate lifestyle changes and promote wellness,*** help client develop plans for managing therapeutic regimen, such as support groups, social and family systems, and financial assistance.

Outcome Criteria

1. Client verbalizes understanding of information presented regarding management of therapeutic regimen.
2. Client demonstrates desire and ability to perform strategies necessary to maintain adequate management of therapeutic regimen.
3. Client verbalizes knowledge of available resources from which he or she may seek assistance as required.

IMPAIRED ADJUSTMENT

Definition: *Inability to modify lifestyle or behavior in a manner consistent with a change in health status.*

Possible Etiologies ("related to")

Low state of optimism
Intense emotional state
Negative attitudes toward health behavior
Absence of intent to change behavior
Multiple stressors
Absence of social support for changed beliefs and practices
Disability or health status change requiring change in lifestyle
Lack of motivation to change behaviors

Defining Characteristics ("evidenced by")

Denial of health status change
Failure to achieve optimal sense of control
Failure to take actions that would prevent further health problems
Demonstration of nonacceptance of health status change

Goals/Objectives

Short-Term Goals

1. Client will discuss with home health nurse the kinds of lifestyle changes that will occur because of the change in health status.
2. With the help of home health nurse, client will formulate a plan of action for incorporating those changes into his or her lifestyle.
3. Client will demonstrate movement toward independence, considering change in health status.

Long-Term Goal

Client will demonstrate competence to function independently to his or her optimal ability, considering change in health status, by time of discharge from home health care.

Interventions with *Selected Rationales*

1. Encourage client to talk about lifestyle before the change in health status. Discuss coping mechanisms that were used at stressful times in the past. ***It is important to identify client's strengths so that they may be used to facilitate adaptation to the change or loss that has occurred.***
2. Encourage client to discuss the change or loss and particularly to express anger associated with it. ***Some individuals may not realize that anger is a normal stage in the grieving process. If it is not released in an appropriate manner, it may be turned inward on the self, leading to pathological depression.***
3. Encourage client to express fears associated with the change or loss or with the alteration in lifestyle that the change or loss has created. ***Change often creates a feeling of disequilibrium, and the individual may respond with fears that are irrational or unfounded. He or she may benefit from feedback that corrects misperceptions about how life will be with the change in health status.***
4. Provide assistance with ADLs as required, but encourage independence to the limit that client's ability will allow. Give positive feedback for activities accomplished independently. ***Independent accomplishments and positive feedback enhance self-esteem and encourage repetition of desired behaviors. Successes also provide hope that adaptive functioning is possible and decrease feelings of powerlessness.***
5. Help client with decision making regarding incorporation of change or loss into lifestyle. Identify problems that the change or loss is likely to create. Discuss alternative solutions, weighing potential benefits and consequences of each alternative. Support client's decision in the selection of an alternative. ***The great amount of anxiety that usually accompanies a major lifestyle change often interferes with an individual's ability to solve problems and to make appropriate decisions. Client may need assistance with this process in an effort to progress toward successful adaptation.***
6. Use role playing ***to decrease anxiety*** as client anticipates stressful situations that might occur in relation to the health status change. ***Role playing decreases anxiety and provides a feeling of security by arming the client with a plan of action with which to respond in an appropriate manner when a stressful situation occurs.***
7. Ensure that client and family are fully knowledgeable regarding the physiology of the change in health status and its necessity for

optimal wellness. Encourage them to ask questions, and provide printed material explaining the change to which they may refer following discharge.

8. Help client identify resources within the community from which he or she may seek assistance in adapting to the change in health status. Examples include self-help, support groups, counselor, and social worker. Encourage client to keep follow-up appointments with physician or to call physician's office before follow-up date if problems or concerns arise.

Outcome Criteria

1. Client is able to perform ADLs independently.
2. Client is able to make independent decisions regarding lifestyle considering change in health status.
3. Client is able to express hope for the future with consideration of change in health status.

SOCIAL ISOLATION

Definition: *Aloneness experienced by the individual and perceived as imposed by others and as a negative or threatening state.*

Possible Etiologies ("related to")

Alterations in mental status
Inability to engage in satisfying personal relationships
Unaccepted social values
Unaccepted social behavior
Inadequate personal resources
Immature interests
Alterations in physical appearance
Altered state of wellness

Defining Characteristics ("evidenced by")

Expresses feelings of aloneness imposed by others
Expresses feelings of rejection
Inappropriate interests for developmental age
Inability to meet expectations of others
Insecurity in public
Absence of supportive significant other(s)
Projects hostility in voice and behavior
Withdrawn; uncommunicative
Seeks to be alone
Preoccupation with own thoughts
Sad, dull affect

Goals/Objectives

Short-Term Goal

Client will verbalize willingness to be involved with others.

Long-Term Goal

Client will participate with others at level of ability or desire.

Interventions with *Selected Rationales*

1. Convey an accepting attitude by making regular visits. ***An accepting attitude increases feelings of self-worth and facilitates trust.***
2. Show unconditional positive regard. ***This conveys your belief in client as a worthwhile human being.***
3. Be honest, and keep all promises. ***Honesty and dependability promote a trusting relationship.***
4. Be cautious with touch until trust has been established. ***A suspicious client may perceive touch as a threatening gesture.***
5. Be with client to offer support during activities that may be frightening or difficult for him or her. ***The presence of a trusted individual provides emotional security for client.***
6. Take walks with client. Help him or her perform simple tasks around the house. ***Increased activity enhances both physical and mental status.***
7. Assess lifelong patterns of relationships. ***Basic personality characteristics will not change. Most individuals keep the same style of relationship development they had in the past.***
8. Help client identify present relationships that are satisfying and activities that he or she considers interesting. ***Only client knows what he or she truly likes, and these personal preferences will facilitate success in reversing social isolation.***
9. Consider the feasibility of a pet. ***There are many documented studies of the benefits of companion pets.***

Outcome Criteria

1. Client demonstrates willingness and desire to socialize with others.
2. Client independently pursues social activities with others.

RISK FOR CAREGIVER ROLE STRAIN

Definition: *Caregiver is vulnerable for felt difficulty in performing the family caregiver role.*

Risk Factors

Caregiver not developmentally ready for caregiver role
Inadequate physical environment for providing care

Unpredictable illness course or instability in the care receiver's health
Psychological or cognitive problems in care receiver
Presence of abuse or violence
Past history of poor relationship between caregiver and care receiver
Marginal caregiver's coping patterns
Lack of respite and recreation for caregiver
Addiction or codependency
Caregiver's competing role commitments
Illness severity of the care receiver
Duration of caregiving required
Family/caregiver isolation

Goals/Objectives

Short-Term Goal

Caregivers will verbalize understanding of ways to facilitate the caregiver role.

Long-Term Goal

Caregivers will demonstrate effective problem-solving skills and develop adaptive coping mechanisms to regain equilibrium.

Interventions with *Selected Rationales*

1. Assess caregivers' ability to anticipate and fulfill client's unmet needs. Provide information to assist caregivers with this responsibility. Ensure that caregivers encourage client to be as independent as possible. ***Caregivers may be unaware of what client can realistically accomplish. They may be unaware of the nature of the illness.***
2. Ensure that caregivers are aware of available community support systems from which they can seek assistance when required. Examples include respite care services, day treatment centers, and adult day-care centers. ***Caregivers require relief from the pressures and strain of providing 24-hour care for their loved one. Studies have shown that abuse arises out of caregiving situations that place overwhelming stress on the caregivers.***
3. Encourage caregivers to express feelings, particularly anger. ***Release of these emotions can serve to prevent psychopathology, such as depression or psychophysiological disorders, from occurring.***
4. Encourage participation in support groups composed of members with similar life situations. Provide information about support groups that may be helpful:
   - National Alliance for the Mentally Ill—(800) 950-NAMI
   - Association on Mental Retardation—(800) 424-3688
   - Association for Retarded Citizens—(301) 565-3842
   - Alzheimer's Disease and Related Disorders Association—(800) 272-3900

Hearing others who are experiencing the same problems discuss ways in which they have coped may help the caregiver adopt more adaptive strategies. Individuals who are experiencing similar life situations provide empathy and support for each other.

Outcome Criteria

1. Caregivers are able to problem-solve effectively regarding care of client.
2. Caregivers demonstrate adaptive coping strategies for dealing with stress of caregiver role.
3. Caregivers express feelings openly.
4. Caregivers express desire to join support group of other caregivers.

INTERNET REFERENCES

- http://www.hcfa.gov/siteindex/
- http://www.nahc.org/Consumer/wihc.html
- http://www.nahc.org/Consumer/hcstats.html

CHAPTER 21

Forensic Nursing

BACKGROUND ASSESSMENT DATA

The International Association of Forensic Nurses and the American Nurses Association (1997) define forensic nursing as "the application of forensic science combined with the bio-psychological education of the registered nurse, in the scientific investigation, evidence collection and preservation, analysis, prevention and treatment of trauma and/or death related medical-legal issues." (p. v)

Hufft and Peternelj-Taylor (1999) offer the following definition: "A nursing specialty that integrates nursing and forensic science to bridge the gap between the health care system and the criminal justice system." (p. 1)

Areas of forensic nursing include:

1. Clinical forensic nursing
2. Sexual assault nurse examiner
3. Forensic psychiatric nursing specialty
4. Correctional/institutional nursing specialty
5. Nurses in general practice

Clinical Forensic Nursing in Trauma Care

Assessment

Lynch (1995) states that forensic nurses who work in trauma care settings may "become the designated clinicians who will evaluate and assess surviving victims of rape, drug and alcohol addiction, domestic violence (including abuse of spouse, children, elderly), assaults, automobile/pedestrian accidents, suicide attempts, occupationally related injuries, incest, medical malpractice and the injuries sustained therefrom, and food and drug tampering."

All traumatic injuries in which liability is suspected are considered within the scope of forensic nursing. Reports to legal agencies are required to ensure follow-up investigation; however, the protection of clients' rights remains a nursing priority.

Several areas of assessment in which the clinical forensic nurse specialist in trauma care may become involved include:

1. **Preservation of Evidence.** Evidence from crime-related and self-inflicted traumas must be safeguarded in a manner consistent with the investigation. Evidence including clothing, bullets, blood stains, hairs, fibers, and small pieces of material such as fragments

of metal, glass, paint, and wood should be saved and documented in all medical accident instances that have legal implications.

2. **Investigation of Wound Characteristics.** Wounds that the nurse must be able to identify include:
   a. ***Sharp-Force Injuries.*** Include stab wounds and other wounds resulting from penetration by a sharp object.
   b. ***Blunt-Force Injuries.*** Include cuts and bruises resulting from the impact of a blunt object against the body.
   c. ***Dicing Injuries.*** Multiple, minute cuts and abrasions caused by contact with shattered glass (e.g., often occur in motor vehicle accidents).
   d. ***Patterned Injuries.*** Specific injuries that reflect the pattern of the weapon used to inflict the injury.
   e. ***Bite-Mark Injuries.*** A type of patterned injury inflicted by human or animal.
   f. ***Defense Wounds.*** Injuries that reflect the victim's attempt to defend himself or herself from attack.
   g. ***Hesitation Wounds.*** Usually superficial, sharp-force wounds; often found perpendicular to the lower part of the body and may reflect self-inflicted wounds.
   h. ***Fast-Force Injuries:*** Usually gunshot wounds; may reflect various patterns of injury.
3. **Deaths in the Emergency Department.** When deaths occur in the emergency department as a result of abuse or accident, evidence must be retained, the death must be reported to legal authorities, and an investigation is conducted (Lynch, 1995). It is therefore essential that the nurse carefully document the appearance, condition, and behavior of the victim upon arrival at the hospital. The information gathered from the client and family (or others accompanying the client) may serve to facilitate the postmortem investigation and may be used during criminal justice proceedings.

The critical factor is the ability to determine whether the cause of death is natural or unnatural. In the emergency department, most deaths are sudden and unexpected. Those that are considered natural most commonly involve the cardiovascular, respiratory, and central nervous systems (Lynch, 1995). Deaths that are considered unnatural include those from trauma, from self-inflicted acts, or from injuries inflicted by another. Legal authorities must be notified of all deaths related to unnatural circumstances.

Common Nursing Diagnoses and Interventions

(For forensic nursing in trauma care)

POST-TRAUMA SYNDROME

Definition: *Sustained maladaptive response to a traumatic, overwhelming event.*

Possible Etiologies ("related to")

Physical and psychosocial abuse
Tragic occurrence involving multiple deaths
Sudden destruction of one's home or community
Epidemics
Rape
Natural or man-made disasters
Serious accidents
Witnessing mutilation, violent death, or other horrors
Serious threat or injury to self or loved ones
Industrial and motor vehicle accidents

Defining Characteristics ("evidenced by")

[Physical injuries related to trauma]
Avoidance
Repression
Difficulty concentrating
Grief; guilt
Intrusive thoughts
Neurosensory irritability
Palpitations
Anger and/or rage; aggression
Intrusive dreams; nightmares; flashbacks
Panic attacks; fear
Gastric irritability
Psychogenic amnesia
Substance abuse

Goals/Objectives

Short-Term Goal

Client's physical wounds will heal without complication.
Client will begin a healthy grief resolution, initiating the process of psychological healing.

Long-Term Goal

Client will demonstrate ability to deal with emotional reactions in an individually appropriate manner.

Interventions with *Selected Rationales*

1. Smith (1987a) relates the importance of communicating the following ideas to the rape victim:
   a. I am very sorry this happened to you.
   b. You are safe here.
   c. I am very glad you are alive.
   d. You are not to blame. You are a victim. It was not your fault. Whatever decisions you made at the time of the victimization were the right ones because you are alive.

   The woman who has been sexually assaulted fears for her life and

must be reassured of her safety. She may also be overwhelmed with self-doubt and self- blame, and these statements instill trust and validate self-worth.

2. Explain every assessment procedure that will be conducted and why. Ensure that data collection is conducted in a caring, non-judgmental manner ***to decrease fear and anxiety and increase trust.***
3. Ledray and Arndt (1994) suggest the following five essential components of a forensic examination of the sexual assault survivor in the emergency department:
   a. Treatment and documentation of injuries. Samples of blood, semen, hair, and fingernail scrapings should be sealed in paper, not plastic, bags, ***to prevent the possible growth of mildew from accumulation of moisture inside the plastic container and the subsequent contamination of the evidence.***
   b. Maintaining the proper chain of evidence. Samples must be properly labeled, sealed, and refrigerated when necessary and kept under observation or properly locked until rendered to the proper legal authority ***in order to ensure the proper chain of evidence and freshness of the samples.***
   c. Treatment and evaluation of sexually transmitted diseases (STDs). If conducted within 72 hours of the attack, several tests and interventions are available for prophylactic treatment of certain STDs.
   d. Pregnancy risk evaluation and prevention. Prophylactic regimens are 97 percent to 98 percent effective if started within 24 hours of the sexual attack and are generally only recommended within 72 hours (AMA, 1999).
   e. Crisis intervention and arrangements for follow-up counseling. ***Because a survivor is often too ashamed or fearful to seek follow-up counseling,*** it may be important for the nurse to obtain the individual's permission to allow a counselor to call her to make a follow-up appointment.
3. In the case of other types of trauma (e.g., gunshot victims; automobile/pedestrian hit-and-run victims), ***ensure that any possible evidence is not lost.*** Clothing that is removed from a victim should not be shaken, and each separate item of clothing should be placed carefully in a paper bag, which should be sealed, dated, timed, and signed.
4. Ensure that the client has adequate privacy for all immediate post-crisis interventions. Try to have as few people as possible providing the immediate care or collecting immediate evidence. ***The post-trauma client is extremely vulnerable. Additional people in the environment increase this feeling of vulnerability and escalate anxiety.***
5. Encourage client to give an account of the trauma/assault. Listen, but do not probe. ***Nonjudgmental listening provides an opportu-***

nity for catharsis that the client needs to begin healing. A detailed account may be required for legal follow-up, and a caring nurse, as client advocate, may help to lessen the trauma of evidence collection.

6. Discuss with client whom to call for support or assistance. Provide information about referrals for aftercare. ***Because of severe anxiety and fear, client may need assistance from others during this immediate postcrisis period. Provide referral information in writing for later reference (e.g., psychotherapist, mental health clinic, community advocacy group).***
7. In the event of a sudden and unexpected death in the trauma care setting, the clinical forensic nurse may be asked to present information associated with an anatomical donation request to the survivors. ***The clinical forensic nurse specialist is an expert in legal issues and has the knowledge and sensitivity to provide coordination between organ/tissue procurement and the medical examiner/coroner system (Lynch, 1995).***

Outcome Criteria

1. Client is no longer experiencing panic anxiety.
2. Client demonstrates some trust in the primary nurse.
3. Client has received immediate attention to physical injuries.
4. Client has initiated behaviors consistent with the grief response.
5. Necessary evidence has been collected and preserved in order to proceed appropriately within the legal system.

Forensic Psychiatric Nursing in Correctional Facilities

Assessment

It was believed that deinstitutionalization increased the freedom of mentally ill individuals in accordance with the principle of "least restrictive alternative." However, because of inadequate community-based services, many of these individuals drifted into poverty and homelessness, increasing their vulnerability to criminalization. Because the bizarre behavior of mentally ill individuals living on the street is sometimes offensive to community standards, law enforcement officials have the authority to protect the welfare of the public, as well as the safety of the individual, by initiating emergency hospitalization. However, legal criteria for commitment are so stringent in most cases that arrest becomes an easier way of getting the mentally ill person off the street if a criminal statute has been violated. It is estimated that between 10 percent and 35 percent of all inmates have some form of psychological disorder or mental disability (Wark, 1998). Some of these individuals are incarcerated as a result of the increasingly popular "guilty but mentally ill" verdict. It is unfortunate that, according to Lego (1995), prisons became the 1990s' "state psychiatric hospitals."

Psychiatric diagnoses commonly identified at the time of incarceration include schizophrenia, affective psychoses, personality disorders, and substance disorders (Rice, Harris, & Quinsey, 1996). Common psychiatric behaviors include hallucinations, suspiciousness, thought disorders, anger/agitation, impulsivity, and denial of problems. In the study by Rice, Harris, and Quinsey, the behavior, "denial of problems," ranked as most significant among this population. Use of substances and medication noncompliance are common obstacles to rehabilitation. Substance abuse has been shown to have a strong correlation with recidivism among the prison population (Rice, Harris, & Quinsey, 1996). Many individuals report that they were under the influence of substances at the time of their criminal actions, and dual diagnoses are common. Detoxification frequency occurs in jails and prisons, and some inmates have died from the withdrawal syndrome because of lack of adequate treatment during this process (Bernier, 1991).

Common Nursing Diagnoses and Interventions
(For forensic nursing in correctional facilities)

DEFENSIVE COPING

Definition: ***Repeated projection of falsely positive self-evaluation based on a self-protective pattern that defends against underlying perceived threats to positive self-regard.***

Possible Etiologies ("related to")

[Low self-esteem]
[Retarded ego development]
[Underdeveloped superego]
[Negative role models]
[Lack of positive feedback]
[Absent, erratic, or inconsistent methods of discipline]
[Dysfunctional family system]

Defining Characteristics ("evidenced by")

Denial of obvious problems or weaknesses
Projection of blame or responsibility
Rationalization of failures
Hypersensitivity to criticism
Grandiosity
Superior attitude toward others
Difficulty establishing or maintaining relationships
Hostile laughter at or ridicule of others
Difficulty in perception of reality
Lack of follow-through or participation in treatment or therapy

Goals/Objectives

Short-Term Goal

Client will verbalize personal responsibility for own actions, successes, and failures.

Long-Term Goal

Client will demonstrate ability to interact with others and adapt to lifestyle goals without becoming defensive, rationalizing behaviors, or expressing grandiose ideas.

Interventions with *Selected Rationales*

1. Recognize and support basic ego strengths. ***Focusing on positive aspects of the personality may help to improve self-concept.***
2. Encourage client to recognize and verbalize feelings of inadequacy and need for acceptance from others and how these feelings provoke defensive behaviors, such as blaming others for own behaviors. ***Recognition of the problem is the first step in the change process toward resolution.***
3. Provide immediate, matter-of-fact, nonthreatening feedback for unacceptable behaviors. ***Client may lack knowledge about how he or she is perceived by others. Direct the behavior in a nonthreatening manner to a more acceptable behavior.***
4. Help client identify situations that provoke defensiveness, and practice more appropriate responses through role playing. ***Role playing provides confidence to deal with difficult situations when they actually occur.***
5. Provide immediate positive feedback for acceptable behaviors. ***Positive feedback enhances self-esteem and encourages repetition of desirable behaviors.***
6. Help client set realistic, concrete goals, and determine appropriate actions to meet those goals. ***Success increases self-esteem.***
7. Evaluate with client the effectiveness of the new behaviors, and discuss any modifications for improvement. ***Because of limited problem-solving ability, assistance may be required to reassess and develop new strategies in the event that certain of the new coping methods prove ineffective.***
8. Use confrontation judiciously ***to help client begin to identify defense mechanisms (e.g., denial and projection) that are hindering development of satisfying relationships and adaptive behaviors.***

Outcome Criteria

1. Client verbalizes and accepts responsibility for own behavior.
2. Client verbalizes correlation between feelings of inadequacy and the need to defend the ego through rationalization and grandiosity.
3. Client does not ridicule or criticize others.

4. Client interacts with others in group situations without taking a defensive stance.

DYSFUNCTIONAL GRIEVING

Definition: ***Extended, unsuccessful use of intellectual and emotional responses by which individuals, families, communities attempt to work through the process of modifying self-concept based upon the perception of loss.***

Possible Etiologies ("related to")

Loss of freedom

Defining Characteristics ("evidenced by")

Anger
[Internalized rage]
[Depressed mood]
Labile affect
[Extreme fear of being alone (fear of abandonment)]
[Acting-out behaviors, such as sexual promiscuity, suicidal gestures, temper tantrums, substance abuse]
[Difficulty expressing feelings]
Alterations in eating habits, sleep patterns, dream patterns, activity level
Prolonged interference with life functioning, with onset or exacerbation of somatic or psychosomatic responses

Goals/Objectives

Short-Term Goal

Client will verbalize feelings of grief related to loss of freedom.

Long-Term Goal

Client will progress satisfactorily through the grieving process.

Interventions with *Selected Rationales*

1. Convey an accepting attitude—one that creates a nonthreatening environment for client to express feelings. Be honest, and keep all promises. ***An accepting attitude conveys to client that you believe he or she is a worthwhile person. Trust is enhanced.***
2. Identify the function that anger, frustration, and rage serve for client. Allow client to express these feelings within reason. ***Verbalization of feelings in a nonthreatening environment may help client come to terms with unresolved grief.***
3. Encourage client to discharge pent-up anger through participation in large-motor activities (e.g., physical exercises, volleyball,

punching bag). ***Physical exercise provides a safe and effective method for discharging pent-up tension.***

4. Anger may be displaced onto the nurse or therapist, and caution must be taken to guard against the negative effects of countertransference. These are very difficult clients who have the capacity for eliciting a whole array of negative feelings from the therapist. These feelings must be acknowledged but not allowed to interfere with the therapeutic process.
5. Explain the behaviors associated with the normal grieving process. Help client to recognize his or her position in this process. ***This knowledge about normal grieving may help facilitate client's progression toward resolution of grief.***
6. Help client understand appropriate ways to express anger. Give positive reinforcement for behaviors used to express anger appropriately. Act as a role model. ***Positive reinforcement enhances self-esteem and encourages repetition of desirable behaviors. It is appropriate to let client know when he or she has done something that has generated angry feelings in you. Role-modeling ways to express anger in an appropriate manner is a powerful learning tool.***
7. Set limits on acting-out behaviors, and explain consequences of violation of those limits. Be supportive yet consistent and firm in working with client. ***Client lacks sufficient self-control to limit maladaptive behaviors; therefore, assistance is required from staff. Without consistency from all staff members working with client, a positive outcome will not be achieved.***
8. Provide a safe and protective environment for client against risk of self-directed violence. ***Depression is the emotion that most commonly precedes suicidal attempts.***

Outcome Criteria

1. Client is able to verbalize ways in which anger and acting-out behaviors are associated with maladaptive grieving.
2. Client expresses anger and hostility outwardly in a safe and acceptable manner.
3. Client has not harmed self or others.

RISK FOR INJURY

Definition: *At risk of injury as a result of [internal or external] environmental conditions interacting with the individual's adaptive and defensive resources.*

Related/Risk Factors ("related to")

[Substance use/detoxification at time of incarceration, exhibiting any of the following:

Substance intoxication
Substance withdrawal
Disorientation
Seizures
Hallucinations
Psychomotor agitation
Unstable vital signs
Delirium
Flashbacks
Panic level of anxiety]

Goals/Objectives

Short-Term Goal

Client's condition will stabilize within 72 hours.

Long-Term Goal

Client will not experience physical injury.

Interventions with *Selected Rationales*

1. Assess client's level of disorientation to determine specific requirements for safety. ***Knowledge of client's level of functioning is necessary to formulate appropriate plan of care.***
2. Obtain a drug history, if possible, to determine:
   a. Type of substance(s) used
   b. Time of last ingestion and amount consumed
   c. Duration and frequency of consumption
   d. Amount consumed on a daily basis
3. Obtain urine sample for laboratory analysis of substance content. ***Subjective history is often not accurate. Knowledge regarding substance ingestion is important for accurate assessment of client condition.***
4. Place client in quiet room, if possible. ***Excessive stimuli increase client agitation.***
5. Institute necessary safety precautions:
   a. Observe client behaviors frequently; assign staff on one-to-one basis if condition is warranted; accompany and assist client when ambulating; use wheelchair for transporting long distances.
   b. Be sure that side rails are up when client is in bed.
   c. Pad headboard and side rails of bed with thick towels to protect client in case of seizure.
   d. Use mechanical restraints as necessary to protect client if excessive hyperactivity accompanies the disorientation.

   Client safety is a nursing priority.
6. Ensure that smoking materials and other potentially harmful objects are stored outside client's access. ***Client may harm self or others in disoriented, confused state.***

7. Monitor vital signs every 15 minutes initially and less frequently as acute symptoms subside. ***Vital signs provide the most reliable information regarding client condition and need for medication during acute detoxification period.***
8. Follow medication regimen as ordered by physician. Common medical intervention for detoxification from the following substances includes:
   a. **Alcohol.** Chlordiazepoxide (Librium) is given orally every 4 to 8 hours in decreasing doses until withdrawal is complete. In clients with liver disease, accumulation of the longer-acting agents, such as chlordiazepoxide (Librium), may be problematic, and the use of the shorter-acting benzodiazepine oxazepam (Serax) is more appropriate. Some physicians may order anticonvulsant medication to be used prophylactically; however, this is not a universal intervention. Multivitamin therapy, in combination with daily thiamine (either orally or by injection), is common protocol.
   b. **Narcotics.** Narcotic antagonists, such as naloxone (Narcan), naltrexone (ReVia), and nalmefene (Revex), are administered for opioid intoxication. Withdrawal is managed with rest and nutritional therapy. Substitution therapy may be instituted to decrease withdrawal symptoms using propoxyphene (Darvon) for weaker effects or methadone (Dolophine) for longer effects.
   c. **Depressants.** Substitution therapy may be instituted to decrease withdrawal symptoms using a long-acting barbiturate, such as phenobarbital (Luminal). Some physicians prescribe oxazepam (Serax) as needed for objective symptoms, gradually decreasing the dosage until the drug is discontinued. Long-acting benzodiazepines are commonly used for substitution therapy when the abused substance is a nonbarbiturate central nervous system depressant.
   d. **Stimulants.** Treatment of stimulant intoxication is geared toward stabilization of vital signs. Intravenous antihypertensives may be used, along with intravenous diazepam (Valium) to control seizures. Minor tranquilizers, such as chlordiazepoxide (Librium), may be administered orally for the first few days while the client is "crashing." Treatment is aimed at reducing drug craving and managing severe depression. Suicide precautions may be required. Therapy with antidepressant medication is not uncommon.
   e. **Hallucinogens and Cannabinols.** Medications are normally not prescribed for withdrawal from these substances. However, in the event of overdose or the occurrence of adverse reactions (e.g., anxiety or panic), diazepam (Valium) or chlordiazepoxide (Librium) may be given as needed to decrease agitation. Should psychotic reactions occur, they may be treated with an-

tipsychotics, such as the phenothiazines, haloperidol, or the newer atypical antipsychotics.

Outcome Criteria

1. Client no longer exhibits any signs or symptoms of substance intoxication or withdrawal.
2. Client shows no evidence of physical injury obtained during substance intoxication or withdrawal.

INTERNET REFERENCES

Additional information related to forensic nursing may be found at the following websites:

- http://www.forensiceducation.com/
- http://www.forensicnurse.org/
- http://www.forensicnurse.org/resource/links.htm

CHAPTER 22

Complementary Therapies

INTRODUCTION

The connection between mind and body, and the influence of each on the other, is well recognized by all clinicians and particularly by psychiatrists. Traditional medicine practiced in the United States is based on scientific methodology. Traditional medicine is also known as *allopathic* medicine, and it is the type historically taught in U.S. medical schools.

The term *alternative medicine* has come to refer to practices that differ from the usual traditional practices in the treatment of disease. A national survey by the American Medical Association's Council on Scientific Affairs revealed that 33 percent of those polled reported at least one alternative treatment during the previous 12 months (Money World, 1997). More than $15 billion a year is spent on alternative medical therapies in the United States (Kaplan & Sadock, 1998).

In 1991, an Office of Alternative Medicine (OAM) was established by the National Institutes of Health (NIH) to study nontraditional therapies and to evaluate their usefulness and their effectiveness. The mission statement of the OAM states, "The NIH Office of Alternative Medicine facilitates research and evaluation of unconventional medical practices and disseminates this information to the public" (Complementary & Alternative Medicine, 1998).

Some health insurance companies and health maintenance organizations appear to be yielding to public pressure by including alternative providers in their networks of providers for such treatments as acupuncture and massage therapy. Chiropractic care has been covered by some third-party payers for many years. Individuals who seek alternative therapy, however, are often reimbursed at lower rates than those who choose traditional practitioners.

Credit, Hartunian, and Nowak (1998) view these treatments not as *alternatives*, but as *complements*, in partnership with traditional medical practice. They acknowledge the superiority of traditional medical intervention in certain situations. However, they do not discount "the body's ability to heal itself with the help of natural, noninvasive therapies that are effective and without harmful side effects." (p. 3.)

Client education is an important part of complementary care. Positive lifestyle changes are encouraged, and practitioners serve as educators as well as treatment specialists (Credit et al, 1998). Complementary medicine is viewed as *holistic* health care, which deals not only with the physical perspective, but also with the emotional and spiritual components of the individual. Dr. Tom Coniglione, former professor of medicine at the Oklahoma University Health Sciences Center, states:

> We must look at treating the "total person" in order to be more efficient and balanced within the medical community. Even finding doctors who are well rounded and balanced has become a criterion in the admitting process for medical students. Medicine has changed from just looking at the "scientist perspective of organ and disease" to the total perspective of lifestyle and real impact/results to the patient. This evolution is a progressive and very positive shift in the right direction (Coniglione, 1998).

Terms such as *harmony* and *balance* are often associated with complementary care. In fact, restoring harmony and balance between body and mind is often the goal of complementary health-care approaches (Credit et al, 1998).

■ TYPES OF COMPLEMENTARY THERAPIES

Herbal Medicine

The use of plants to heal is probably as old as humankind. Virtually every culture in the world has relied on herbs and plants to treat illness. Clay tablets from about 4000 BC reveal that the Sumerians had apothecaries for dispensing medicinal herbs, and the *Pen Tsao*, a Chinese text written around 3000 BC, contained some 1000 herbal formulas that had probably been used as remedies for thousands of years (Guinness, 1993). When the Pilgrims came to America in the 1600s, they brought with them a variety of herbs to be established and used for medicinal purposes; they soon discovered that the Native Americans also had their own varieties of plants used for healing.

Many people are seeking a return to herbal remedies, because they view these remedies as being less potent than prescription drugs and as being free of adverse side effects. However, because the Food and Drug Administration (FDA) classifies herbal remedies as dietary supplements or food additives, their labels cannot indicate medicinal uses. They are not subject to FDA approval, and they lack uniform standards of quality control.

Several organizations have been established to attempt regulation and control of the herbal industry. They include the Council for Responsible Nutrition, the American Herbal Association, and the American Botanical Council. The Commission E of the German Federal Health Agency is the group responsible for researching and regulating the safety and efficacy of herbs and plant medicines in Germany. All 380 German Commission E monographs of herbal medicines have been translated into English and compiled into one text (Blumenthal, 1998). This is an invaluable reference for practitioners of holistic medicine.

Until more extensive testing has been completed on people and animals, the use of herbal medicines must be approached with caution and responsibility. The notion that because something is "natural," it is therefore completely safe, is a myth. In fact, some of the plants from which prescription drugs are derived are highly toxic in their "natural" state (Guinness, 1993). Also, because of lack of regulation and standardization, ingredients may be adulterated, and methods of manufacture may alter potency. For example, dried herbs lose potency rapidly because of exposure to air. Guinness offers the following points for practitioners and individuals considering the use of herbal medicines:

1. **Be careful of your sources.** Because of the lack of government scrutiny, the purity and potency of the herbal medicines cannot be guaranteed. The buyer must be careful to select reputable brands.
2. **Choose the most reliable forms.** Tinctures and freeze-dried products have been prepared to retard spoilage and prevent loss of potency.
3. **More is not better.** Always take the recommended dosages at the suggested intervals. Adverse effects can occur from overdosing with herbal medicines, just as they do with prescription pharmaceuticals.
4. **Monitor your reactions.** Discontinue the herbal medication at the first sign of allergic or other adverse reaction or, after a reasonable amount of time, if there seems to be no significant indication that it is producing the desired effect.
5. **Take no risks.** Do not self-medicate with herbal remedies for serious illnesses or injuries. Do not take herbal medications without a physician's approval if you are pregnant or lactating, very young or very old, or taking other medications.

Table 22–1 lists information about common herbal remedies, with possible implications for psychiatric/mental health nursing. Botanical names, medicinal uses, and safety profiles are included.

Acupressure and Acupuncture

Acupressure and acupuncture are healing techniques based on the ancient philosophies of traditional Chinese medicine, dating back to 3000 BC. The main concept behind Chinese medicine is that healing energy (*chi*) flows through the body along specific pathways called *meridians.* It is believed that these meridians of chi connect various parts of the body in a way similar to the way in which lines on a road map link various locations. The pathways link a conglomerate of points, called *acupoints.* Therefore, it is possible to treat a part of the

TABLE 22–1 **Herbal Remedies**

Common Names (Botanical Name)	Medicinal Uses/ Possible Action	Safety Profile
Black cohosh (*Cimicifuga racemosa*)	May provide relief of menstrual cramps; improved mood; calming effect. Extracts from the roots are thought to have action similar to that of estrogen.	Generally considered safe in low doses. Toxic in large doses, causing dizziness, nausea, headaches, stiffness, and trembling. Should not take with heart problems, concurrently with antihypertensives, or during pregnancy.
Cascara sagrada (*Rhamnus purshiana*)	Relief of constipation.	Generally recognized as safe; sold as over-the-counter drug in the U.S. Should not be used during pregnancy.
Chamomile (*Matricaria chamomilla*)	As a tea, is effective as a mild sedative in the relief of insomnia. May also aid digestion, relieve menstrual cramps, and settle upset stomach.	Generally recognized as safe when consumed in reasonable amounts.
Echinacea (*Echinacea angustifolia*) (*Echinacea purpurea*)	Stimulates immune system; may have value in fighting infections and easing the symptoms of colds and flu.	Considered safe in reasonable doses. Observe for side effects of allergic reaction.
Fennel (*Foeniculum vulgare*)(*Foeniculum officinale*)	Used to ease stomachaches and to aid digestion. Taken in a tea or in extracts to stimulate the appetites of anorexics (1–2 tsp. seeds steeped in boiling water for making tea).	Generally recognized as safe when consumed in reasonable amounts.
Feverfew (*Tanacetum parthenium*)	Prophylaxis and treatment of migraine headaches. Effective in either the fresh leaf or freeze-dried forms (2–3 fresh leaves [or equivalent] per day.)	A small percentage of individuals may experience the adverse effect of temporary mouth ulcers. Considered safe in reasonable doses.

TABLE 22–1 **Herbal Remedies**

Common Names (Botanical Name)	Medicinal Uses/ Possible Action	Safety Profile
Ginger *(Zingiber officinale)*	Ginger tea to ease stomachaches and to aid digestion. Two powdered gingerroot capsules have been shown to be effective in preventing motion sickness.	Generally recognized as safe.
Ginkgo *(Ginkgo biloba)*	Used to treat senility, short-term memory loss, and peripheral insufficiency. Has been shown to dilate blood vessels. Usual dosage is 120 mg/day.	Safety has been established with recommended dosages. Possible side effects include headache, GI problems, and dizziness. Contraindicated for pregnancy and lactation and for patients with bleeding disorder. Possible compound effect with concomitant use of aspirin or anticoagulants.
Ginseng *(Panax ginseng)*	The ancient Chinese believed this herb increased wisdom and longevity. Current studies support a possible positive effect on the cardiovascular system. Action not known.	Generally considered safe. Side effects may include headache, insomnia, anxiety, skin rashes, diarrhea. Avoid concomitant use with anticoagulants.
Hops *(Humulus lupulus)*	Used in cases of nervousness, mild anxiety, and insomnia. Also may relieve the cramping associated with diarrhea. May be taken as a tea, in extracts, or capsules.	Generally recognized as safe when consumed in recommended dosages.

(*Continued*)

TABLE 22–1 **Herbal Remedies** (Continued)

Common Names (Botanical Name)	**Medicinal Uses/ Possible Action**	**Safety Profile**
Kava-Kava *(Piper methysticum)*	Used to reduce anxiety while promoting mental acuity. Dosage range: 150–300 mg bid.	Generally considered safe. May cause scaly skin rash when taken at the higher dosage range for long periods. Concurrent use with CNS depressants may produce additive tranquilizing effects. Recent indication of potential liver toxicity. FDA is investigating.
Passion flower *(Passiflora incarnata)*	Used in tea, capsules, or extracts to treat nervousness and insomnia. Depresses the CNS to produce a mild sedative effect.	Generally recognized as safe in recommended doses.
Peppermint *(Mentha piperita)*	Used as a tea to relieve upset stomachs and headaches and as a mild sedative. Pour boiling water over 1 tbsp. dried leaves and steep to make tea.	Considered safe when consumed in normal quantities.
Psyllium *(Plantago ovata) (Plantago major)*	Psyllium seeds are a popular bulk laxative commonly used for chronic constipation.	Approved as an over-the-counter drug in the United States.
Skullcap *(Scutellaria lateriflora)*	Used as a sedative for mild anxiety and nervousness.	Considered safe in reasonable amounts.
St. John's Wort *(Hypericum perforatum)*	Used in the treatment of mild to moderate depression. May block reuptake of serotonin/norepinephrine and have a mild monoamine oxidase inhibiting effect. Effective dose: 900 mg/day. May also have antiviral, antibacterial, and anti-inflammatory properties.	Generally recognized as safe when taken at recommended dosages. Side effects include mild GI irritation that is lessened with food; photosensitivity when taken in high dosages over long periods. Do not take with other psychoactive medications.

TABLE 22–1 **Herbal Remedies**

Common Names (Botanical Name)	Medicinal Uses/ Possible Action	Safety Profile
Valerian (*Valeriana officinalis)*	Used to treat insomnia. Produces restful sleep without morning "hangover." The root may be used to make a tea, or capsules are available in a variety of dosages. Mechanism of action is similar to that of benzodiazepines but without addicting properties. Daily dosage range: 100–1000 mg.	Generally recognized as safe when taken at recommended dosages. Side effects may include mild headache or upset stomach. Taking doses higher than recommended may result in severe headache, nausea, morning grogginess, and blurry vision. Should not be taken concurrently with CNS depressants.

Sources: Adapted from Guinness (1993); Kaplan & Sadock (1998); Institute for Natural Resources (1998); Yeager, 1998; and PDR for Herbal Medicines (2000).

body distant to another, because they are linked by a meridian. Credit and associates (1998) state, "The goal of traditional Chinese medicine is to keep the body in balance and harmony through the free flow of chi. Disease is a result of blockages in this energy current."

In acupressure, the fingers, thumbs, palms, or elbows are used to apply pressure to the acupoints. This pressure is thought to dissolve any obstructions in the flow of healing energy and to restore the body to a healthier functioning. In acupuncture, hair-thin, sterile, disposable, stainless-steel needles are inserted into acupoints to dissolve the obstructions along the meridians. The needles may be left in place for a specified amount of time, they may be rotated, or a mild electric current may be applied. An occasional tingling or numbness is experienced, but little to no pain is associated with the treatment (Credit et al, 1998).

The Western medical philosophy regarding acupressure and acupuncture is that they stimulate the body's own painkilling chemicals—the morphine-like substances known as *endorphins.* The treatment has been found to be effective in the treatment of asthma, headaches, dysmenorrhea, cervical pain, insomnia, anxiety, depression, substance abuse, stroke rehabilitation, nausea of pregnancy, postoperative and chemotherapy-induced nausea and vomiting, tennis elbow, fibromyalgia, low back pain, and carpal tunnel syndrome (Kaplan & Sadock, 1998; National Institutes of Health, 1997). A recent study suggests that acupuncture may aid in the treatment of cocaine dependence (Avants et al, 2000).

Acupuncture is gaining wide acceptance in the United States by patients and physicians. This treatment can be administered at the same time other techniques are being used, such as conventional Western techniques, although it is essential that all health-care providers have knowledge of all treatments being received. Acupuncture should be administered by a physician or an acupuncturist who is board certified by the National Commission for the Certification of Acupuncturists, which requires more than 1000 hours of acupuncture training. Currently, 34 states have set licensure standards for acupuncturists (Institute for Natural Resources, 1998).

Diet and Nutrition

The value of nutrition in the healing process has long been underrated. Lutz & Przytulski (1994) state:

> Today many diseases are linked to lifestyle behaviors such as smoking, lack of adequate physical activity, and poor nutritional habits. Health care providers, in their role as educators, emphasize the relationship between lifestyle and risk of contracting disease. People are increasingly managing their health problems and making personal commitments to lead healthier lives. Nutrition is, in part, a preventive science. How and what one eats is a lifestyle choice. (p. 5)

Individuals select the foods they eat based on a number of factors, not the least of which is enjoyment. Eating must serve social and cultural as well as nutritional needs. The U.S. Departments of Agriculture (USDA) and Health and Human Services (USDHHS) have collaborated on a set of guidelines to help individuals understand what types of foods to eat in order to promote health and prevent disease. Following is a list of these guidelines (USDA/USDHHS, 1995):

1. **Eat a Variety of Foods.** No single food can supply all nutrients in the amounts needed for good health. A variety of foods should be selected from the Food Guide Pyramid (Fig. 22–1). Most of the daily servings of food should be selected from the food groups that are the largest in the figure and closest to the base of the pyramid. A range of servings is suggested for each group of foods. Smaller, sedentary persons should select the lower number of servings. The higher number of servings are meant for larger, more active individuals. Table 22–2 provides a summary of information about essential vitamins and minerals.
2. **Balance the Food You Eat with Physical Activity—Maintain or Improve Your Weight.** Many individuals gain weight with age, increasing their chances of developing a number of health problems associated with excess weight. These problems include high blood pressure, heart disease, stroke, diabetes, certain types of cancer, arthritis, breathing problems, and other illnesses. Thirty minutes or more of moderate physical activity, such as walking, 3 to 5 days

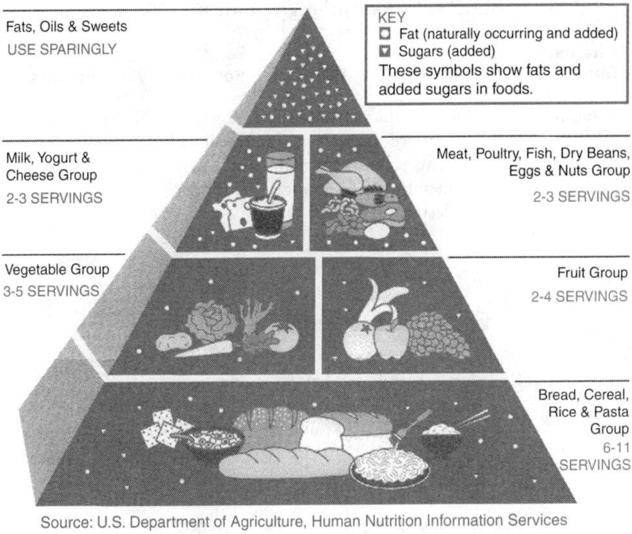

Figure 22–1 The Food Pyramid.

TABLE 22–2 **Essential Vitamins and Minerals**

Vitamin/ Mineral	Function	RDA*	Food Sources	Comments
Vitamin A	Prevention of night blindness; calcification of growing bones; resistance to infection	Men:1000 μg Women: 800 μg	Liver, butter, cheese, whole milk, egg yolk, fish liver oil, green leafy vegetables, carrots	May be of benefit in prevention of cancer due to antioxidant properties associated with control of free radicals that damage DNA and cell membranes.
Vitamin D	Promotes absorption of calcium and phosphorus in small intestine; prevention of rickets	Men:5 μg Women: 5 μg	Fortified milk and dairy products; egg yolk, fish liver oils, liver, oysters; formed in skin by exposure to sunlight	Without vitamin D, very little dietary calcium can be absorbed.

(Continued)

TABLE 22–2 **Essential Vitamins and Minerals**

Vitamin/ Mineral	Function	RDA*	Food Sources	Comments
Vitamin E	Antioxidant that prevents cell membrane destruction	Men: 10 mg Women: 8 mg	Vegetable oils, wheat germ, whole grain or fortified cereals, green leafy vegetables	As an antioxidant, may have implications in prevention of Alzheimer's disease, heart disease, breast cancer.
Vitamin K	Synthesis of prothrombin and other clotting factors; normal blood coagulation	Men: 80 μg Women: 65 μg	Formed in intestines by bacteria; also found in green leafy vegetables, meats, dairy products	
Vitamin C	Formation of collagen in connective tissues; a powerful antioxidant; facilitates iron absorption; aids in release of epinephrine from adrenal glands during stress	Men and women: 60 mg	Citrus fruits, tomatoes, potatoes, green leafy vegetables, strawberries	As an antioxidant, may have implications in the prevention of cancer, cataracts, heart disease. It may stimulate immune system to fight various types of infection.
Vitamin B_1 (Thiamine)	Essential for normal functioning of nervous tissue; coenzyme in carbohydrate metabolism	Men: 1.5 mg Women: 1.1 mg	Whole grains, legumes, nuts, egg yolk, meat, green leafy vegetables	Large doses may improve mental performance in people with Alzheimer's disease.

TABLE 22–2 **Essential Vitamins and Minerals**

Vitamin/ Mineral	Function	RDA*	Food Sources	Comments
Vitamin B_2 (Riboflavin)	Coenzyme in metabolism of protein and carbohydrate	Men: 1.7 mg Women: 1.3 mg	Meat, dairy products, whole or enriched grains, legumes	May help in prevention of cataracts; high-dose therapy may be effective in migraine prophylaxis (Schoenen et al, 1998).
Vitamin B_3 (Niacin)	Coenzyme in metabolism of protein and carbohydrate	Men: 19 mg Women: 15 mg	Milk, eggs, meats, legumes, whole grain and enriched cereals	High doses of niacin have been successful in decreasing levels of cholesterol in some individuals.
Vitamin B_6 (Pyridoxine)	Coenzyme in synthesis and catabolism of amino acids. Essential for metabolism of tryptophan to niacin	Men:2 mg Women: 1.6 mg	Meat, fish, grains, legumes, bananas, figs	May decrease depression in some individuals by increasing levels of serotonin; deficiencies may contribute to memory problems; also used in the treatment of migraines and premenstrual discomfort.
Vitamin B_{12}	Necessary in formation of DNA and production of red blood cells; associated with folic acid metabolism	Men and women: 2 μg	Found in animal products (e.g., meats, eggs, dairy products)	Deficiency may contribute to memory problems. Vegetarians can get this vitamin from fortified foods. Intrinsic factor must be present in the stomach for absorption of vitamin B_{12}.

(*Continued*)

TABLE 22–2 **Essential Vitamins and Minerals**

Vitamin/ Mineral	Function	RDA*	Food Sources	Comments
Folic Acid (Folate)	Necessary in formation of DNA and production of red blood cells	Men: 200 µg Women: 180 µg	Meat, green leafy vegetables, beans, peas, oranges, cantaloupe	Important in women of childbearing age to prevent fetal neural tube defects; may contribute to prevention of heart disease and colon cancer
Calcium	Necessary in formation of bones and teeth; neuron and muscle functioning; blood clotting	Men and women: 800 mg	Dairy products, green leafy vegetables, sardines, oysters, salmon	Calcium has been associated with prevention of headaches, muscle cramps, osteoporosis, and premenstrual problems. Requires vitamin D for absorption.
Phosphorus	Necessary in formation of bones and teeth; a component of DNA, RNA, adenosine diphosphate, and adenosine triphosphate; helps control acid-base balance in the blood	Men and women: 800 mg	Milk, cheese, fish, meat	

TABLE 22–2 **Essential Vitamins and Minerals**

Vitamin/ Mineral	Function	RDA*	Food Sources	Comments
Magnesium	Protein synthesis and carbohydrate metabolism; muscular relaxation following contraction; bone formation	Men: 350 mg Women: 280 mg	Green vegetables, legumes, seafood, milk	May aid in prevention of asthmatic attacks and migraine headaches. Deficiencies may contribute to insomnia and premenstrual problems.
Iron	Synthesis of hemoglobin and myoglobin; cellular oxidation	Men and women: 10 mg (women who breastfeed and women of childbearing age: 15 mg)	Meats, egg yolks, shellfish, dark green leafy vegetables, dried fruit	Iron deficiencies can result in headaches and feeling chronically fatigued.
Iodine	Aids in synthesis of T_3 and T_4	Men and women: 150 μg	Iodized salt, seafood	Exerts strong controlling influence on overall body metabolism.
Selenium	Works with vitamin E to protect cellular compounds from oxidation	Men: 70 μg Women: 55 μg	Seafood, low-fat meats, whole grains, dairy products, legumes	As an antioxidant combined with vitamin E, may have some anticancer effect. Deficiency has also been associated with depressed mood.

(*Continued*)

TABLE 22–2 **Essential Vitamins and Minerals**

Vitamin/ Mineral	Function	RDA*	Food Sources	Comments
Zinc	Involved in synthesis of DNA and RNA; energy metabolism and protein synthesis; wound healing; increased immune functioning; necessary for normal smell and taste sensation.	Men and women: 15 mg	Meat, seafood, grains, legumes	An important source for prevention of infection and improvement in wound healing.

* Recommended dietary allowances

SOURCES: Adapted from Yeager (1998); Lutz & Przytulski (2001); Scanlon & Sanders (1999); Institute for Natural Resources (1998)

each week can help to increase calorie expenditure and maintain a healthy weight.

3. **Choose a Diet with Plenty of Grain Products, Vegetables, and Fruits.** Consumption of these foods is associated with a substantially lower risk for many chronic diseases, including certain types of cancer. These foods are emphasized in this guideline because they are an excellent source of vitamins, minerals, and complex carbohydrates (starch and dietary fiber). They are also low in fat, depending on how they are prepared.
4. **Choose a Diet Low in Fat, Saturated Fat, and Cholesterol.** Heart disease and some types of cancer (e.g., breast and colon) have been linked to high-fat diets. Some dietary fat is required for good health. Fats supply energy and essential fatty acids and promote absorption of the fat-soluble vitamins A, D, E, and K. However, fats should comprise no more than 30 percent of the total daily calorie intake. Individuals should choose foods with mono- and polyunsaturated fat sources and keep daily cholesterol intake below 300 mg.
5. **Choose a Diet Moderate in Sugars.** Many foods that contain sugars supply unnecessary calories and few nutrients. Tooth decay is a significant health problem resulting from eating too much sugar. Scientific evidence indicates that diets high in sugar do not cause hyperactivity or diabetes. A study by Dr. W.B. Grant of the Atmospheric Sciences Division of NASA's Langley Research Center reports that sugar may be the highest dietary risk factor for heart disease in women 35 years and older (*Sunday Oklahoman,*

1998). He states, "Fructose metabolizes into triglycerides, then is incorporated into very low density lipoprotein cholesterol." Sugars should be used in moderation by most healthy people and sparingly by people with low calorie needs.

6. **Choose a Diet Moderate in Salt and Sodium.** Sodium and sodium chloride (salt) occur naturally in foods, usually in small amounts. Most foods are prepared with some salt, and some is added during processing. Studies with many diverse populations have established that a high intake of salt is associated with high blood pressure. It is therefore important for individuals at risk for high blood pressure to consume less salt in their diets (as well as increase physical activity and control weight).
7. **Drink Alcoholic Beverages in Moderation.** High levels of alcohol intake raise the risk for high blood pressure, stroke, heart disease, and certain cancers. It also may lead to accidents, violence, suicides, and birth defects. Too much alcohol may cause cirrhosis of the liver, inflammation of the pancreas, and damage to the brain and heart. Heavy drinkers also are at risk of malnutrition because alcohol contains calories that may substitute for those in more nutritious foods. The USDA/USDHHS (1995) report defines "moderation" as follows:

    No more than one drink per day for women, and no more than two drinks per day for men. Count as a drink:
    - 12 ounces of regular beer (150 calories)
    - 5 ounces of wine (100 calories)
    - 1.5 ounces of 80-proof distilled spirits (100 calories)

Good nutrition can help with adaptation to the inevitable stresses of life by promoting a healthy body and a feeling of well-being. Knowledge of good nutrition is learned and not necessarily something that comes naturally. Nurses are in an ideal situation for providing individuals with this type of information.

Chiropractic Medicine

Chiropractic is probably the most widely used form of alternative healing in the United States. It was developed in the late 1800s by a self-taught healer named David Palmer. It was later reorganized and expanded by his son Joshua, a trained practitioner. Palmer's objective was to find a cure for disease and illness that did not rely on drugs, which he considered harmful (Guinness, 1993). Palmer's theory of chiropractic medicine was that energy flows from the brain to all parts of the body through the spinal cord and spinal nerves. When vertebrae of the spinal column become displaced, they may press on a nerve and interfere with normal nerve transmission. Palmer named the displacement of these vertebrae *subluxation*, and he alleged that the way to restore normal function was to manipulate the vertebrae back into their normal positions. These manipulations are called *adjustments* (Guinness, 1993).

Adjustments are usually performed by hand, although some chiropractors have special treatment tables equipped to facilitate these manipulations. Other processes used to facilitate the outcome of the spinal adjustment by providing muscle relaxation include massage tables, application of heat or cold, and ultrasound treatments.

The chiropractor takes a medical history and performs a clinical examination, which usually includes x-rays of the spine. Today's chiropractors may practice "straight" therapy; that is, the only therapy provided is that of subluxation adjustments. *Mixer* is a term applied to a chiropractor who combines adjustments with adjunct therapies, such as exercise, heat treatments, or massage.

Individuals seek treatment from chiropractors for many types of ailments and illnesses; the most common type is back pain. In addition, chiropractors treat clients with headaches, sciatica, shoulder pain, tennis and golfer's elbow, leg and foot pain, hand and wrist pain, allergies, asthma, stomach disorders, and menstrual problems (Guinness, 1993). Some chiropractors are employed by professional sports teams as their team physicians.

Chiropractors are licensed to practice in all 50 states, and treatment is covered by government and most private insurance plans. They treat approximately 20 million people in the United States annually (Kaplan & Sadock, 1998).

Therapeutic Touch and Massage

Therapeutic Touch

The technique of therapeutic touch was developed in the 1970s by Dolores Krieger, a nurse associated with the New York University School of Nursing. This therapy is based on the philosophy that the human body projects a field of energy around it. When this field of energy becomes blocked, pain or illness occurs. Practitioners of therapeutic touch use this technique to correct the blockages, thereby relieving the discomfort and improving health.

Based on the premise that the energy field extends beyond the surface of the body, the practitioner need not actually touch the client's skin. The therapist's hands are passed over the client's body, remaining two to four inches from the skin. The goal is to repattern the energy field (Credit et al, 1998) by performing slow, rhythmic, sweeping hand motions over the entire body. Heat should be felt where the energy is blocked. The therapist "massages" the energy field in that area, smoothing it out, and thus correcting the obstruction. Therapeutic touch is thought to reduce pain and anxiety and promote relaxation and health maintenance. It has been useful in the treatment of chronic health conditions.

Massage

Massage is the technique of manipulating the muscles and soft tissues of the body. Chinese physicians prescribed massage for the treatment of disease more than 5000 years ago. The Eastern style focuses on balancing the body's vital energy (chi) as it flows through pathways (meridians), as described earlier in the discussion of acupressure and acupuncture. The Western style of massage affects muscles, connective tissues (e.g., tendons and ligaments), and the cardiovascular system. The Swedish massage, which is probably the best-known Western style, uses a variety of gliding and kneading strokes along with deep circular movements and vibrations to relax the muscles, improve circulation, and increase mobility (Guinness, 1993).

Massage has been shown to be beneficial in anxiety, chronic back and neck pain, arthritis, sciatica, migraine headaches, muscle spasms, insomnia, pain of labor and delivery, stress-related disorders, and whiplash. Massage is contraindicated in certain conditions, such as high blood pressure, acute infection, osteoporosis, phlebitis, skin conditions, and varicose veins. It also should not be performed over the site of a recent injury, bruise, or burn.

Massage therapists require specialized training in a program accredited by the American Massage Therapy Association and must pass the National Certification Examination for Therapeutic Massage and Bodywork.

Yoga

Yoga is thought to have developed in India some 5000 years ago and is attributed to an Indian physician and Sanskrit scholar named Patanjali. The ultimate goal of yoga is to unite the human soul with the universal spirit (Guinness, 1993). Yoga has been found to be especially helpful in relieving stress and in improving overall physical and psychological wellness. Proper breathing is a major component of yoga. It is believed that yoga breathing—a deep, diaphragmatic breathing—increases oxygen to brain and body tissues, thereby easing stress and fatigue and boosting energy.

Another component of yoga is meditation. Individuals who practice the meditation and deep breathing associated with yoga find that they are able to achieve a profound feeling of relaxation.

The most familiar type of yoga practiced in Western countries is hatha yoga. Hatha yoga uses body postures, along with the meditation and breathing exercises, to achieve a balanced, disciplined workout that releases muscle tension, tones the internal organs, and energizes the mind, body, and spirit to allow natural healing to occur (Credit et al, 1998). The complete routine of poses is designed to work all parts of the body, stretching and toning muscles and keeping joints flexible. Studies have shown that yoga has provided beneficial effects to some individuals with back pain, stress, migraine, insomnia, high blood pressure, rapid heart rates, and limited mobility (Guinness, 1993).

Pet Therapy

The therapeutic value of pets is no longer just theory. Evidence has shown that animals can directly influence a person's mental and physical well-being. Many pet-therapy programs have been established across the country, and the numbers are increasing regularly.

Several studies have provided information about the positive results of human interaction with pets. Some of these include the following:

1. One year following heart attack, clients who have pets have one-fifth the death rate of those who do not (Friedmann & Thomas, 1995).
2. Petting a dog or cat has been shown to lower blood pressure. In one study, volunteers experienced a 7.1–mm Hg drop in systolic and an 8.1–mm Hg decrease in diastolic blood pressure when they talked to and petted their dogs, as opposed to reading aloud or resting quietly (Whitaker, 2000).
3. Bringing a pet into a nursing home or hospital has been shown to enhance a client's mood and social interaction (Sobel & Ornstein, 1996). Some researchers believe that animals actually may retard the aging process among those who live alone. Loneliness often results in premature death, and having a pet mitigates the effects of loneliness and isolation.

Whitaker (2000) suggests:

> Though owning a pet doesn't make you immune to illness, pet owners are, on the whole, healthier than those who don't own pets. Study after study shows that people with pets have fewer minor health problems, require fewer visits to the doctor and less medication, and have fewer risk factors for heart disease, such as high blood pressure or cholesterol levels. (p. 7)

It may never be known precisely why animals affect humans the way they do, but for those who have pets to love, it comes as no surprise. Pets provide unconditional, nonjudgmental love and affection, which can be the perfect antidote for a depressed mood or a stressful situation. The role of animals in the human healing process still requires more research, but its validity is now widely accepted in both the medical and lay communities.

■ SUMMARY

Complementary therapies help the practitioner view the client in a holistic manner. Most complementary therapies consider the mind and body connection and strive to enhance the body's own natural healing powers. The OAM within NIH has established a list of alternative therapies to be used in practice and for investigative purposes. More than $15 billion a year is spent on alternative medical therapies in the United States.

This chapter examined herbal medicine, acupressure, acupuncture, diet and nutrition, chiropractic medicine, therapeutic touch, massage, yoga, and pet therapy. Nurses must be familiar with these therapies, as more and more clients seek the healing properties of these complementary strategies to traditional care.

INTERNET REFERENCES

- http://www.herbalgram.org
- http://www.herbmed.org
- http://www.eatright.org
- http://www.chiropractic.org
- http://www.pawssf.org
- http://www.superdog.com/therapy.htm
- http://www.holisticmed.com/www/acupuncture.html
- http://www.americanyogaassociation.org

CHAPTER 23

Loss and Bereavement

■ BACKGROUND ASSESSMENT DATA

Loss is the experience of separation from something of personal importance. Loss is anything that is perceived as such by the individual. The separation from loved ones or the giving up of treasured possessions, for whatever reason; the experience of failure, either real or perceived; or life events that create change in a familiar pattern of existence—all can be experienced as loss, and all can trigger behaviors associated with the grieving process. Loss and bereavement are universal events encountered by all beings who experience emotions. Following are examples of some notable forms of loss:

1. A significant other (person or pet) through death, divorce, or separation for any reason.
2. Illness or debilitating conditions. Examples include (but are not limited to) diabetes, stroke, cancer, rheumatoid arthritis, multiple sclerosis, Alzheimer's disease, hearing or vision loss, and spinal cord or head injuries. Some of these conditions not only incur a loss of physical and/or emotional wellness but may also result in the loss of personal independence.
3. Developmental/maturational changes or situations, such as menopause, andropause, infertility, "empty nest" syndrome, aging, impotence, and hysterectomy.
4. A decrease in self-esteem, if one is unable to meet self-expectations or the expectations of others (even if these expectations are only perceived by the individual as unfulfilled). This includes a loss of potential hopes and dreams.
5. Personal possessions that symbolize familiarity and security in a person's life. Separation from these familiar and personally valued external objects represents a loss of material extensions of the self.

Some texts differentiate the terms *mourning* and *grief* by describing mourning as the psychological process (or stages) through which the individual passes on the way to successful adaptation to the loss of a valued object. Grief is thought of as the subjective states that accompany mourning, or the emotional work involved in the mourning process. For purposes of this text, grief work and the process of mourning are collectively referred to as the *grief response.*

Theoretical Perspectives on Loss and Bereavement (Symptomatology)

Stages of Grief

Behavior patterns associated with the grief response include many individual variations. However, sufficient similarities have been observed to warrant characterization of grief as a syndrome that has a predictable course with an expected resolution. Early theorists, including Kübler-Ross (1969), Bowlby (1961), and Engel (1964), described behavioral stages through which individuals advance in their progression toward resolution. A number of variables influence one's progression through the grief process. Some individuals may reach acceptance, only to revert back to an earlier stage; some may never complete the sequence; and some may never progress beyond the initial stage. A comparison of the similarities among these three models is presented in Table 23–1.

TABLE 23–1 **Stages of the Normal Grief Response: A Comparison of Models by Elisabeth Kübler-Ross, John Bowlby, and George Engel**

Kübler-Ross	Bowlby	Engel	Possible Time Dimension	Behaviors
I. Denial	I. Numbness/Protest	I. Shock/Disbelief	Occurs immediately on experiencing loss. Usually lasts no more than 2 weeks.	Individual refuses to acknowledge that loss has occurred.
II. Anger	II. Disequilibrium	II. Developing awareness	In most cases, begins within hours of loss. Peaks within 2 to 4 weeks.	Anger is directed toward self or others. Ambivalence and guilt may be felt toward the lost object.
III. Bargaining				The individual fervently seeks alternatives to improve current situation.

(Continued)

TABLE 23–1 **Stages of the Normal Grief Response: A Comparison of Models by Elisabeth Kübler-Ross, John Bowlby, and George Engel** (Continued)

Kübler-Ross	Bowlby	Engel	Possible Time Dimension	Behaviors
		III. Restitution		Attends to various rituals associated with the culture in which loss has occurred.
IV. Depression	III. Disorganization and despair	IV. Resolution of loss	A year or more.	The actual work of grieving. Preoccupation with lost object. Feelings of helplessness and loneliness occur in response to realization of loss. Feelings associated with loss are confronted.
V. Acceptance	IV. Reorganization	V. Recovery		Resolution is complete. Bereaved person experiences a reinvestment in new relationships and new goals. Terminally ill persons express readiness to die.

A more contemporary grief specialist, J. William Worden (1991), offers a set of tasks that must be processed in order to complete the grief response. He suggests that it is possible for a person to accomplish some of these tasks and not others, resulting in an incomplete bereavement and thus impairing further growth and development.

ELISABETH KÜBLER-ROSS

These well-known stages of the grief process were identified by Kübler-Ross in her extensive work with dying patients. Behaviors associated with each of these stages can be observed in individuals experiencing the loss of any concept of personal value.

Stage I: Denial. The individual does not acknowledge that the loss has occurred. He or she may say, "No, it can't be true!" or "It's just not possible." This stage may protect the individual against the psychological pain of reality.

Stage II: Anger. This is the stage when reality sets in. Feelings associated with this stage include sadness, guilt, shame, helplessness, and hopelessness. Self-blame or blaming of others may lead to feelings of anger toward the self and others. The anxiety level may be elevated, and the individual may experience confusion and a decreased ability to function independently. He or she may be preoccupied with an idealized image of what has been lost. Numerous somatic complaints are common.

Stage III: Bargaining. The individual attempts to strike a bargain with God for a second chance or for more time. The person acknowledges the loss or impending loss but holds out hope for additional alternatives, as evidenced by such statements as, "If only I could ..." or "If only I had ...".

Stage IV: Depression. The individual mourns for what has been or will be lost. This is a very painful stage, during which the individual must confront feelings associated with having lost someone or something of value (called *reactive* depression). An example might be the individual who is mourning a change in body image. Feelings associated with an impending loss (called *preparatory* depression) are also confronted. Examples include permanent lifestyle changes related to the altered body image or even an impending loss of life itself. Regression, withdrawal, and social isolation may be observed behaviors with this stage. Therapeutic intervention should be available but not imposed and with guidelines for implementation based on client readiness.

Stage V: Acceptance. The individual has worked through the behaviors associated with the other stages and either accepts or is resigned to the loss. Anxiety decreases, and methods for coping with the loss have been established. The client is less preoccupied with what has been lost and increasingly interested in other aspects of the environment. If this is an impending death of self, the individual is ready to die. The person may become very quiet and withdrawn, seemingly devoid of feelings. These behaviors are an attempt to facilitate the passage by slowly disengaging from the environment.

JOHN BOWLBY

John Bowlby hypothesized four stages in the grief process. He implied that these behaviors can be observed in all individuals who have experienced the loss of something or someone of value, even in babies as young as 6 months.

Stage I: Numbness or Protest. This stage is characterized by a feeling of shock and disbelief that the loss has occurred. Reality of the loss is not acknowledged.

Stage II: Disequilibrium. The individual has a profound urge to recover what has been lost. Behaviors associated with this stage include a preoccupation with the loss, intense weeping and expressions of anger toward the self and others, and feelings of ambivalence and guilt associated with the loss.

Stage III: Disorganization and Despair. Feelings of despair occur in response to the realization that the loss has occurred. Activities of daily living become increasingly disorganized, and behavior is characterized by restlessness and aimlessness. Efforts to regain productive patterns of behavior are ineffective, and the individual experiences fear, helplessness, and hopelessness. Somatic complaints are common. Perceptions of visualizing or being in the presence of what has been lost may occur. Social isolation is common, and the individual may feel a great deal of loneliness.

Stage IV: Reorganization. The individual accepts or becomes resigned to the loss. New goals and patterns of organization are established. The individual begins a reinvestment in new relationships and indicates a readiness to move forward within the environment. Grief subsides and recedes into valued remembrances.

George Engel

Stage I: Shock and Disbelief. The initial reaction to a loss is a stunned, numb feeling and refusal by the individual to acknowledge the reality of the loss. Engel states that this stage is an attempt by the individual to protect the self "against the effects of the overwhelming stress by raising the threshold against its recognition or against the painful feelings evoked thereby."

Stage II: Developing Awareness. This stage begins within minutes to hours of the loss. Behaviors include excessive crying and regression to a state of helplessness and a childlike manner. Awareness of the loss creates feelings of emptiness, frustration, anguish, and despair. Anger may be directed toward the self or toward others in the environment who are held accountable for the loss.

Stage III: Restitution. The various rituals associated with loss within a culture are performed. Examples include funerals, wakes, special attire, a gathering of friends and family, and religious practices customary to the spiritual beliefs of the bereaved. Participation in these rituals is thought to assist the individual to accept the reality of the loss and to facilitate the recovery process.

Stage IV: Resolution of the Loss. This stage is characterized by a preoccupation with the loss. The concept of the loss is idealized, and the individual may even imitate admired qualities of a person who has been lost. Preoccupation with the loss gradually decreases over a year or more, and the individual eventually begins to reinvest feelings in others.

Stage V: Recovery. Obsession with the loss has ended, and the individual is able to go on with his or her life.

J. William Worden

Worden views the bereaved as active and self-determining rather than passive participants in the grief process. He proposes that bereavement includes a set of tasks that must be reconciled in order to complete the grief process. Worden's four tasks of mourning include the following:

Task I: Accepting the Reality of the Loss. When something of value is lost, it is common for individuals to refuse to believe that the loss has occurred. Behaviors include misidentifying individuals in the environment for their lost loved one, retaining possessions of the lost loved one as though he or she has not died, and removing all reminders of the lost loved one so as not to have to face the reality of the loss. Worden states: "Coming to an acceptance of the reality of the loss takes time since it involves not only an intellectual acceptance but also an emotional one. The bereaved person may be intellectually aware of the finality of the loss long before the emotions allow full acceptance of the information as true." (p. 12) Belief and denial are intermittent while grappling with this task. It is thought that traditional rituals such as the funeral help some individuals move toward acceptance of the loss.

Task II: Working Through the Pain of Grief. Pain associated with a loss includes physical pain and emotional pain. This pain must be acknowledged and worked through. To avoid or suppress it serves only to delay or prolong the grieving process. People accomplish this by refusing to allow themselves to think painful thoughts, by idealizing or avoiding reminders of what has been lost, and by using alcohol or drugs. The intensity of the pain and the manner in which it is experienced are different for all individuals, but the commonality is that the pain *must* be experienced. Failure to do so generally results in some form of depression that commonly requires therapy, which then focuses on working through the pain of grief that the individual failed to work through at the time of the loss. In this very difficult Task II, individuals must "indulge the pain of loss—to feel it and to know that one day it will pass." (p. 14)

Task III: Adjusting to an Environment that has Changed Because of the Loss. It usually takes a number of months for a bereaved person to realize what his or her world will be like without what has been lost. In the case of a lost loved one, how the environment changes will depend on the types of roles that person fulfilled in life. In the case of a changed lifestyle, the individual will be required to make adaptations to his or her environment in terms of the changes as they are presented in daily life. In addition, those individuals who had defined their identity through what was lost will require an adjustment to their own sense of self. Worden states, "The coping strategy of redefining the loss in such a way that it can redound to the benefit of the survivor is often part of the successful completion of Task III." (p. 15)

If the bereaved person experiences failures in his or her attempt to adjust in an environment without the valued person or thing, feelings of low self-esteem may result. Regressed behaviors and feelings of helplessness and inadequacy are not uncommon. Worden states:

> [Another] area of adjustment may be to one's sense of the world. Loss through death can challenge one's fundamental life values and philosophical beliefs—beliefs that are influenced by our families, peers, education, and religion as well as life experiences. The bereaved person searches for meaning in the loss and its attendant life changes in order to make sense of it and to regain some control of his or her life. (pp. 15–16)

To be successful in Task III, bereaved individuals must develop new skills to cope and adapt to their new environment without what was lost. Successful achievement of this task determines the outcome of the mourning process—continued growth or a state of arrested development.

Task IV: Emotionally Relocating What Was Lost and Moving on with Life. This task allows for the bereaved person to identify a special place for what was lost. Individuals need not purge from their history or find a replacement for what was lost; instead, there is a kind of continued presence of the lost concept in the life of the bereaved. The lost concept is *relocated* in the life of the bereaved. Successful completion of Task IV involves letting go of past attachments and forming new ones. However, there is also the recognition that although the relationship between the bereaved and what was lost is changed, it is nonetheless still a relationship. Worden states:

> One never loses memories of a significant relationship. For many people Task IV is the most difficult one to accomplish. They get stuck at this point in their grieving and later realize that their life in some way stopped at the point the loss occurred. (pp. 17–18)

Worden relates the story of a teenage girl who had a difficult time adjusting to the death of her father. After 2 years, when she began to finally fulfill some of the tasks associated with successful grieving, she wrote these words that express rather clearly what bereaved people in Task IV are struggling with: "There are other people to be loved, and it doesn't mean that I love Dad any less." (p. 18)

Length of the Grief Process

Stages of grief allow bereaved persons an orderly approach to the resolution of mourning. Each stage presents tasks that must be overcome through a painful experiential process. Engel (1964) states that successful resolution of the grief response is thought to have occurred when a bereaved individual is able "to remember comfortably and realistically both the pleasures and disappointments of [what is lost]." The duration of the grief process depends on the individual and can last for a number of years without being maladaptive. The acute phase of normal grieving usually lasts 6 to 8 weeks—longer in older adults—but complete resolution of the grief response may take much longer. Kaplan and Sadock (1998) state:

> Traditionally, grief lasts about six months to one year, as the grieving person experiences the calendar year at least once without the lost person. Some signs and symptoms of grief may persist much longer than one or two years, and a survivor may have various grief-related feelings, symptoms, and behavior throughout life. In general, the acute grief symptoms gradually lessen, and within one or two months the grieving person is able to eat, sleep, and return to functioning. (p. 71)

A number of factors influence the eventual outcome of the grief response. The grief response can be more difficult if:

- The bereaved person was strongly dependent on or perceived what was lost as an important means of physical and/or emotional support.
- The relationship with what was lost was highly ambivalent. A love-hate relationship may instill feelings of guilt that can interfere with the grief work.
- The individual has experienced a number of recent losses. Grief tends to be cumulative, and if previous losses have not been resolved, each succeeding grief response becomes more difficult.
- The loss is that of a young person. Grief over loss of a child is often more intense than it is over the loss of an elderly person.
- The state of the person's physical or psychological health is unstable at the time of the loss.
- The bereaved person perceives (whether real or imagined) some responsibility for the loss.

The grief response may be facilitated if:

- The individual has the support of significant others to assist him or her through the mourning process.
- The individual has the opportunity to prepare for the loss. Grief work is more intense when the loss is sudden and unexpected. The experience of *anticipatory grieving* is thought to facilitate the grief response that occurs at the time of the actual loss.

Worden (1991) states:

> There is a sense in which mourning can be finished, when people regain an interest in life, feel more hopeful, experience gratification again, and adapt to new roles. There is also a sense in which mourning is never finished. [People must understand] that mourning is a long-term process, and the culmination [very likely] will not be to a pre-grief state. (pp. 18–19)

Anticipatory Grief

Anticipatory grieving is the experiencing of the feelings and emotions associated with the normal grief response before the loss actually occurs. One dissimilar aspect relates to the fact that conventional grief tends to diminish in intensity with the passage of time. Conversely, anticipatory grief may increase in intensity as the expected loss becomes more imminent.

Although anticipatory grief is thought to facilitate the actual mourning process, there may be some problems. In the case of a dying person, difficulties can arise when the family members complete the process of anticipatory grief and detachment from the dying person occurs prematurely. The person who is dying experiences feelings of loneliness and isolation as the psychological pain of imminent death is faced without family support. Kaplan and Sadock (1998) describe another example of difficulty associated with premature completion of the grief response: "Once anticipatory grief has been expended, the bereaved person may find it difficult to reestablish a previous relationship; this phenomenon is experienced with the return of persons long gone (for example, to war or confined to concentration camps) and of persons thought to have been dead." (p. 71)

Anticipatory grieving may serve as a defense for some individuals to ease the burden of loss when it actually occurs. It may prove to be less functional for others who, because of interpersonal, psychological, or sociocultural variables, are unable in advance of the actual loss to express the intense feelings that accompany the grief response.

Maladaptive Responses to Loss

When is the grieving response considered to be maladaptive? Three types of pathological grief reactions have been described. These are delayed or inhibited grief, an exaggerated or distorted grief response, and chronic or prolonged grief.

Delayed or Inhibited Grief

This type refers to the absence of evidence of grief when it ordinarily would be expected. Many times, cultural influences, such as the expectation to keep a "stiff upper lip," cause the delayed response.

This type of grief is potentially pathological because the person is simply not dealing with the reality of the loss. He or she remains fixed in the denial stage of the grief process, sometimes for many years. When this occurs, the grief response may be triggered, sometimes many years later, when the individual experiences a subsequent loss. Sometimes the grief process is triggered spontaneously or in response to a seemingly insignificant event. Overreaction to another person's loss may be one manifestation of delayed grief.

The recognition of delayed grief is critical because, depending on the profoundness of the loss, the failure of the mourning process may prevent assimilation of the loss and thereby delay a return to a satisfying living. Delayed grieving most commonly occurs because of ambivalent feelings toward what was lost, outside pressure to resume normal function, or perceived lack of internal and external resources to cope with a profound loss.

Distorted (Exaggerated) Grief Response

In the distorted grief reaction, all of the symptoms associated with normal grieving are exaggerated. Feelings of sadness, helplessness, hopelessness, powerlessness, anger, and guilt as well as numerous somatic complaints render the individual dysfunctional in terms of management of daily living. Murray and Zentner (1997) describe an exaggerated grief reaction in the following way: "an intensification of grief to the point that the person is overwhelmed, demonstrates prolonged maladaptive behavior, manifests excessive symptoms and extensive interruptions in healing, and does not progress to integration of the loss, finding meaning in the loss, and resolution of the mourning process." (p. 800)

When the exaggerated reaction occurs, the individual remains fixed in the anger stage. This anger may be directed toward others in the environment to whom the individual may be attributing the loss. However, many times the anger is turned inward on the self. When this occurs, depression is the result. Depressive mood disorder is a type of exaggerated grief reaction.

Chronic or Prolonged Grieving

Some authors have discussed a chronic or prolonged grief response as a type of maladaptive grief response. Care must be taken in making this determination because, as was stated previously, duration of the grief response is highly individual. An adaptive response may take years for some people. A prolonged process may be considered maladaptive when certain behaviors are exhibited. Prolonged grief may be a problem when behaviors are in evidence such as maintaining personal possessions aimed at keeping a lost loved one alive (as though he or she will eventually reenter the life of the bereaved) or disabling behaviors that prevent the bereaved from adaptively performing activities of daily living. Another example is of a widow who refused to participate in family gatherings following the death of her husband. For many years until her own death, she took a sandwich to the cemetery on holidays, sat on the tombstone, and ate her "holiday meal" with her husband. Other bereaved individuals have been known to set a place at the table for the deceased loved one long after the completed mourning process would have been expected.

Normal Versus Maladaptive Grieving

Several authors have identified one crucial difference between normal and maladaptive grieving: the loss of self-esteem. Kaplan, Sadock, and Grebb (1994) assert that "marked feelings of worthlessness" are indicative of depression rather than uncomplicated bereavement. Eisendrath (1996) affirms, "Grief is usually accompanied by intact self-esteem, whereas depression is marked by a sense of guilt and worthlessness." (p. 939) It is thought that this major difference between normal grieving and maladaptive grieving (the feeling of worthlessness or low self-esteem) ultimately precipitates depression.

Concepts of Death—Developmental Issues

Children

Birth to Age 2. Infants are unable to recognize and understand death, but they can experience the feelings of loss and separation. Infants who are separated from their mother may become quiet, lose weight, and sleep less. Children at this age will likely sense changes in the atmosphere of the home where a death has occurred. They often react to the emotions of adults by becoming more irritable and crying more.

Ages 3 to 5. Preschoolers and kindergartners have some understanding about death but often have difficulty distinguishing between fantasy and reality. They believe death is reversible, and their thoughts about death may include magical thinking. For example, they may believe that their thoughts or behaviors caused a person to become sick or to die.

Children of this age are capable of understanding at least some of what they see and hear from adult conversations or media reports. They become frightened if they feel a threat to themselves or to their loved ones. They are concerned with safety issues and require a great deal of personal reassurance that they will be protected. Regressive behaviors, such as loss of bladder or bowel control, thumbsucking, and temper tantrums, are not uncommon. Changes in eating and sleeping patterns also may occur.

Ages 6 to 9. Children at this age begin to understand the finality of death. They are able to understand a more detailed explanation of why or how the person died, although death is often associated with old age or with accidents. They may believe that death is contagious and avoid association with individuals who have experienced a loss by death. Death is often personified in the form of a bogeyman or a monster—someone who takes people away or someone whom they can avoid if they try hard enough. It is difficult for them to conceive of their own death. Normal grief reactions at this age include regressive and aggressive behaviors, withdrawal, school phobias, somatic symptoms, and clinging behaviors.

Ages 10 to 12. Preadolescent children are able to understand that death is final and eventually affects everyone, including themselves. They are interested in the physical aspects of dying and the final disposition of the body. They may ask questions about how death will affect them personally. Feelings of anger, guilt, and depression are common. Peer relationships and school performance may be disrupted. There may be a preoccupation with the loss and a withdrawal into the self. They will require reassurance of their own safety and self-worth.

Adolescents

Adolescents are usually able to view death on an adult level. They understand death to be universal and inevitable; however, they have difficulty tolerating the intense feelings associated with the death of a loved one. They may or may not cry. They may withdraw into themselves or attempt to go about usual activities in an effort to avoid dealing with the pain of the loss. Some teens exhibit acting-out behaviors, such as aggression and defiance. It is often easier for adolescents to discuss their feelings with peers than with their parents or other adults. Some adolescents may show regressive behaviors, whereas others react by trying to take care of their loved ones who are also grieving. In general, individuals of this age group have an attitude of immortality. Although they understand that their own death is inevitable, the concept is so far-reaching as to be imperceptible.

Adults

The adult's concept of death is influenced by cultural and religious backgrounds (Murray & Zentner, 1997). Behaviors associated with grieving in the adult were discussed in the section on "Theoretical Perspectives on Loss and Bereavement."

Elderly Persons

Bateman (1999) states:

> For the older adult, the later years have been described by philosophers and poets as the "season of loss." Loss of one's occupational role upon retirement, loss of control and competence, loss in some life experiences, loss of material possessions, and loss of dreams, loved ones, and friends must be understood and accepted if the older adult is to adapt effectively. (p. 144)

By the time individuals reach their 60s and 70s, they have experienced numerous losses, and mourning has become a life-long process. Those who are most successful at adapting earlier in life will similarly cope better with the losses and grief inherent in aging (Cath & Sadavoy, 1991). Unfortunately, with the aging process comes a convergence of losses, the timing of which makes it impossible for the aging individual to complete the grief process in response to one loss before another occurs. Because grief is cumulative, this can result in bereavement overload; the person is less able to adapt and reintegrate, and mental and physical health is jeopardized (Halstead, 1999). Bereavement overload has been implicated as a predisposing factor in the development of depressive disorder in the elderly person.

Depression is a common symptom in the grief response to significant losses. It is important to understand the difference between the depression of normal grieving and the disorder of clinical depression. Some of these differences are presented in Table 23–2.

TABLE 23–2 **Normal Grief Reactions Versus Symptoms of Clinical Depression**

Normal Grief	Clinical Depression
Self-esteem intact	Self-esteem disturbed
May express anger openly	Usually does not express anger directly
Experiences a mixture of "good and bad days"	Persistent state of dysphoria
Able to experience moments of pleasure	Anhedonia prevalent
Accepts comfort and support from others	Does not respond to social interaction and support from others
Maintains feeling of hope	Feelings of hopelessness prevail
May express guilt feelings over some aspect of the loss	Has generalized feelings of guilt
Relates feelings of depression to specific loss experienced	Does not relate feelings to a particular experience
May experience transient physical symptoms	Expresses chronic physical complaints

Source: Adapted from Periyakoil (2001) and Wolfelt (1988).

Common Nursing Diagnoses and Interventions (For the individual who is grieving)

RISK FOR DYSFUNCTIONAL GRIEVING

Definition: *[Risk for] extended, unsuccessful use of intellectual and emotional responses by which individuals, families, communities attempt to work through the process of modifying self-concept based upon the perception of loss.*

Risk Factors ("related to")

Actual or perceived object loss (e.g., people, possessions, job, status, home, ideals, parts and process of the body)
Denial of loss
Interference with life functioning
Labile affect
Reliving of past experiences with little or no reduction (diminishment) of intensity of the grief
[Feelings of sadness, anger, guilt, self-reproach, anxiety, loneliness, fatigue, helplessness, shock, yearning, and numbness]

Goals/Objectives

Short-Term Goals

1. Client will acknowledge awareness of the loss.
2. Client will express feelings about the loss.
3. Client will verbalize own position in the grief process.

Long-Term Goal

Client will progress through the grief process in a healthful manner toward resolution.

Interventions with *Selected Rationales*

1. Assess client's stage in the grief process. ***Accurate baseline data are required to provide appropriate assistance.***
2. Develop trust. Show empathy, concern, and unconditional positive regard. ***Developing trust provides the basis for a therapeutic relationship.***
3. Help client actualize the loss by talking about it. "When did it happen? How did it happen?" and so forth. ***Reviewing the events of the loss can help client come to full awareness of the loss.***
4. Help client identify and express feelings. ***Until client can recognize and accept personal feelings regarding the loss, grief work cannot progress.*** Some of the more problematic feelings include:
   a. Anger. The anger may be directed at the deceased or at God, displaced on others, or retroflected inward on the self. Encourage client to examine this anger and validate the appropriateness of this feeling. ***Many people will not admit to angry feelings, believing it is inappropriate and unjustified. Expression of this emotion is necessary to prevent fixation in this stage of grief.***
   b. Guilt. Client may feel that he or she did not do enough to prevent the loss. Help client by reviewing the circumstances of the loss and the reality that it could not be prevented. ***Feelings of guilt prolong resolution of the grief process.***
   c. Anxiety and helplessness. Help client recognize the way that life was managed before the loss. Help client put the feelings of helplessness into perspective by pointing out ways that he or she effectively managed situations without help from others. Role-play life events and assist with decision-making situations. ***Client may have fears that he or she may not be able to carry on alone.***
5. Interpret normal behaviors associated with grieving, and provide client with adequate time to grieve. ***Understanding of the grief process will help prevent feelings of guilt generated by these responses. Individuals need adequate time to accommodate to the loss and all its ramifications. This involves getting past birthdays and anniversaries of which the deceased was a part.***

6. Provide continuing support. If this is not possible by the nurse, then offer referrals to support groups. Support groups of individuals going through the same experiences can be very helpful for the grieving individual. ***The availability of emotional support systems facilitates the grief process.***
7. Identify pathological defenses that client may be using (e.g., drug/alcohol use, somatic complaints, social isolation). Help client understand why these are not healthy defenses and how they delay the process of grieving. ***The bereavement process is impaired by behaviors that mask the pain of the loss.***
8. Encourage client to make an honest review of the relationship with what was lost. Keeping a journal is a facilitative tool with this intervention. ***Only when client is able to recognize positive and negative aspects related to the loss will the grieving process be complete.***

Outcome Criteria

1. Client is able to express feelings about the loss.
2. Client verbalizes stages of the grief process and behaviors associated with each.
3. Client acknowledges own position in the grief process and recognizes the appropriateness of the associated feelings and behaviors.

RISK FOR SPIRITUAL DISTRESS

Definition: *At risk for an altered sense of harmonious connectedness with all of life and the universe in which dimensions that transcend and empower the self may be disrupted.*

Risk Factors ("related to")

Loss of loved one
Situational losses
Maturational losses
Low self-esteem
Natural disasters
[Loss of any concept of value to the individual]

Goals/Objectives

Short-Term Goal

Client will identify meaning and purpose in life, moving forward with hope for the future.

Long-Term Goal

Client will express achievement of support and personal satisfaction from spiritual practices.

Interventions with *Selected Rationales*

1. Be accepting and nonjudgmental when client expresses anger and bitterness toward God. Stay with client. ***The nurse's presence and nonjudgmental attitude increase client's feelings of self-worth and promote trust in the relationship.***
2. Encourage client to ventilate feelings related to meaning of own existence in the face of current loss. ***Client may believe he or she cannot go on living without lost object. Catharsis can provide relief and put life back into realistic perspective.***
3. Encourage client as part of grief work to reach out to previously used religious practices for support. Encourage client to discuss these practices and how they provided support in the past. ***Client may find comfort in religious rituals with which he or she is familiar.***
4. Ensure client that he or she is not alone when feeling inadequate in the search for life's answers. ***Validation of client's feelings and assurance that they are shared by others offer reassurance and an affirmation of acceptability.***
5. Contact spiritual leader of client's choice, if he or she requests. ***These individuals serve to provide relief from spiritual distress and often can do so when other support persons cannot.***

Outcome Criteria

1. Client verbalizes increased sense of self-concept and hope for the future.
2. Client verbalizes meaning and purpose in life that reinforces hope, peace, and contentment.
3. Client expresses personal satisfaction and support from spiritual practices.

■ INTERNET REFERENCES

Additional references related to bereavement may be located at the following websites:

- http://www.journeyofhearts.org
- http://www.nhpco.org
- http://www.aarp.org/griefandloss/
- http://www.hospicefoundation.org
- http://www.bereavement.org
- http://www.partnershipforcaring.org/
- http://www.aahpm.org
- http://www.hpna.org

UNIT FOUR

PSYCHOTROPIC MEDICATIONS

CHAPTER 24

Antianxiety Agents

CHEMICAL CLASS: ANTIHISTAMINES

Examples

Generic Name	Trade Name	Half-life	Pregnancy Category	Available Forms (mg)
Hydroxyzine	Atarax	3 h	C	Tabs: 10, 25, 50, 100 Syrup: 10 mg/5 mL
	Vistaril	3 h	C	Caps: 25, 50, 100 Oral suspension: 25 mg/5 mL Injection: 25 mg/mL, 50 mg/mL

Indications

- Anxiety disorders
- Temporary relief of anxiety symptoms
- Allergic reactions producing pruritic conditions
- Antiemetic
- Reduction of narcotic requirement, alleviation of anxiety, and control of emesis in preoperative/postoperative and prepartum/postpartum clients

Action

- Exerts central nervous system (CNS)–depressant activity at the subcortical level of the CNS
- Have anticholinergic, antihistaminic, and antiemetic properties

Contraindications and Precautions

Contraindicated in:

- Hypersensitivity
- Pregnancy and lactation

Use cautiously in:

- Elderly or debilitated patients (dosage reduction recommended)
- Hepatic or renal dysfunction
- Concomitant use of other CNS depressants

Adverse Reactions and Side Effects

- Dry mouth
- Drowsiness
- Pain at intramuscular site

Interactions

- Additive CNS depression with other **CNS depressants** (e.g., **alcohol, other anxiolytics, opioid analgesics**, and **sedative/hypnotics**) and with **herbal depressants** (e.g., **kava, valerian**).
- Additive anticholinergic effects with other **drugs possessing anticholinergic properties** (e.g., **antihistamines, antidepressants, atropine, haloperidol, phenothiazines**) and **herbal products** such as **angel's trumpet, jimson weed,** and **scopolia.**

Route and Dosage

Intramuscular

- **Anxiety:** *Adults*—50 to 100 mg 4 times/day
- **Pruritus:** *Adults*—25 mg 3 or 4 times/day
- **Pre- and postoperative sedative:** *Adults*—50 to 100 mg; *children*—0.6 mg/kg
- **Antiemetic/adjunctive therapy to analgesia:** *Adults*—25 to 100 mg; *children*—1.1 mg/kg

Oral

- **Anxiety:** *Adults*—50 to 100 mg 4 times/day; ***children (>6 years)***—50 to 100 mg/d in divided doses; ***children (<6 years)***—50 mg/d in divided doses
- **Pruritus:** *Adults*—25 mg 3 or 4 times/day; ***children (>6 years)***—50 to 100 mg/d in divided doses; ***children (<6 years)***—50 mg/d in divided doses
- **Pre- and postoperative sedative:** *Adults*—50 to 100 mg; *children*—0.6 mg/kg

CHEMICAL CLASS: BENZODIAZEPINES

Examples

Generic (Trade) Name	Controlled/ Pregnancy Categories	Half-life	Indications	Available Forms (mg)
Alprazolam (Xanax)	C-IV/D	6–26 h	Anxiety disorders Anxiety symptoms Panic disorder *Unlabeled use:* Premenstrual syndrome	Tabs: 0.25, 0.5, 1.0, 2.0 Oral solution: 1 mg/mL
Chlordiazepoxide (Librium)	C-IV/D	5–30 h	Anxiety disorders Anxiety symptoms Acute alcohol withdrawal Preoperative sedation	Caps: 5, 10, 25 Injection: 100 mg/amp
Clonazepam (Klonopin)	C-IV/C	18–50 h	Petit mal, akinetic and myoclonic seizures Panic disorder *Unlabeled uses:* Acute manic episodes Neuralgias Uncontrolled leg movements during sleep Adjunct therapy in schizophrenia	Tabs: 0.5, 1.0, 2.0
Clorazepate (Tranxene)	C-IV/UK	40–50 h	Anxiety disorders Anxiety symptoms Acute alcohol withdrawal Partial seizures	Tabs/Caps: 3.75, 7.5, 15 Single-dose tabs: 11.25, 22.5

Generic (Trade) Name	Controlled/ Pregnancy Categories	Half-life	Indications	Available Forms (mg)
Diazepam (Valium)	C-IV/D	20–80 h	Anxiety disorders Anxiety symptoms Skeletal muscle relaxant Status epilepticus Preoperative sedation *Unlabeled use:* Panic attacks	Tabs: 2, 5, 10 Oral solution: 5 mg/5 mL, 5 mg/mL Injection: 5 mg/mL
Lorazepam (Ativan)	C-IV/D	10–20 h	Anxiety disorders Anxiety symptoms Insomnia Preoperative sedation *Unlabeled uses:* Status epilepticus Chemotherapy-induced nausea and vomiting	Tabs: 0.5, 1.0, 2.0 Oral solution: 2 mg/mL Injection: 2 mg/mL, 4 mg/mL
Oxazepam (Serax)	C-IV/D	5–20 h	Anxiety disorders Anxiety symptoms Acute alcohol withdrawal	Tabs: 15 Caps: 10, 15, 30

Action

Benzodiazepines are thought to potentiate the effects of gamma-aminobutyric acid, a powerful inhibitory neurotransmitter, thereby producing a calmative effect. The activity may involve the spinal cord, brain stem, cerebellum, limbic system, and cortical areas.

Contraindications and Precautions

Contraindicated in:

- Hypersensitivity
- Narrow-angle glaucoma
- Preexisting CNS depression

- Pregnancy and lactation
- Shock
- Coma

Use cautiously in:

- Elderly or debilitated patients (reduced dosage recommended)
- Hepatic and renal impairment
- History of drug abuse/dependence
- Depressed/suicidal patients
- Children

Adverse Reactions and Side Effects

- Drowsiness
- Dizziness
- Ataxia
- Dry mouth
- Blurred vision
- Hypotension
- Tolerance
- Physical and psychological dependence

Interactions

- Additive CNS depression with other **CNS depressants** (e.g., **alcohol, other anxiolytics, opioid analgesics,** and **sedative/hypnotics**) and with **herbal depressants** (e.g., **kava, valerian**).
- **Cimetidine, oral contraceptives, disulfiram, fluoxetine, isoniazid, ketoconazole, metoprolol, propoxyphene, propranolol,** and **valproic acid** may enhance effects of benzodiazepines.
- Benzodiazepines may decrease the efficacy of **levodopa.**
- Sedative effects of benzodiazepines may be decreased by **theophylline.**

Route and Dosage

Alprazolam (Xanax)

- **Anxiety disorders and anxiety symptoms:** PO: 0.25 to 0.5 mg 3 times/day. Maximum daily dose 4 mg in divided doses. In elderly or debilitated patients: 0.25 mg 2 or 3 times/day. Gradually increase if needed and tolerated.
- **Panic disorder:** PO: Initial dose: 0.5 mg 3 times/day. Increase dose at intervals of 3 to 4 days in increments of no more than 1 mg/d.
- **Premenstrual syndrome:** PO: 0.25 mg 3 times/day.

Chlordiazepoxide (Librium)

- **Mild to moderate anxiety:** PO: 5 or 10 mg 3 or 4 times/day.
- **Severe anxiety:** PO: 20 or 25 mg 3 or 4 times/day; IM: 50 to 100 mg initially, then 25 to 50 mg 3 or 4 times/day, if necessary.

- **Preoperative sedation:** PO: 5 to 10 mg 3 or 4 times/day; IM: 50 to 100 mg 1 hour before surgery.
- **Acute alcohol withdrawal:** PO: 50 to 100 mg; repeat as needed up to 300 mg/day. IM: 50 to 100 mg initially; repeat in 2 to 4 hours if necessary.

Clonazepam (Klonopin)

- **Seizures:** *Adults*—PO: 0.5 mg 3 times/day; may increase by 0.5 to 1 mg every 3rd day. Total daily maintenance dose not to exceed 20 mg; ***children (<10 years or 30 kg)***—PO: Initial daily dose 0.01 to 0.03 mg/kg/d (not to exceed 0.05 mg/kg/d) given in two to three equally divided doses; increase by not more than 0.25 to 0.5 mg every 3rd day until therapeutic blood levels are reached (not to exceed 0.2 mg/kg/d). **Therapeutic serum concentrations of clonazepam are 20 to 80 ng/mL.**
- **Panic disorder:** PO: 0.125 mg 2 times/day. Increase after 3 days toward target dose of 1 mg/d (some patients may require up to 4 mg/d).
- **Acute manic episode:** PO: 0.75 to 6 mg/d.
- **Neuralgia:** PO: 2 to 4 mg/d.
- **Uncontrolled leg movements during sleep:** PO: 0.5 to 2 mg/night.
- **Adjunct therapy in schizophrenia:** PO: 0.5 to 2 mg/d.

Clorazepate (Tranxene)

- **Anxiety disorders/anxiety symptoms:** *Adults*—PO: 7.5 to 15 mg 2 to 4 times/day. Adjust gradually to dose within range of 15 to 60 mg/d. May also be given in a single daily dose at bedtime. Initial dose: 15 mg. Adjust dosage within range of 11.25 to 22.5 mg.
- **Geriatric or debilitated patients:** PO: 3.75 to 15 mg/d.
- **Acute alcohol withdrawal:** PO: *Day 1:* 30 mg initially, followed by 15 mg 2 to 4 times/day; *Day 2:* 45 to 90 mg in divided doses; *Day 3:* 22.5 to 45 mg in divided doses; *Day 4:* 15 to 30 mg in divided doses. Thereafter, gradually reduce the daily dose to 7.5 to 15 mg.
- **Partial seizures:** *Adults*—PO: 7.5 mg 3 times/day. Can increase by no more than 7.5 mg/d at weekly intervals (daily dose not to exceed 90 mg); ***children (9 to 12 years)***—PO: 7.5 mg 2 times/day initially; may increase by 7.5 mg/wk (not to exceed 60 mg/d).

Diazepam (Valium)

- **Antianxiety/adjunct anticonvulsant:** *Adults*—PO: 2 to 10 mg 2 to 4 times/day; ***children (>6 months)***—PO: 1 to 2.5 mg 3 to 4 times/day.
- **Moderate to severe anxiety:** *Adults*—IM or IV: 2 to 10 mg. Repeat in 3 to 4 hours if necessary.

- **Skeletal muscle relaxant:** *Adults*—PO: 2 to 10 mg 3 or 4 times/day *or* 15 to 30 mg of extended-release form once daily; *geriatric or debilitated patients*—PO: 2 to 2.5 mg 1 to 2 times/day initially. Increase gradually as needed and tolerated; *children (>6 mo.)*—PO: 0.12 to 0.8 mg/kg/d divided into 3 to 4 equal doses.
- **Acute alcohol withdrawal:** PO: 10 mg 3 to 4 times/day in first 24 hours; decrease to 5 mg 3 or 4 times/day. IM or IV: 10 mg initially, then 5 to 10 mg in 3 to 4 hours as needed.
- **Status epilepticus/acute seizure activity:** *Adults*—IV (IM route may be used if IV is unavailable): 5 to 10 mg; may repeat every 10 to 15 minutes to a total of 30 mg; may repeat regimen again in 2 to 4 hours; *children (≥5 years):* IM or IV: 1 mg every 2 to 5 minutes to a maximum of 10 mg; may repeat in 2 to 4 hours if necessary; *children (1 month to 5 years)*—IM or IV: 0.2 to 0.5 mg every 2 to 5 minutes to a maximum of 5 mg.
- **Preoperative sedation :** *Adults*—IM: 10 mg.

■ CHEMICAL CLASS: PROPANEDIOLS

Example

Generic (Trade) Name	Controlled/Pregnancy Categories	Half-life	Available Forms (mg)
Meprobamate (Miltown)	C-IV/D	6–17 h	Tabs: 200, 400

Indications

- Anxiety disorders
- Temporary relief of anxiety symptoms

Action

- Depress multiple sites in the CNS, including the thalamus and limbic system.
- Appear to inhibit multineuronal spinal reflexes.

Contraindications and Precautions

Contraindicated in:

- Hypersensitivity to the drug
- Combination with other CNS depressants
- Children younger than 6 years
- Pregnancy and lactation
- Acute intermittent porphyria

Use cautiously in:

- Elderly or debilitated clients
- Hepatic or renal dysfunction
- Individuals with a history of drug abuse/addiction
- Clients with a history of seizure disorders
- Depressed/suicidal clients

Adverse Reactions and Side Effects

- Palpitations, tachycardia
- Drowsiness, dizziness, ataxia
- Nausea, vomiting, diarrhea
- Reduced seizure threshold
- Tolerance
- Physical and psychological dependence

Interactions

- Additive CNS depression with other **CNS depressants** (e.g., **alcohol, other anxiolytics, opioid analgesics,** and **sedative-hypnotics**) and with **herbal depressants** (e.g., **kava, valerian**).

Route and Dosage

- **Anxiety disorders/anxiety symptoms***: Adults*—PO: 1.2 to 1.6 g/d in 3 to 4 divided doses; maximum daily dose: 2.4 g; ***children*** *(>6 years)*—PO: 100 to 200 mg 2 or 3 times/day.

■ CHEMICAL CLASS: AZASPIRODECANEDIONES

Example

Generic Name	Trade Name	Pregnancy Category	Half-life	Available Forms (mg)
Buspirone HCl	BuSpar	B	2–11 h	Tabs: 5, 10, 15, 30

Indications

- Generalized anxiety states

Unlabeled Use

- Symptomatic management of premenstrual syndrome

Actions

- Unknown
- May produce desired effects through interactions with serotonin, dopamine, and other neurotransmitter receptors
- Delayed onset (a lag time of 7 to 10 days between onset of therapy and subsiding of anxiety symptoms)
- Cannot be used on a PRN basis

Contraindications and Precautions

Contraindicated in:

- Hypersensitivity to the drug
- Severe hepatic or renal impairment

Use cautiously in:

- Elderly or debilitated clients
- Pregnancy and lactation
- Children

- Buspirone will not block the withdrawal syndrome in clients with a history of chronic benzodiazepine or other sedative/hypnotic use. Clients should be withdrawn gradually from these medications before beginning therapy with buspirone.

Adverse Reactions and Side Effects

- Drowsiness, dizziness
- Excitement, nervousness
- Fatigue, headache
- Nausea, dry mouth
- Incoordination, numbness

Interactions

- Increased effects of buspirone with **erythromycin, itraconazole,** and **nefazodone.**
- Increased serum concentrations of **haloperidol** when used concomitantly with buspirone.
- Use of buspirone with a **monoamine oxidase inhibitor** may result in elevated blood pressure.
- Increased risk of hepatic effects when used concomitantly with **trazodone.**
- Additive effects when used with certain **herbal products** (e.g., **kava, valerian**).

Route and Dosage

- **Anxiety:** *Adults*—PO: 5 mg 3 times/day. Increase by 5 mg/d every 2 to 3 days as needed (not to exceed 60 mg/d). Usual dose is 20 to 30 mg/d in divided doses.

■ NURSING DIAGNOSES RELATED TO ALL ANTIANXIETY AGENTS

1. Risk for injury related to seizures, panic anxiety, acute agitation from alcohol withdrawal (indications); abrupt withdrawal from the medication after long-term use; effects of medication intoxication or overdose.
2. Anxiety (specify) related to threat to physical integrity or self-concept.
3. Risk for activity intolerance related to medication side effects of sedation, confusion, lethargy.
4. Disturbed sleep pattern related to situational crises, physical condition, severe level of anxiety.
5. Deficient knowledge related to medication regimen.

■ NURSING IMPLICATIONS FOR ANTIANXIETY AGENTS

1. Instruct client not to drive or operate dangerous machinery while taking the medication.

2. Advise client receiving long-term therapy not to stop taking the drug abruptly. Abrupt withdrawal can be life-threatening (with the exception of buspirone). Symptoms include depression, insomnia, increased anxiety, abdominal and muscle cramps, tremors, vomiting, sweating, convulsions, and delirium.
3. Instruct client not to drink alcohol or take other medications that depress the CNS while taking this medication.
4. Assess mood daily. ***May aggravate symptoms in depressed persons.*** Take necessary precautions for potential suicide.
5. Monitor lying and standing blood pressure and pulse every shift. Instruct client to arise slowly from a lying or sitting position.
6. Withhold drug and notify the physician should paradoxical excitement occur.
7. Have client take frequent sips of water, ice chips, suck on hard candy, or chew sugarless gum to relieve dry mouth.
8. Have client take drug with food or milk to prevent nausea and vomiting.
9. Symptoms of sore throat, fever, malaise, easy bruising, or unusual bleeding should be reported to the physician immediately. They may be indications of blood dyscrasias.
10. Ensure that client taking buspirone (BuSpar) understands there is a lag time of 7 to 10 days between onset of therapy and subsiding of anxiety symptoms. Client should continue to take the medication during this time. (NOTE: This medication is not recommended for PRN administration because of this delayed therapeutic onset. There is no evidence that buspirone creates tolerance or physical dependence as do the CNS depressant anxiolytics.)

■ CLIENT/FAMILY EDUCATION RELATED TO ALL ANTIANXIETY AGENTS

- Do not drive or operate dangerous machinery. Drowsiness and dizziness can occur.
- Do not stop taking the drug abruptly. Can produce serious withdrawal symptoms, such as depression, insomnia, anxiety, abdominal and muscle cramps, tremors, vomiting, sweating, convulsions, and delirium.
- ***(With buspirone only):*** Be aware of lag time between start of therapy and subsiding of symptoms. Relief is usually evident within 7 to 10 days. Take the medication regularly, as ordered, so that it has sufficient time to take effect.
- Do not consume other CNS depressants (including alcohol).
- Do not take nonprescription medication without approval from physician.
- Rise slowly from sitting or lying position to prevent a sudden drop in blood pressure.

- Report to physician immediately symptoms of sore throat, fever, malaise, easy bruising, unusual bleeding, or motor restlessness.
- Be aware of risks of taking these drugs during pregnancy. (Congenital malformations have been associated with use during the first trimester.) If pregnancy is suspected or planned, the client should notify the physician of the desirability to discontinue the drug.
- Be aware of possible side effects. Refer to written materials furnished by health-care providers regarding the correct method of self-administration.
- Carry card or piece of paper at all times stating names of medications being taken.

INTERNET REFERENCES

- http://www.mentalhealth.com/fr30.html
- http://www.nimh.nih.gov/publicat/medicate.cfm
- http://www.fadavis.com/townsend

CHAPTER 25

Antidepressants

■ CHEMICAL CLASS: TRICYCLICS

Examples

Generic (Trade) Name	Pregnancy Category/ Half-life	Indications	Therapeutic Plasma Level Range (ng/mL)	Available Forms (mg)
Amitriptyline (Elavil)	D/31–46 h	Depression *Unlabeled uses:* Chronic pain (migraine, neuropathy, neuralgia, arthritis, tic douloureux) Dermatological disorders	110–250 (including metabolite)	Tabs: 10, 25, 50, 75, 100, 150 Injection: 10/mL
Amoxapine (Asendin)	C/8 h	Depression Depression with anxiety *Unlabeled uses:* Chronic pain (see amitriptyline)	200–500	Tabs: 25, 50, 100, 150
Clomipramine (Anafranil)	C/19–37 h	Obsessive-compulsive disorder *Unlabeled uses:* Premenstrual symptoms	80–100	Caps: 25, 50, 75
Desipramine (Norpramin)	C/12–24 h	Depression *Unlabeled uses:* Chronic pain (see amitriptyline) Cocaine withdrawal Premenstrual symptoms Dermatological disorders	125–300	Tabs: 10, 25, 50, 75, 100, 150

(*Continued on following page*)

Generic (Trade) Name	Pregnancy Category/ Half-life	Indications	Therapeutic Plasma Level Range (ng/mL)	Available Forms (mg)
Doxepin (Sinequan)	C/8–24 h	Depression or anxiety Depression or anxiety associated with alcoholism Depression or anxiety associated with organic disease Psychotic depressive disorders with anxiety *Unlabeled uses:* Chronic pain (see amitriptyline) Peptic ulcer disease Dermatological disorders	100–200 (including metabolite)	Caps: 10, 25, 50, 75, 100, 150 Oral concentrate: 10/mL
Imipramine (Tofranil)	D/11–25 h	Depression Childhood enuresis *Unlabeled uses:* Chronic pain (see amitriptyline) Cocaine withdrawal	200–350 (including metabolite)	HCl tabs: 10, 25, 50 Pamoate caps: 75, 100, 125, 150
Nortriptyline (Aventyl; Pamelor)	D/18–44 h	Depression *Unlabeled uses:* Chronic pain (see amitriptyline) Premenstrual symptoms Dermatological disorders	50–150	Caps: 10, 25, 50, 75 Oral solution: 10/5 mL
Protriptyline (Vivactil)	C/67–89 h	Depression *Unlabeled uses:* Chronic pain (see amitriptyline)	100–200	Tabs: 5, 10
Trimipramine (Surmontil)	C/7–30 h	Depression *Unlabeled uses:* Peptic ulcer disease	180 (includes active metabolite)	Caps: 25, 50, 100

Action

- Inhibit reuptake of norepinephrine or serotonin at the presynaptic neuron.

Contraindications and Precautions:

Contraindicated in:

- Hypersensitivity to tricyclics
- Concomitant use with monoamine oxidase (MAO) inhibitors
- Acute recovery period following myocardial infarction
- Narrow angle glaucoma
- Pregnancy and lactation (safety not established)

Use cautiously in:

- Patients with history of seizures
- Urinary retention
- Benign prostatic hypertrophy
- Cardiovascular disorders
- Hepatic or renal insufficiency
- Psychotic patients
- Elderly or debilitated patients

Adverse Reactions and Side Effects

- Drowsiness
- Dry mouth
- Blurred vision
- Orthostatic hypotension
- Tachycardia
- Constipation
- Urinary retention
- Blood dyscrasias
- Nausea and vomiting
- Photosensitivity

Interactions

- Increased effects of tricyclic antidepressants with **bupropion, cimetidine, haloperidol, selective serotonin reuptake inhibitors,** and **valproic acid.**
- Decreased effects of tricyclic antidepressants with **carbamazepine, barbiturates,** and **rifamycins.**
- Hyperpyretic crisis, convulsions, and death can occur with **MAO inhibitors.**
- Coadministration with **clonidine** may produce hypertensive crisis.
- Decreased effects of **levodopa** and **guanethidine** with tricyclic antidepressants.
- Potentiation of pressor response with direct-acting **sympathomimetics.**
- Increased anticoagulation effects with **dicumarol.**

Route and Dosage

Amitriptyline (Elavil)

- **Depression:** PO: 75 mg/d in divided doses. May gradually increase to 150 mg/d.
- Hospitalized patients may require up to 300 mg/d. ***Adolescent and elderly patients***—10 mg 3 times/day and 20 mg at bedtime. IM: ***Adults*** 20 to 30 mg 4 times/day.
- **Chronic pain:** PO: 75 to 300 mg/d.
- **Dermatological disorders:** PO: 10 to 50 mg/d.

Amoxapine (Asendin)

- **Depression/depression with anxiety:** PO: 50 mg 2 or 3 times/day. May increase to 100 mg 2 or 3 times/day by end of 1st week. ***Elderly patients***—25 mg 2 or 3 times/day. May increase to 50 mg 2 or 3 times/day by end of 1st week.
- **Chronic pain:** PO: 100 to 300 mg/d.

Clomipramine (Anafranil)

- **Obsessive-compulsive disorder:** PO: ***Adults***—25 mg/d. Gradually increase to 100 mg during first 2 weeks, given in divided doses. May increase gradually over several weeks to maximum of 250 mg/d. ***Children and adolescents***—25 mg/d. Gradually increase during first 2 weeks to daily dose of 3 mg/kg or 100 mg, whichever is smaller. Maximum daily dose: 200 mg.

Desipramine (Norpramin)

- **Depression:** PO: 100 to 200 mg/d in divided doses or as a single daily dose. May increase to maximum dose of 300 mg/d. ***Elderly and adolescents***—25 to 100 mg/d in divided doses or as a single daily dose. Maximum dose: 150 mg/d.
- **Chronic pain:** PO: 75 to 300 mg/d.
- **Cocaine withdrawal:** PO: 50 to 200 mg/d.
- **Premenstrual symptoms:** PO: 100 to 150 mg/d for depression.
- **Dermatological disorders:** PO: 100 to 150 mg/d.

Doxepin (Sinequan)

- **Depression:** PO: (Mild to moderate illness) 75 mg/d. Increase to maximum dose of 150 mg/d. (Mild symptoms associated with organic illness): 25 to 50 mg/d. (Severe symptoms): 50 mg 3 times/day; gradually increase to 300 mg/d.
- **Chronic pain:** PO: 30 to 300 mg/d.
- **Peptic ulcer disease:** PO: 50 to 150 mg/d.
- **Dermatological disorders:** PO: 10 to 30 mg/d.

Imipramine (Tofranil)

- **Depression:** PO: 75 mg/d. Increase to maximum of 200 mg/d. Hospitalized patients may require up to 300 mg/d. ***Adolescent and geriatric patients***—30 to 40 mg/d. Increase to maximum of 100 mg/d.

- **Childhood enuresis (children ≥6 years of age):** PO: 25 mg/d 1 hour before bedtime. May increase after 1 week to 50 mg/night if <12 years of age; up to 75 mg/night if >12 years of age. Maximum dose 2.5 mg/kg/d.
- **Chronic pain:** PO: 75 to 300 mg/d.
- **Cocaine withdrawal:** PO: 150 to 300 mg/d.

Nortriptyline (Aventyl; Pamelor)

- **Depression:** PO: 25 mg 3 or 4 times/day. The total daily dose may be given at bedtime. ***Elderly and adolescent patients***—30 to 50 mg daily in divided doses or total daily dose may be given once/day.
- **Chronic pain:** PO: 50 to 150 mg/d.
- **Premenstrual symptoms:** PO: 50 to 125 mg/d.
- **Dermatological disorders:** PO: 20 to 75 mg/d.

Protriptyline (Vivactil)

- **Depression:** PO: 15 to 40 mg/d divided into 3 or 4 doses. Maximum daily dose: 60 mg. ***Adolescent and elderly patients***—Initially, 50 mg/d, with gradual increments up to 100 mg/d.
- **Chronic pain:** PO: 15 to 60 mg/d.

Trimipramine (Surmontil)

- **Depression:** PO: 75 mg/d. Increase gradually to 150 to 200 mg/d. Hospitalized patients may require up to 300 mg/d. ***Adolescent and elderly patients***—Initially, 50 mg/d, with gradual increments up to 100 mg/d.
- **Peptic ulcer disease:** PO: 25 to 50 mg/d.

■ CHEMICAL CLASS: HETEROCYCLICS

Examples

Generic (Trade) Name	Pregnancy Category/ Half-life	Indications	Therapeutic Plasma Level Range (ng/mL)	Available Forms (mg)
Bupropion (Wellbutrin; Zyban)	B/8–24 h	Depression Smoking cessation (Zyban) *Unlabeled use:* Attention deficit hyperactivity disorder (ADHD)	Not well established	Tabs: 75, 100 Tabs (SR): 100, 150
Maprotiline (Ludiomil)	B/21–25 h	Depression Depression with anxiety	200–300 (including metabolite)	Tabs: 25, 50, 75

(*Continued on following page*)

Generic (Trade) Name	Pregnancy Category/ Half-life	Indications	Therapeutic Plasma Level Range (ng/mL)	Available Forms (mg)
Mirtazapine (Remeron)	C/20–40 h	Depression	Not well established	Tabs: 15, 30
Trazodone (Desyrel)	C/4–9 h	Depression *Unlabeled uses:* Aggressive behavior Alcohol dependence Panic disorder or agoraphobia with panic attacks Insomnia	800–1600	Tabs: 50, 100, 150, 300

Action

Maprotiline and mirtazapine enhance central noradrenergic and serotonergic activity. Trazodone selectively inhibits serotonin uptake at synapses in the brain, thereby potentiating its effects. Bupropion blocks the uptake of serotonin and norepinephrine and inhibits the reuptake of dopamine.

Contraindications and Precautions

Contraindicated in:

- Hypersensitivity to the drug
- Concomitant use with, or within 2 weeks of use of, MAO inhibitors
- Known or suspected seizure disorder (maprotiline; bupropion)
- Acute phase of myocardial infarction
- Bulimia or anorexia nervosa (bupropion)

Use cautiously in:

- Urinary retention
- Hepatic, renal, or cardiovascular disease
- Suicidal patients
- Pregnancy and lactation (safety not established)
- Elderly and debilitated patients

Adverse Reactions and Side Effects

- Dry mouth
- Sedation; dizziness
- Tachycardia
- Headache
- Nausea/vomiting
- Priapism (trazadone)
- Seizures (maprotiline; bupropion)
- Constipation

Interactions

- Additive effects of **CNS depressants** when taken with mirtazapine or trazodone.
- Increased risk of seizures with concurrent use of maprotiline and **phenothiazines** and with bupropion and **other drugs that lower seizure threshold**.
- Prothrombin time is altered with concurrent use of **warfarin** and trazodone.
- Serotonin syndrome may occur with concurrent use of trazodone and selective serotonin reuptake inhibitors (**SSRIs**) or **venlafaxine**.
- Acute toxicity of bupropion is enhanced with concurrent use of **monoamine oxidase inhibitors** (**MAOIs**).
- May cause hypertension, seizures, and death when used with **MAOIs;** should not be taken within 14 days of MAOI therapy.

Route and Dosage

Bupropion (Wellbutrin; Zyban)

- **Depression:** PO: ***Adults***—100 mg 2 times/day. May increase to 100 mg given 3 times/day. No single dose of bupropion should exceed 150 mg. To prevent the risk of seizures, administer 4 to 6 hours between doses. Sustained release tabs may be given as a single 150-mg dose in the morning. May increase to twice a day (total 300 mg), with 8 hours between doses.
- **Smoking cessation (Zyban):** PO: 150 mg (SR tabs) twice daily, with an interval of 8 hours between doses. Continue treatment for 7 to 12 weeks. Some patients may need treatment for as long as 6 months.
- **ADHD:** PO: 3 mg/kg/d.

Maprotiline (Ludiomil)

- **Depression/depression with anxiety:** PO: ***Adults***—Initial dose: 75 mg/d. After 2 weeks, may increase gradually in 25 mg increments. Maximum daily dose: 150 to 225 mg. ***Elderly patients***—50 to 75 mg/d.

Mirtazapine (Remeron)

- **Depression:** PO: Initial dose: 15 mg/d administered in a single dose, preferably in the evening prior to sleep. May increase dose at intervals of 1 to 2 weeks up to a maximum dose of 45 mg/d. WARNING: At least 14 days should elapse between discontinuation of an MAOI and initiation of therapy with mirtazapine. In addition, allow at least 14 days after stopping mirtazapine before starting an MAOI.

Trazodone (Desyrel)

- **Depression:** PO: Initial dose: 150 mg/d in divided doses. May increase by 50 mg/d every 3 to 4 days to a maximum dose of 400 mg/d in divided doses. May need to administer a major portion of the dose at bedtime due to sedative effect.

- **Aggressive behavior:** PO: trazodone 50 mg twice daily and tryptophan 500 mg twice daily have been successful in treatment of aggressive behavior.
- **Alcohol dependence:** PO: 50 to 100 mg/d of trazodone have resulted in decreased cravings for alcohol, depression, and anxiety in patients with alcoholism.
- **Panic disorder or agoraphobia with panic attacks:** PO: 300 mg/d.
- **Insomnia:** PO: 25 to 75 mg/d at bedtime.

■ CHEMICAL CLASS: SELECTIVE SEROTONIN REUPTAKE INHIBITORS (SSRIs)

Examples

Generic (Trade) Name	Pregnancy Category/ Half-life	Indications	Therapeutic Plasma Level Range	Available Forms (mg)
Citalopram (Celexa)	C/ ~35 h	Treatment of depression *Unlabeled uses:* Alcoholism treatment Panic disorder Premenstrual dysphoria Social phobia Trichotillomania	Not well established	Tabs: 10, 20, 40 Oral solution: 10/5 mL
Escitalopram (Lexapro)	C/27–32 h	Major depressive disorder	Not well established	Tabs: 5, 10, 20
Fluoxetine (Prozac; Prozac Weekly; Sarafem)	C/1–16 days (including metabolite)	Treatment of depression Obsessive-compulsive disorder Bulimia nervosa Premenstrual disorder *Unlabeled uses:* Alcoholism Anorexia nervosa ADHD Bipolar II disorder	Not well established	Caps: 10, 20, 40 Conc: 20 mg/5 mL Caps, delayed release (weekly dosage): 90

(*Continued on following page*)

Generic (Trade) Name	Pregnancy Category/ Half-life	Indications	Therapeutic Plasma Level Range	Available Forms (mg)
		Borderline personality disorder Narcolepsy Kleptomania Migraine/tension headaches Post-traumatic stress disorder (PTSD) Schizophrenia Trichotillomania Social phobia Chronic rheumatoid pain Panic disorder Peripheral neuropathy		
Fluvoxamine (Luvox)	C/13.6–15.6 h	Obsessive-compulsive disorder	Not well established	Tabs: 50, 100
Paroxetine (Paxil)	C/21 h	Major depressive disorder Panic disorder Obsessive-compulsive disorder Social anxiety disorder Generalized anxiety disorder PTSD	Not well established	Tabs and Caps: 10, 20, 30, 40 Oral Suspension: 10/5 mL Tabs (CR): 12.5, 25, 37.5
Sertraline (Zoloft)	26–104 h (including metabolite)	Major depressive disorder Obsessive-compulsive disorder Panic disorder PTSD Premenstrual dysphoria	Not well established	Tabs: 25, 50, 100

Action

Selectively inhibit the central nervous system neuronal uptake of serotonin (5-HT), thereby potentiating its activity.

Contraindications and Precautions

Contraindicated in:

- Hypersensitivity to SSRIs
- Concomitant use with, or within 14 days' use of, MAO inhibitors
- **Fluvoxamine:** concomitant use with cisapride

Use cautiously in:

- Patients with history of seizures
- Underweight or anorexic patients
- Hepatic or renal insufficiency
- Elderly or debilitated patients
- Suicidal patients
- Pregnancy and lactation

Adverse Reactions and Side Effects

- Headache
- Insomnia
- Nausea
- Diarrhea
- Constipation
- Sexual dysfunction
- Somnolence
- Dry mouth
- Serotonin syndrome (if taken concurrently with other medications that increase levels of serotonin, e.g., MAOIs, tryptophan, amphetamines, other antidepressants, buspirone, lithium, or dopamine agonists). Symptoms of serotonin syndrome include diarrhea, cramping, tachycardia, labile blood pressure, diaphoresis, fever, tremor, shivering, restlessness, confusion, disorientation, mania, myoclonus, hyperreflexia, ataxia, seizures, cardiovascular shock, and death.

Interactions

- Toxic, sometimes fatal, reactions have occurred with concomitant use of MAOIs.
- Increased effects of SSRIs with **cimetidine, L-tryptophan,** and **lithium.**
- Concomitant use of SSRIs may increase effects of **hydantoins, tricyclic antidepressants, benzodiazepines, beta blockers, carbamazepine, clozapine, haloperidol, phenothiazines, St. John's wort, sumatriptan, sympathomimetics, tacrine, theophylline,** and **warfarin.**
- Concomitant use of SSRIs may decrease effects of **buspirone** and **digoxin.**

Route and Dosage

Citalopram (Celexa)

- **Depression:** PO: Initial dose: 20 mg/d as a single daily dose. May increase in increments of 20 mg at intervals of no less than

1 week. Recommended maximum dose: 40 mg/d. ***Elderly clients***—20 mg/d.
- **Alcoholism treatment:** PO: 20 to 30 mg/d.
- **Panic disorder:** PO: 20 to 30 mg/d.

Escitalopram (Lexapro)
- **Depression:** PO: Initial dose: 10 mg/d as a single daily dose. May increase to 20 mg/d after 1 week. ***Elderly clients***—PO: 10 mg/d.

Fluoxetine (Prozac; Sarafem)
- **Depression and obsessive-compulsive disorder:** PO: Initial dose: 20 mg/d in the morning. May increase dose after several weeks if clinical improvement is not observed. Doses >20 mg may be administered on a once-daily (morning) or twice-daily (morning and noon) schedule. Maximum dose: 80 mg/d.
- **Bulimia nervosa:** PO: 60 mg/d administered in the morning. May need to titrate up to this target dose in some clients.
- **Premenstrual dysphoric disorder (Sarafem):** PO: Initial dose: 20 mg/d. Maximum: 80 mg/d.
- **Alcoholism:** PO: 40 to 80 mg/d.
- **Anorexia nervosa:** PO: 20 to 80 mg/d.
- **ADHD:** PO: 20 to 60 mg/d.
- **Bipolar II disorder:** PO: 20 to 80 mg/d.
- **Borderline personality disorder:** PO: 5 to 80 mg/d.
- **Narcolepsy:** PO: 20 to 40 mg/d.
- **Kleptomania:** PO: 60 to 80 mg/d.
- **Migraine/tension headaches:** PO: 20 mg every other day to 40 mg/d.
- **PTSD:** PO: 10 to 80 mg/d.
- **Schizophrenia:** PO: 20 to 60 mg/d.
- **Trichotillomania:** PO: 20 to 80 mg/d.
- **Social phobia:** PO: 10 to 60 mg/d.
- **Chronic rheumatoid pain:** PO: 20 mg/d.
- **Panic disorder:** PO: 10 to 70 mg/d.
- **Diabetic peripheral neuropathy:** PO: 5 to 40 mg/d.

Fluvoxamine (Luvox)
- **Obsessive-compulsive disorder:** PO: ***Adults***—Initial dose: 50 mg at bedtime. May increase dose in 50-mg increments every 4 to 7 days. Maximum dose: 300 mg. Administer daily doses >100 mg in 2 divided doses. If unequal, give larger dose at bedtime. ***Children 8 to 17 years***—Initial dose 25 mg single dose at bedtime. May increase the dose in 25-mg increments every 4 to 7 days to a maximum dose of 200 mg/d for children up to 11 years of age. Maximum dose for adolescents: 300 mg/d. Divide daily doses >50 mg into 2 doses.

Paroxetine (Paxil)
- **Depression:** PO (immediate release): Initial dose: 20 mg/d in the morning. May increase dose in 10-mg increments at inter-

vals of at least 1 week to a maximum of 50 mg/d. (controlled release): Initial dose: 25 mg/d in the morning. May increase dose in 12.5-mg increments at intervals of at least 1 week to a maximum of 62.5 mg/d.

- **Panic disorder:** PO (immediate release): Initial dose: 10 mg/d in the morning. May increase dose in 10-mg increments at intervals of at least 1 week to a target dose of 40 mg/d. Maximum dose: 60 mg/d. (controlled release): Initial dose: 12.5 mg/d in the morning. May increase dose in 12.5-mg/d increments at intervals of at least 1 week to a maximum dose of 75 mg/d.
- **Obsessive-compulsive disorder:** PO: (immediate release): 20 mg/d in the morning. May increase dose in 10-mg/d increments at intervals of at least 1 week. Recommended dose: 40 mg/d. Maximum dose: 60 mg/d.
- **Social anxiety disorder:** PO: (immediate release): 20 mg/d in the morning. Usual range is 20 to 60 mg/d.
- **Generalized anxiety disorder and PTSD:** PO: (immediate release): 20 mg/d in the morning. Usual range is 20 to 50 mg/d. Change doses in increments of 10 mg/d at intervals of at least 1 week.

Sertraline (Zoloft)

- **Depression and obsessive-compulsive disorder:** PO: 50 mg/d (either morning or evening). May increase dose at 1-week intervals to a maximum of 200 mg/d.
- **Panic disorder and PTSD:** PO: Initial dose: 25 mg/d. After 1 week, increase dose to 50 mg/d. For patients not responding, may increase dose at 1 week intervals to a maximum of 200 mg/d.
- **Premenstrual dysphoric disorder:** PO: 50 mg/d given on each day of the menstrual cycle or only during each day of the luteal phase of the menstrual cycle. For patients not responding, may increase dose in 50-mg increments per menstrual cycle up to 150 mg/d when dosing throughout the cycle or 100 mg/d when dosing only during the luteal phase.

■ CHEMICAL CLASS: NONSELECTIVE REUPTAKE INHIBITORS

Examples

Generic (Trade) Name	Pregnancy Category/ Half-life(h)	Indications	Therapeutic Plasma Level Ranges	Available Forms (mg)
Nefazodone (Serzone)	C/2–4	Treatment of depression	Not well established	Tabs: 50, 100, 150, 200, 250

(*Continued on following page*)

Generic (Trade) Name	Pregnancy Category/ Half-life(h)	Indications	Therapeutic Plasma Level Ranges	Available Forms (mg)
Venlafaxine (Effexor)	C/5–11 (includes metabolite)	Treatment of depression Generalized anxiety disorder (extended release)	Not well established	Tabs: 25, 37.5, 50, 75, 100 Caps XR: 37.5, 75, 150

Action

- Inhibit neuronal reuptake of serotonin and norepinephrine.
- Venlafaxine is also a weak inhibitor of dopamine reuptake.

Contraindications and Precautions

Contraindicated in:

- Hypersensitivity to the drug
- Children and pregnancy (safety not established)
- Concomitant (or within 14 days) use with MAOIs
- ***Nefazodone:*** concomitant use with cisapride, pimozide, carbamazepine, or triazolam

Use cautiously in:

- Hepatic and renal insufficiency
- Elderly and debilitated patients
- Patients with history of drug abuse
- Suicidal patients
- Patients with history of or existing cardiovascular disease
- Patients with history of mania
- Patients with history of seizures

Adverse Reactions and Side Effects

- Headache
- Dry mouth
- Nausea
- Somnolence
- Dizziness
- Insomnia
- Asthenia
- Constipation

Interactions

- Concomitant use with **MAOIs** results in serious, sometimes fatal, effects resembling neuroleptic malignant syndrome.
- Increased sedative-hypnotic effects when used concomitantly with **St. John's wort**.

- Increased effects of **haloperidol** when used concomitantly with these drugs.
- Increased risk of serotonin syndrome when used concomitantly with **sumatriptan**, **sibutramine**, or **trazodone**.
- Increased effects of **benzodiazepines**, **buspirone**, **carbamazepine**, **digoxin**, and **HMG-CoA reductase inhibitors** when taken with nefazodone.

Route and Dosage

Nefazodone (Serzone)

- **Depression:** PO: Initial dose: 200 mg/d in 2 divided doses. May increase dose in increments of 100 to 200 mg/d at intervals of at least 1 week. Usual effective dose range: 300 to 600 mg/d. ***Elderly and debilitated patients***—100 mg/d in 2 divided doses.

Venlafaxine (Effexor)

- **Depression:** PO: Initial dose (with immediate-release tabs): 75 mg/d in 2 or 3 divided doses, taken with food. May increase in increments up to 75 mg/d at intervals of at least 4 days. Maximum dose: 225 mg/d.
- **Depression and generalized anxiety disorder:** PO: Initial dose (with extended-release caps): 75 mg/d with food given in the morning or in the evening at the same time each day. May increase dose in increments of up to 75 mg/d at intervals of at least 4 days to a maximum of 225 mg/d.

■ CHEMICAL CLASS: SELECTIVE NOREPINEPHRINE REUPTAKE INHIBITOR

NOTE: This drug is not classified as an antidepressant. Its therapeutic classification is as an agent for ADHD (other agents for ADHD are discussed in Chapter 30). Atomoxetine is included in this chapter because of its particular chemical classification.

Example

Generic (Trade) Name	Pregnancy Category/ Half-life	Indications	Therapeutic Plasma Level Range	Available Forms (mg)
Atomoxetine (Strattera)	C/5.2 h	Treatment of ADHD	Not well established	Caps: 10, 18, 25, 40, 60

Action

The exact mechanism by which atomoxetine produces its therapeutic effects in ADHD is unknown, but it is thought to be related to selective inhibition of the presynaptic norepinephrine transporter.

Contraindications and Precautions

Contraindicated in:

- Hypersensitivity
- Concurrent use of an MAOI or use of an MAOI within 2 weeks
- Narrow angle glaucoma

Use cautiously in:

- Clients with hypertension or tachycardia
- Clients with cardiovascular or cerebrovascular disease
- Pregnancy and lactation
- Elderly and debilitated clients
- Hepatic and renal insufficiency

Adverse Reactions and Side Effects

- Headache
- Nausea and vomiting
- Upper abdominal pain
- Dry mouth
- Decreased appetite; weight loss
- Constipation
- Insomnia
- Sexual dysfunction
- Urinary hesitancy and/or retention
- Increased blood pressure and heart rate
- Irritability

Interactions

- Concomitant use with **albuterol** increases cardiovascular effects.
- Use with **MAOIs** increases risk of neuroleptic malignant syndrome. Separate doses of MAOIs and atomoxetine by 14 days.
- **Pressor agents** potentiate effects on blood pressure.
- Coadministration with strong CYP 2D6 inhibitors (e.g., **paroxetine, fluoxetine, quinidine**) may increase atomoxetine plasma concentration.

Route and Dosage

Atomoxetine (Strattera)

- **ADHD: Adults, adolescents, and children weighing more than 70 kg (154 lb):** PO: Initial dose: 40 mg/d. Increase after a minimum of 3 days to a target total daily dose of 80 mg, as a single dose in the morning or 2 evenly divided doses in the morning and late afternoon or early evening. After 2 to 4 weeks, total dose may be increased to a maximum of 100 mg, if needed.
- **ADHD: Children weighing 70 kg (154 lb) or less:** PO: Initial dose: 0.5 mg/kg/d. Increase after a minimum of 3 days to a target total daily dose of about 1.2 mg/kg taken either as a single dose in the morning or 2 evenly divided doses in the morning

and late afternoon or early evening. Maximum daily dose: 1.4 mg/kg or 100 mg daily, whichever is less.

- **Adjusted dosing: hepatic impairment:** In clients with moderate hepatic impairment, reduce to 50% of normal dose. In clients with severe hepatic impairment, reduce to 25% of normal dose.
- **Adjusted dosing: Coadministration with strong CYP 2D6 inhibitors:** ***Adults, adolescents, and children over 70 kg body weight***—Initiate dose at 40 mg/d and increase to the usual target dose of 80 mg/d only if symptoms fail to improve after 4 weeks and the initial dose is well tolerated. ***Children and adolescents up to 70 kg body weight***—Initiate dose at 0.5 mg/kg/d and increase to the usual target dose of 1.2 mg/kg/d only if symptoms fail to improve after 4 weeks and the initial dose is well tolerated.

CHEMICAL CLASS: MONOAMINE OXIDASE INHIBITORS (MAOIs)

Examples

Generic (Trade) Name	Pregnancy Category/ Half-life	Indications	Therapeutic Plasma Level Range	Available Forms (mg)
Isocarboxazid (Marplan)	C/Not established	Treatment of depression	Not well established	Tabs: 10
Phenelzine (Nardil)	C/Not established	Treatment of depression	Not well established	Tabs: 15
Tranylcypromine (Parnate)	C/2.4–2.8 h	Treatment of depression	Not well established	Tabs: 10

Action

Inhibition of the enzyme monamine oxidase, resulting in an increase in the concentration of endogenous epinephrine, norepinephrine, and serotonin in storage sites throughout the nervous system.

Contraindications and Precautions

Contraindicated in:

- Hypersensitivity
- Pheochromocytoma
- Hepatic or renal insufficiency
- History of or existing cardiovascular disease
- Hypertension
- History of severe or frequent headaches

- Concomitant use with guanethidine
- Concomitant use with other antidepressants (e.g., tricyclics, SSRIs, heterocyclics, venlafaxine, nefazodone, or other MAOIs)
- Children younger than 16 years of age
- Pregnancy and lactation (safety not established)

Use cautiously in:

- Patients with a history of seizures
- Diabetes mellitus
- Suicidal patients
- Schizophrenia
- Agitated or hypomanic patients
- History of angina pectoris or hyperthyroidism

Adverse Reactions and Side Effects

- Dizziness
- Headache
- Orthostatic hypotension
- Constipation
- Nausea
- Disturbances in cardiac rate and rhythm
- Blurred vision
- Dry mouth
- Weight gain
- Hypomania

Interactions

- Serious, potentially fatal adverse reactions may occur with concurrent use of other **antidepressants, carbamazepine, cyclobenzaprine, maprotiline, furazolidone, procarbazine,** or **selegiline.** Avoid using within 2 weeks of each other (5 weeks after therapy with fluoxetine).
- Hypertensive crisis may occur with **amphetamines, methyldopa, levodopa, dopamine, epinephrine, norepinephrine, guanethidine, guanadrel, reserpine,** or **vasoconstrictors.**
- Hypertension or hypotension, coma, convulsions, and death may occur with **opioids** (avoid use of **meperidine** within 14 to 21 days of MAOI therapy).
- Concurrent use with **dextromethorphan** or **tryptophan** may produce hypertension, excitation, and hyperpyrexia.
- Hypertension may occur with concurrent use of **buspirone**; avoid using within 10 days of each other.
- Excess central nervous system stimulation and hypertension may occur with **methylphenidate.**
- Additive hypotension may occur with **antihypertensives** or **spinal anesthesia.**
- Additive hypoglycemia may occur with **insulins** or **oral hypoglycemic agents.**

- **Doxapram** may increase pressor response.
- Serotonin syndrome may occur with concomitant use of **St. John's wort.**
- Hypertensive crisis may occur with ingestion of foods or other products containing high concentrations of **tyramine** (see Nursing Implications).
- Consumption of foods or beverages with high **caffeine** content increases the risk of hypertension and arrhythmias.

Route and Dosage

Isocarboxazid (Marplan)

- **Depression:** PO: Initial dose: 10 mg twice daily. May increase dose by 10 mg every 2 to 4 days to 40 mg by end of 1st week. If needed, may continue to increase dose by increments of up to 20 mg/wk. Maximum dose: 60 mg/d divided into 2 to 4 doses. Gradually reduce to smallest effective dose.

Phenelzine (Nardil)

- **Depression:** PO: Initial dose: 15 mg 3 times/day. Increase to 60 to 90 mg/d in divided doses until therapeutic response is achieved. Then gradually reduce to smallest effective dose (15 mg/d or every other day).

Tranylcypromine (Parnate)

- **Depression:** PO: 30 mg/d in 2 divided doses. After 2 weeks, may increase by 10 mg/d; at 1- to 3-week intervals, up to 60 mg/d.

■ NURSING DIAGNOSES RELATED TO ALL ANTIDEPRESSANTS

1. Risk for suicide related to depressed mood
2. Risk for injury related to side effects of sedation, lowered seizure threshold, orthostatic hypotension, priapism, photosensitivity, arrhythmias, and hypertensive crisis
3. Social isolation related to depressed mood
4. Risk for constipation related to side effects of the medication

■ NURSING IMPLICATIONS FOR ANTIDEPRESSANTS

The plan of care should include monitoring for the following side effects from antidepressant medications. Nursing implications are designated by an asterisk (*).

1. **May occur with all chemical classes:**
   a. **Dry mouth**
      *Offer the client sugarless candy, ice, frequent sips of water.
      *Strict oral hygiene is very important.
   b. **Sedation**
      *Request an order from the physician for the drug to be given at bedtime.

*Request that the physician decrease the dose or perhaps order a less sedating drug.

*Instruct the client not to drive or use dangerous equipment while experiencing sedation.

c. **Nausea**

*Medication may be taken with food to minimize gastrointestinal distress.

d. **Discontinuation syndrome**

*All classes of antidepressants have varying potentials to cause discontinuation syndromes. Abrupt withdrawal following long-term therapy with SSRIs and venlafaxine may result in dizziness, lethargy, headache, and nausea. Fluoxetine is less likely to result in withdrawal symptoms because of its long half-life. Abrupt withdrawal from tricyclics may produce hypomania, akathisia, cardiac arrhythmias, and panic attacks. The discontinuation syndrome associated with MAOIs includes confusion, hypomania, and worsening of depressive symptoms. All antidepressant medication should be tapered gradually to prevent withdrawal symptoms (Haddad, 2001).

*Atomoxetine (Strattera) is not associated with a discontinuation syndrome and need not be tapered.

2. **Most commonly occur with tricyclics or heterocyclics:**

a. **Blurred vision**

*Offer reassurance that this symptom should subside after a few weeks.

*Instruct client not to drive until vision is clear.

*Clear small items from routine pathway to prevent falls.

b. **Constipation**

*Order foods high in fiber; increase fluid intake if not contraindicated; and encourage client to increase physical exercise, if possible.

c. **Urinary retention**

*Instruct client to report hesitancy or inability to urinate.

*Monitor intake and output.

*Various methods to stimulate urination may be tried, such as running water in the bathroom or pouring water over the perineal area.

d. **Orthostatic hypotension**

*Instruct client to rise slowly from a lying or sitting position.

*Monitor blood pressure (lying and standing) frequently, and document and report significant changes.

*Avoid long hot showers or baths.

e. **Reduction of seizure threshold**

*Clients with history of seizures should be observed closely.

*Institute seizure precautions as specified in hospital procedure manual.

*Bupropion (Wellbutrin) should be administered in doses of

no more than 150 mg and should be given at least 4 hours apart. Bupropion has been associated with a relatively high incidence of seizure activity in anorectic and cachectic clients.

f. **Tachycardia; arrhythmias**
   *Carefully monitor blood pressure and pulse rate and rhythm, and report any significant change to the physician.

g. **Photosensitivity**
   *Ensure that client wears protective sunscreens, clothing, and sunglasses while outdoors.

3. **Most commonly occur with SSRIs:**

a. **Insomnia; agitation**
   *Take dose early in the day.
   *Avoid caffeinated food and drinks.
   *Teach relaxation techniques for use before bedtime.

b. **Headache**
   *Administer anaglesics as prescribed.
   *May need to switch to another SSRI or to another class of antidepressants.

c. **Anorexia; weight loss**
   *Ensure that client is provided with caloric intake sufficient to maintain desired weight.
   *Caution should be taken in prescribing these drugs for anorectic clients.
   *Weigh client daily or every other day, at the same time and on the same scale if possible.

d. **Sexual dysfunction**
   ****Males***—May report abnormal ejaculation or impotence.
   ****Females***—May experience delay or loss of orgasm.
   *If side effect becomes intolerable, a switch to another antidepressant may be necessary.

e. **Serotonin syndrome**
   *Discontinue offending agent immediately.
   *The physician will prescribe medications to block serotonin receptors, relieve hyperthermia and muscle rigidity, and prevent seizures. Artificial ventilation may be required.
   *Symptomatic measures, such as cooling blankets to decrease fever, may be instituted.

4. **Most commonly occur with MAOIs:**

a. **Hypertensive crisis**
   *This occurs if the individual consumes foods or other substances containing tyramine while receiving MAOI therapy. Foods that should be avoided include aged cheeses, raisins, fava beans, red wines, smoked and processed meats, caviar, pickled herring, soy sauce, monosodium glutamate (MSG), beer, chocolate, yogurt, and bananas. Drugs that should be avoided include other antidepressants (tricyclics, heterocyclics, SSRIs, NSRIs), sympathomimetics (including over-

the-counter cough and cold preparations), stimulants (including over-the-counter diet drugs), antihypertensives, meperidine and other opioid narcotics, and antiparkinsonian agents such as levodopa.

*Symptoms of hypertensive crisis include severe occipital headache, palpitations, nausea and vomiting, nuchal rigidity, fever, sweating, marked increase in blood pressure, chest pain, and coma.

*Treatment of hypertensive crisis: Discontinue drug immediately; monitor vital signs; administer short-acting antihypertensive medication as ordered by physician; use external cooling measures to control hyperpyrexia.

5. **Miscellaneous side effects:**
   a. **With trazodone (Desyrel): Priapism**

   *This is a rare side effect, but it has occurred in some men taking trazodone.

   *If the client complains of prolonged or inappropriate penile erection, withhold medication dose, and notify the physician immediately.

   *This can become very problematic, requiring surgical intervention and, if not treated successfully, can result in impotence.

■ CLIENT/FAMILY EDUCATION RELATED TO ALL ANTIDEPRESSANTS

- Continue to take the medication even though the symptoms have not subsided. The therapeutic effect may not be seen for as long as 4 weeks. If after this time no improvement is noted, the physician may prescribe a different medication.
- Use caution when driving or operating dangerous machinery. Drowsiness and dizziness can occur. If these side effects become persistent or interfere with activities of daily living, report them to the physician. Dosage adjustment may be necessary.
- Do not stop taking the drug abruptly. Doing so might produce uncomfortable and/or dangerous withdrawal symptoms.
- Use sunscreens, and wear protective clothing when spending time outdoors. The skin may be sensitive to sunburn.
- Report occurrence of any of the following symptoms to the physician immediately: sore throat, fever, malaise, unusual bleeding, easy bruising, persistent nausea and vomiting, severe headache, rapid heart rate, difficulty urinating, anorexia or weight loss, seizure activity, stiff or sore neck, and chest pain.
- Rise slowly from a sitting or lying position to prevent a sudden drop in blood pressure.
- Take frequent sips of water, chew sugarless gum, or suck on hard candy if dry mouth is a problem. Good oral care (frequent brushing, flossing) is very important.

- Do not consume the following foods or medications while taking MAOIs: aged cheese, wine (especially chianti), beer, chocolate, colas, coffee, tea, sour cream, smoked and processed meats, chicken or beef liver, soy sauce, pickled herring, yogurt, raisins, caviar, broad beans, cold remedies, diet pills. To do so could cause a life-threatening hypertensive crisis.
- Avoid smoking while receiving tricyclic therapy. Smoking increases the metabolism of tricyclics, requiring an adjustment in dosage to achieve the therapeutic effect.
- Do not drink alcohol while taking antidepressant therapy. Antidepressants potentiate the effects of each other.
- Do not consume other medications (including over-the-counter medications) without the physician's approval while receiving antidepressant therapy. Many medications contain substances that, in combination with antidepressant medication, could precipitate a life-threatening hypertensive crisis.
- Notify physician immediately if inappropriate or prolonged penile erections occur while taking trazodone (Desyrel). If the erection persists longer than 1 hour, seek emergency department treatment. This condition is rare, but it has occurred in some men who have taken trazodone. If measures are not instituted immediately, impotence can result.
- Do not "double up" on medication if a dose of bupropion (Wellbutrin) is missed, unless advised to do so by the physician. Taking bupropion in divided doses will decrease the risk of seizures and other adverse effects.
- Be aware of possible risks of taking antidepressants during pregnancy. Safe use during pregnancy and lactation has not been fully established. These drugs are believed to cross the placental barrier readily; if so, the fetus could experience adverse effects of the drug. Inform the physician immediately if pregnancy occurs, is suspected, or is planned.
- Be aware of the side effects of antidepressants. Refer to written materials furnished by health-care providers for safe self-administration.
- Carry a card or other identification at all times describing the medications being taken.

INTERNET REFERENCES

- http://www.mentalhealth.com/fr30.html
- http://www.nimh.nih.gov/publicat/medicate.cfm
- http://www.fadavis.com/townsend

CHAPTER 26

Mood-Stabilizing Drugs

CHEMICAL CLASS: ANTIMANIC

Examples

Generic (Trade) Name	Pregnancy Category/ Half-life	Indications	Therapeutic Plasma Level Range	Available Forms (mg)
Lithium carbonate (Eskalith; Lithane; Lithobid)	D/10–50 h	Manic episodes associated with bipolar disorder Maintenance therapy to prevent or diminish intensity of subsequent manic episodes Depression associated with bipolar disorder	Acute mania: 1.0–1.5 mEq/L Maintenance: 0.6–1.2 mEq/L	Caps: 150, 300, 600 Tabs: 300 Tabs (SR): 300, 450
Lithium citrate		*Unlabeled uses:* Major depression Neutropenia Cluster or migraine headaches (prophylaxis) Alcohol dependence		Syrup: 8 mEq (as citrate equivalent to 300 mg lithium carbonate)/5 mL

Action

Not fully understood, but antimanic effects may be the result of increases in norepinephrine reuptake and increased serotonin receptor sensitivity.

Contraindications and Precautions

Contraindicated in:

- Hypersensitivity
- Cardiovascular or renal disease

- Dehydration
- Sodium depletion
- Pregnancy and lactation

Use Cautiously in:

- Elderly patients
- Any extent of cardiac, renal, or thyroid disease
- Diabetes mellitus
- Urinary retention
- Children younger than 12 years (safety not established)

Adverse Reactions and Side Effects

- Drowsiness, dizziness, headache
- Dry mouth, thirst
- Gastrointestinal upset
- Fine hand tremors
- Hypotension, arrhythmias, pulse irregularities
- Polyuria, dehydration
- Weight gain
- Hypothyroidism
- Arrhythmia

Interactions

- Increased renal excretion of lithium with **acetazolamide, osmotic diuretics,** and **theophylline.**
- Decreased renal excretion of lithium with **nonsteroidal anti-inflammatory drugs** (NSAIDs) and **thiazide diuretics.**
- Increased risk of neurotoxicity with **carbamazepine, haloperidol,** and **methyldopa.**
- Increased serum lithium levels with **fluoxetine** and **loop diuretics.**
- Increased effects of **neuromuscular blocking agents** and **tricyclic antidepressants** with lithium.
- Decreased pressor sensitivity of **sympathomimetics** when used with lithium.
- Use with **phenothiazines** may result in neurotoxicity, decreased phenothiazines concentration, or increased lithium concentration.
- Concurrent use with **verapamil** may result in decreased lithium levels or lithium toxicity.

Route and Dosage

- **Acute mania:** PO: 600 mg 3 times/day or 900 mg twice daily for the slow release form. Serum levels should be taken twice weekly at the initiation of therapy and until therapeutic level has been achieved.
- **Long-term (maintenance) use:** PO: 300 mg 3 to 4 times/day. Serum levels should be monitored in uncomplicated cases during maintenance therapy every 1 to 2 months.

■ CHEMICAL CLASS: ANTICONVULSANTS

Examples

Generic (Trade) Name	Pregnancy Category/ Half-life	Indications	Therapeutic Plasma Level Range	Available Forms (mg)
Carbamazepine (Tegretol)	D/25–65 h (initial) 12–17 h (repeated doses)	Epilepsy Trigeminal neuralgia *Unlabeled uses:* Bipolar disorder Resistant schizophrenia Post-traumatic stress disorder Management of alcohol, cocaine, and benzodiazepine withdrawal Restless legs syndrome	4-12 μg/mL	Tabs: 100, 200 Tabs XR: 100, 200, 400 Caps XR: 200, 300 Suspension: 100/5 mL
Clonazepam (C-IV) (Klonopin)	C/18–50 h	Petit mal, akinetic, and myoclonic seizures Panic disorder *Unlabeled uses:* Acute manic episodes Multifocal tic disorders Uncontrolled leg movements during sleep Schizophrenia (adjunctive therapy) Neuralgias	20-80 ng/mL	Tabs: 0.5, 1, 2
Valproic acid (Depakene; Depakote)	D/5–20 h	Epilepsy Manic episodes Migraine prophylaxis	50-150 μg/mL	Caps: 250 Syrup: 250 /5 mL Tabs (DR): 125, 250, 500 Tabs (ER): 500

(*Continued on following page*)

Generic (Trade) Name	Pregnancy Category/ Half-life	Indications	Therapeutic Plasma Level Range	Available Forms (mg)
Valproic acid (cont'd)				Caps (sprinkle): 125 Injection: 100/mL in 5 mL vial
Lamotrigine (Lamictal)	C/~ 33 h	Epilepsy *Unlabeled use:* Bipolar disorder	Not established	Tabs: 25, 100, 150, 200 Tabs (chewable): 2, 5, 25
Gabapentin (Neurontin)	C/5–7 h	Epilepsy *Unlabeled uses:* Bipolar disorder Migraine prophylaxis Neuropathic pain Tremors associated with multiple sclerosis	Not established	Caps: 100, 300, 400 Tabs: 600, 800 Oral solution: 250/5 mL
Topiramate (Topamax)	C/21 h	Epilepsy *Unlabeled uses:* Bipolar disorder Cluster headaches	Not established	Tabs: 25, 100, 200 Caps (sprinkle): 15, 25

Action

Action in the treatment of bipolar disorder is unclear.

Contraindications and Precautions

Contraindicated in:

- Hypersensitivity
- Lactation

Carbamazepine

- Concomitant use with monoamine oxidase inhibitors

Clonazepam

- Glaucoma

Valproic acid; clonazepam

- Severe liver disease

Use Cautiously in:

- Elderly and debilitated patients
- Patients with hepatic, renal, or cardiac disease
- Pregnancy

Clonazepam
- Patients with history of drug abuse/addiction or depression/suicidal ideation

Adverse Reactions and Side Effects

Clonazepam
- Drowsiness, ataxia
- Dependence, tolerance
- Blood dyscrasias

Carbamazepine
- Drowsiness, ataxia
- Nausea, vomiting
- Blood dyscrasias

Valproic acid
- Drowsiness, dizziness
- Nausea, vomiting
- Prolonged bleeding time

Gabapentin
- Drowsiness, dizziness, ataxia
- Nystagmus

Lamotrigine
- Ataxia, dizziness, headache
- Nausea, vomiting
- Risk of severe rash

Topiramate
- Drowsiness, dizziness, fatigue, ataxia
- Impaired concentration, nervousness
- Vision changes
- Nausea, weight loss

Interactions

The effects of:	Are increased by:	Are decreased by:	Concurrent use may result in:
Clonazepam	**CNS depressants, cimetidine, hormonal contraceptives, disulfiram, fluoxetine, isoniazid, ketoconazole, metoprolol, propoxyphene, propranolol, valproic acid**	**Rifampin, barbiturates, theophylline** (↓ sedative effects), **phenytoin**	Increased **phenytoin** levels; decreased efficacy of **levodopa**

(*Continued on following page*)

The effects of:	Are increased by:	Are decreased by:	Concurrent use may result in:
Carbamazepine	Verapamil, diltiazem, propoxyphene, erythromycin, clarithromycin, SSRIs, antidepressants, cimetidine, danazol	Cisplatin, doxorubicin, felbamate, rifampin, phenobarbital, phenytoin, primidone, theophylline	Decreased levels of **corticosteroids, doxycycline, felbamate, quinidine, warfarin, estrogen-containing contraceptives, barbiturates, cyclosporine, benzodiazepines, theophylline, lamotrigine, valproic acid, bupropion, haloperidol**
Valproic acid	Chlorpromazine, cimetidine, erythromycin, felbamate, salicylates	Rifampin, carbamazepine, cholestyramine, lamotrigine, phenobarbital, phenytoin	Increased effects of **tricyclic antidepressants, carbamazepine, CNS depressants, ethosuximide, lamotrigine, phenobarbital, phenytoin, warfarin and other anti-platelet agents, zidovudine**
Gabapentin	Cimetidine, CNS depressants	Antacids	
Lamotrigine	Folate inhibitors, valproic acid	Primidone, phenobarbital, phenytoin, rifamycin, succinimides	Decreased levels of **valproic acid**
Topiramate		Phenytoin, carbamazepine, valproic acid	Increased risk of CNS depression with **alcohol** or other **CNS depressants.** Increased risk of kidney stones with **carbonic anhydrase inhibitors.** Increased effects of **phenytoin.** Decreased effects of **oral contraceptives and valproic acid.**

Route and Dosage

Clonazepam (Klonopin)

- **Seizures: *Adults***—PO: 0.5 mg 3 times/day; may increase by 0.5 to 1 mg every 3rd day. Maximum daily dose: 20 mg. ***Children <10 years or 30 kg***—PO: Initial daily dose 0.01 to 0.03 mg/kg/d (not to exceed 0.05 mg/kg/d) given in 2 to 3 divided doses; increase by no more than 0.25 to 0.5 mg every 3rd day until therapeutic blood levels are reached (not to exceed 0.2 mg/kg/d).
- **Panic disorder:** PO: 0.125 mg twice daily; increase after 3 days toward target dose of 1 mg/d. Some patients may require up to 4 mg/d.
- **Bipolar disorder, mania:** PO: 0.75 to 16 mg/d.
- **Multifocal tic disorders:** PO: 1.5 to 12 mg/d.
- **Uncontrolled leg movements during sleep:** PO: 0.5 to 2 mg/night.
- **Schizophrenia (adjunct therapy):** PO: 0.5 to 2 mg/d.
- **Neuralgias:** PO: 2 to 4 mg/d.

Carbamazepine (Tegretol)

- **Seizure disorders: *Adults and children >12 years***—PO: 200 mg 2 times/day or 100 mg 4 times/day of suspension. Increase by 200 mg/d every 7 days until therapeutic levels are achieved. Maximum dose: 1000 mg/d in children 12 to 15 years; 1200 mg/d in patients >15 years. ***Children 6 to 12 years***—PO: 100 mg 2 times/day (50 mg 4 times/day of suspension). Increase by 100 mg weekly until therapeutic levels are obtained. Maximum daily dose: 1000 mg. ***Children <6 years***—PO: 10 to 20 mg/kg/d in 2 to 3 divided doses. May increase by 100 mg/d at weekly intervals. Maximum daily dose: 400 mg.
- **Trigeminal neuralgia:** PO: Initial dose 100 mg 2 times/day. May increase by up to 200 mg/d using 100-mg increments every 12 hours. Maximum daily dose: 1200 mg.
- **Bipolar disorder, mania:** PO: Initial dose 200 to 600 mg/d in 3 to 4 divided doses. May increase by up to 200 mg/d every 7 days until therapeutic levels are achieved. Maintenance dose averages ~ 1000 mg/d. Range: 200 to 1600 mg/d. Doses higher than 1600 mg/d are not recommended.
- **Resistant schizophrenia:** PO: Dosage same as seizure disorders.
- **Management of alcohol withdrawal:** PO: 200 mg 4 times/day up to 1000 mg/d.
- **Management of cocaine and benzodiazepine withdrawal:** PO: 200 mg 2 times/day up to 800 mg/d.
- **Restless leg syndrome:** PO: 100 to 300 mg at bedtime.

Valproic Acid (Depakene; Depakote)

- **Epilepsy:** PO: Initial dose: 5 to 15 mg/kg/d. Increase by 5 to 10 mg/kg/wk until therapeutic levels are reached. Maximum recommended dosage: 60 mg/kg/d. When daily dosage exceeds 250 mg, give in 2 divided doses.

- **Manic episodes:** PO (delayed-release tabs): Initial dose: 750 mg/d in divided doses. Titrate rapidly to desired clinical effect or trough plasma levels of 50 to 125 μg/mL. Maximum recommended dose: 60/mg/kg/d.
- **Migraine prophylaxis:** PO (delayed-release tabs): 250 mg 2 times/day. Some patients may require up to 1000 mg/d. No evidence that higher doses lead to greater efficacy.

Lamotrigine (Lamictal)

- **Epilepsy:** ***Adults and children >12 years***—Adjunctive therapy with carbamazepine, phenobarbital, phenytoin, or primidone: PO: 50 mg as a single daily dose for 2 weeks, then 50 mg 2 times/day for next 2 weeks; then increase by 100 mg/d on a weekly basis to maintenance dose of 300 to 500 mg/d in 2 doses. If valproic acid is also being taken, the initial dose should be 25 mg every other day for 2 weeks, then 25 mg once daily for next 2 weeks; then increase by 25 to 50 mg/d every 1 to 2 weeks to maintenance dose of 50 to 75 mg 2 times/day (not to exceed 200 mg/d). ***Children 2 to 12 years***—Indicated only as adjunctive therapy for generalized seizures of Lennox-Gastaut syndrome. Refer to manufacturer's dosing recommendations. Safety and efficacy for other uses in patients <16 years of age have not been established.
- **Bipolar disorder:** PO: 25 mg/d for the first 2 weeks, then 50 mg/d for weeks 3 and 4. After that, 50 mg can be added per week as clinically indicated. **When administered concomitantly with valproic acid:** 12.5 mg/d or 25 mg every other day for 2 weeks, then 25 mg/d for weeks 3 and 4.

Gabapentin (Neurontin)

- **Epilepsy:** ***Adults and children >12 years***—PO: Initial dose: 300 mg 3 times/day. Titration may be continued until desired results have been achieved (range is 900 to 1800 mg/d in 3 divided doses). Doses should not be more than 12 hours apart. Doses up to 3600 mg have been well tolerated. ***Children 3 to 12 years***—Initial dose: 10 to 15 mg/kg/d in 3 divided doses. Titrate dosage over 3 days to 25 to 35 mg/kg/d in 3 divided doses for children ≥5 years (40 mg/kg/d for children ages 3 and 4). Dosage interval should not exceed 12 hours. Dosages up to 50 mg/kg/d have been used.
- **Bipolar disorder:** PO: 900 to 1800 mg/d in 3 divided doses.

Topiramate (Topamax)

- **Epilepsy:** ***Adults and children ≥17 years***—PO: Initial dose: 25 to 50 mg/d. Gradually increase by 25 to 50 mg weekly up to 200 mg 2 times/day. Doses >400 mg/d have not been shown to improve responses. ***Children 2 to 17 years***—PO: 5 to 9 mg/kg/d in 2 divided doses; initiate with 25 mg (or less, based on 1 to 3 mg/kg) nightly for 7 days, then increase at 1- to 2-week intervals in increments of 1 to 3 mg/kg/d in 2 divided doses. Titration should be based on clinical outcome.

- **Bipolar disorder:** PO: Initial dose: 25 to 50 mg/d. Increase to target range of 125 to 400 mg/d.

CHEMICAL CLASS: CALCIUM CHANNEL BLOCKERS

Example

Generic (Trade) Name	Pregnancy Category/ Half-life	Indications	Therapeutic Plasma Level Range	Available Forms (mg)
Verapamil (Calan; Isoptin)	C/3–7 h (initially) 4.5–12 h (repeated dosing)	Angina Arrhythmias Hypertension *Unlabeled uses:* Bipolar mania Migraine headache prophylaxis	80-300 ng/mL	Tabs: 40, 80, 120 Tabs (XR; SR): 120, 180, 240 Caps SR: 120, 180, 240, 360 Caps XR: 100, 120, 180, 200, 240, 300 Injection: 2.5/mL

Action

Action in the treatment of bipolar disorder is unclear.

Contraindications and Precautions

Contraindicated in:

- Hypersensitivity
- Severe left ventricular dysfunction
- Heart block
- Hypotension
- Cardiogenic shock
- Congestive heart failure

Use cautiously in:

- Liver or renal disease
- Cardiomyopathy
- Intracranial pressure
- Elderly patients
- Pregnancy and lactation (safety not established)

Adverse Reactions and Side Effects

- Drowsiness
- Dizziness
- Headache
- Hypotension
- Bradycardia
- Nausea
- Constipation

Interactions

- Additive hypotension with **fentanyl,** other **antihypertensives, nitrates, alcohol,** or **quinidine.**
- Antihypertensive effects may be decreased with **NSAIDS.**
- Concurrent use may increase serum levels of **digoxin.**
- Concurrent use with **beta blockers, digoxin, disopyramide,** or **phenytoin** may result in bradycardia, conduction defects, or chronic heart failure.
- Concurrent use may decrease the metabolism of and increase the risk of toxicity from **cyclosporine, prazosin, quinidine,** or **carbamazepine.**
- May decrease the effectiveness of **rifampin.**
- Increases the muscle-paralyzing effects of **nondepolarizing neuromuscular-blocking agents.**
- Verapamil effectiveness may be decreased by coadministration with **vitamin D compounds** and **calcium.**
- May alter serum **lithium** levels.

Route and Dosage

- **Angina:** PO: 80 to 120 mg 3 times/day.
- **Arrhythmias:** PO: 240 to 320 mg/d in 3 or 4 divided doses.
- **Hypertension:** PO: 40 to 80 mg 3 times/day. Maximum recommended daily dose: 360 mg.
- **Bipolar mania:** PO: 80 to 320 mg/d in divided doses.
- **Migraine prophylaxis:** PO (tabs SR; XR): 120 to 240 mg/d.

■ CHEMICAL CLASS: THIENOBENZODIAZEPINE

Example

Generic (Trade) Name	Pregnancy Category/ Half-life	Indications	Available Forms (mg)
Olanzapine (Zyprexa)	C/21–54 h	Treatment of schizophrenia Acute manic episodes	Tabs: 2.5, 5, 7.5, 10, 15, 20 Tabs (orally disintegrating): 5, 10, 15, 20

Action

- Efficacy in schizophrenia is achieved through a combination of dopamine and serotonin type 2 ($5HT_2$) antagonism.
- Mechanism of action in the treatment of acute manic episodes is unknown.

Contraindications and Precautions

Contraindicated in:

- Hypersensitivity
- Lactation

Orally disintegrating tablets only:

- Phenylketonuria (orally disintegrating tablets contain aspartame)

Use cautiously in:

- Hepatic insufficiency
- Elderly clients (reduce dosage)
- Pregnancy and children (safety not established)
- Cardiovascular or cerebrovascular disease
- History of glaucoma
- History of seizures
- History of attempted suicide
- Prostatic hypertrophy

Adverse Reactions and Side Effects

- Drowsiness, dizziness, weakness
- Dry mouth, constipation, increased appetite
- Orthostatic hypotension, tachycardia
- Restlessness
- Rhinitis
- Tremor

Interactions

- Decreased effects of olanzapine with **carbamazepine, omeprazole,** or **rifampin.**
- Increased serum levels of olanzapine with **fluvoxamine.**
- Increased CNS effects with concomitant use of **alcohol** and other **CNS depressants.**
- May antagonize the effects of **levodopa** and other **dopamine agonists.**

Route and Dosage

- **Schizophrenia:** PO: Initial dose: 5 to 10 mg once daily. May increase at weekly intervals by 5 mg/d (not to exceed 20 mg/d).
- **Bipolar mania:** PO: Initial dose: 10 to 15 mg once daily. May increase every 24 hours by 5 mg/d (not to exceed 20 mg/d).
- **Elderly and debilitated patients:** PO: Initial dose: 5 mg/d. When indicated, use caution with dose escalation.

NURSING DIAGNOSES RELATED TO ALL MOOD-STABILIZING DRUGS

1. Risk for injury related to manic hyperactivity.
2. Risk for self-directed or other-directed violence related to unresolved anger turned inward on the self or outward on the environment.
3. Risk for injury related to lithium toxicity.
4. Risk for activity intolerance related to side effects of drowsiness and dizziness.

NURSING IMPLICATIONS FOR MOOD-STABILIZING DRUGS

1. Assess for changes in mood, particularly mood swings.
2. For the client on lithium therapy, assess for signs of lithium toxicity: ataxia, blurred vision, severe diarrhea, persistent nausea and vomiting, and tinnitus.
3. Instruct client to take medication on a regular basis, even when feeling well. Discontinuation can result in return of symptoms.
4. Ensure that client does not drive or operate dangerous machinery until response is stabilized. Drowsiness and dizziness can occur.
5. Ensure that client on lithium therapy receives sufficient dietary sodium intake and 2500 to 3000 mL of water per day.
6. Notify the physician if vomiting or diarrhea occur. These symptoms in client on lithium therapy can result in increased risk of toxicity.
7. Some clients may gain weight on this therapy. Help client plan appropriate diet from the Food Guide Pyramid to ensure that weight gain does not become a problem. Include adequate sodium and other nutrients while decreasing the number of calories.
8. Administer the medication with food if nausea becomes a problem.

CLIENT/FAMILY EDUCATION RELATED TO MOOD-STABILIZING DRUGS

- Do not drive or operate dangerous machinery. Drowsiness or dizziness can occur.
- Do not stop taking the drug abruptly; can produce serious withdrawal symptoms. The physician will administer orders for tapering the drug when therapy is to be discontinued.
- Report the following symptoms to the physician immediately: *Client taking anticonvulsant:* unusual bleeding, spontaneous bruising, sore throat, fever, malaise, skin rash, dark urine, and yellow skin or eyes. *Client taking calcium channel blocker:* irregular heartbeat, shortness of breath, swelling of the hands and feet, pronounced dizziness, chest pain, profound mood swings, and severe and persistent headache. *Client taking lithium:* ataxia,

blurred vision, severe diarrhea, persistent nausea and vomiting, tinnitus, excessive urine output, increasing tremors, and mental confusion. *Client taking olanzapine:* high fever; muscle rigidity; altered mental state; and abnormal, involuntary movements of the face, head, or extremities.

- For the client on lithium: ensure that the diet contains adequate sodium. Drink 6 to 8 glasses of water each day. Avoid drinks that contain caffeine (that have a diuretic effect). Have serum lithium level checked every 1 to 2 months, or as advised by physician.
- Avoid consuming alcoholic beverages and nonprescription medications without approval from physician.
- Carry card at all times identifying the name of medications being taken.

INTERNET REFERENCES

- http://www.rxlist.com
- http://www.nimh.nih.gov/publicat/medicate.cfm
- http://www.fadavis.com/townsend

CHAPTER 27

Antipsychotic Agents

■ CHEMICAL CLASS: PHENOTHIAZINES

Examples

Generic (Trade) Name	Pregnancy Categories/ Half-life	Indications	Available Forms (mg)
Chlorpromazine (Thorazine)	UK/8–35 h	Psychotic disorders Pediatric behavioral disorders Nausea and vomiting Intractable hiccups Preoperative sedation Acute intermittent porphyria	Tabs: 10, 25, 50, 100, 200 Caps (SR): 30, 75, 150 Syrup: 10/5 mL Concentration: 30/mL, 100/mL Suppositories: 25, 100 Injection: 25/mL
Fluphenazine (Prolixin)	C/HCl: 15 h Decanoate: 6.8–9.6 days	Psychotic disorders	Tabs: 1, 2.5, 5, 10 Elixir: 2.5/5 mL Concentrate: 5/mL Injection: 2.5/mL Injection (Decanoate): 25 mL
Mesoridazine (Serentil)	C/24–48 h	Refractory schizophrenia	Tabs: 10, 25, 50, 100 Concentrate: 25/mL Injection: 25/mL
Perphenazine (Trilafon)	C/8–21 h	Psychotic disorders Nausea and vomiting *Unlabeled uses:* Intractable hiccups	Tabs: 2, 4, 8, 16 Concentrate: 16/5 mL Injection: 5/mL

(Continued on following page)

Generic (Trade) Name	Pregnancy Categories/ Half-life	Indications	Available Forms (mg)
Prochlor-perazine (Compazine)	C/Unknown	Psychotic disorders Nonpsychotic anxiety Nausea and vomiting *Unlabeled uses:* Migraine headache	Tabs: 5, 10 Caps (SR): 10, 15 Suppositories: 2.5, 5, 25 Syrup: 5/5mL Injection: 5/mL
Thioridazine (Mellaril)	C/21–24 h	Psychotic disorders Psychoneurotic manifestations Pediatric behavioral disorders	Tabs: 10, 15, 25, 50, 100, 150, 200 Concentrate: 30/mL; 100/mL Suspension: 25/5 mL; 100/5 mL
Trifluoperazine (Stelazine)	C/Unknown	Schizophrenia Nonpsychotic anxiety	Tabs: 1, 2, 5, 10 Concentrate: 10/mL Injection: 2/mL

Action

- These drugs are thought to work by blocking postsynaptic dopamine receptors in the basal ganglia, hypothalamus, limbic system, brainstem, and medulla.
- They also demonstrate varying affinity for cholinergic, $alpha_1$-adrenergic, and histaminic receptors.
- Antipsychotic effects may also be related to inhibition of dopamine-mediated transmission of neural impulses at the synapses.

Contraindications and Precautions

Contraindicated in:

- Hypersensitivity (cross-sensitivity may exist among phenothiazines)
- In comatose or severely central nervous system (CNS)–depressed clients
- Poorly controlled seizure disorders
- Clients with blood dyscrasias
- Clients with liver, renal, or cardiac insufficiency
- Coadministration with **pimozide**

Use cautiously in:

- Severely ill or elderly clients
- Diabetes mellitus
- History of glaucoma

- Epilepsy
- Respiratory insufficiency
- Prostatic hypertrophy
- Pregnancy and lactation (safety has not been established)

Adverse Reactions and Side Effects

- Dry mouth
- Blurred vision
- Constipation
- Urinary retention
- Nausea
- Skin rash
- Sedation
- Orthostatic hypotension
- Photosensitivity
- Decreased libido
- Amenorrhea
- Retrograde ejaculation
- Gynecomastia
- Weight gain
- Reduction of seizure threshold
- Agranulocytosis
- Extrapyramidal symptoms
- Tardive dyskinesia
- Neuroleptic malignant syndrome

Interactions

- Additive effects with other **anticholinergics, antihypertensives,** and **CNS-active drugs.**
- Coadministration with phenothiazines may decrease the effects of **CNS stimulants, bromocriptine,** and **guanethidine.**
- Additive QT prolongation effect with **pimozide.**
- Decreased pharmacological effects of phenothiazines with **antacids** (aluminum salts), **anticholinergics,** and **barbiturates.**
- Increased plasma levels of both drugs with coadministration of **phenothiazines** and **propranolol.**
- Decreased pressor effects of **epinephrine** and **norepinephrine.**
- Increased effects of **valproic acid, tricyclic antidepressants.**
- Coadministration with **lithium** may cause disorientation, unconsciousness, and extrapyramidal symptoms.
- Coadministration with **meperidine** may produce excessive sedation and hypotension.

Route and Dosage

Chlorpromazine (Thorazine)

- **Psychotic disorders:** ***Adults***—PO: 25 mg 3 times/day. Increase gradually until effective dose is reached, usually 400 mg/d. IM:

Initial dose: 25 mg. May give additional 25 to 50 mg in 1 hour. Increase gradually over several days (up to 400 mg every 4 to 6 hours in severe cases).

- **Pediatric behavioral disorders:** ***Children >6 months***—PO: 0.5 mg/kg every 4 to 6 hours, as needed. Rectal: 1 mg/kg every 6 to 8 hours, as needed. IM: 0.5 mg/kg every 6 to 8 hours (not to exceed 40 mg/d in children 6 months to 5 years or 75 mg/d in children 5 to 12 years).
- **Nausea and vomiting:** ***Adults***—PO: 10 to 25 mg every 4 to 6 hours. Rectal: 50 to 100 mg every 6 to 8 hours. IM: 25 mg initially, may repeat 25 to 50 mg every 3 to 4 hours. ***Children >6 months***—PO: 0.55 mg/kg every 4 to 6 hours. Rectal: 1.1 mg/kg every 6 to 8 hours. IM: 0.55 mg/kg every 6 to 8 hours (not to exceed 40 mg/d in children up to 5 years or 75 mg/d in children 5 to 12 years).
- **Intractable hiccups:** ***Adults***—PO: 25 to 50 mg 3 or 4 times daily. If symptoms persist for 2 to 3 days, give 25 to 50 mg IM.
- **Preoperative sedation:** ***Adults***—PO: 25 to 50 mg 2 to 3 hours before surgery. IM: 12.5 to 25 mg 1 to 2 hours before surgery. ***Children***—PO: 0.5 mg/kg 2 to 3 hours before surgery, or IM: 0.5 mg/kg 1 to 2 hours before surgery.
- **Acute intermittent porphyria:** ***Adults***—PO: 25 to 50 mg 3 or 4 times/day, or IM: 25 mg 3 or 4 times/day until patient can take PO.

Fluphenazine (Prolixin)

- **Psychotic disorders:** ***Adults***—PO: Initial dose: 2.5 to 10 mg/d in divided doses every 6 to 8 hours. Maintenance dose: 1 to 5 mg/d. IM: 1.25 to 2.5 mg every 6 to 8 hours. ***Elderly or debilitated patients***—PO, IM: 1 to 2.5 mg/d initially.
- **Decanoate formulation:** ***Adults***—IM, SC: Initial dose: 12.5 to 25 mg. May be repeated every 1 to 4 weeks. Dose may be slowly increased in 12.5-mg increments as needed (not to exceed 100 mg/dose).

Mesoridazine (Serentil)

- **Schizophrenia:** ***Adults***—PO: 50 mg 3 times/day. Usual optimum daily dose range: 100 to 400 mg. IM: Initial dose: 25 mg. May repeat dose in 30 to 60 minutes. Usual optimum dose range: 25 to 200 mg/d.

Perphenazine (Trilafon)

- **Psychotic disorders:** ***Adults***—PO: *Outpatients:* 4 to 8 mg 3 times/day. Reduce as soon as possible to minimum effective dose. *Hospitalized patients:* 8 to 16 mg 2 to 4 times/day, not to exceed 64 mg/d. IM: 5 mg every 6 hours, not to exceed 30 mg/d.
- **Nausea and vomiting and intractable hiccups:** ***Adults***—PO: 8 to 16 mg daily in divided doses, up to 24 mg, if necessary. IM:

5 mg repeated every 6 hours as necessary, not to exceed 30 mg/d. ***Children >12 years***—PO: May receive the lowest limit of the adult dose.

Prochlorperazine (Compazine)

- **Psychotic disorders:** ***Adults and children >12 years***—PO: 5 to 10 mg 3 to 4 times/day. May be increased every 2 to 3 days (up to 150 mg/d). IM: 10 to 20 mg every 2 to 4 hours for up to 4 doses, then 10 to 20 mg every 4 to 6 hours. ***Children 2 to 12 years***—PO/Rectal: 2.5 mg 2 or 3 times/day. ***Children 2 to 5 years***—Do not exceed total daily dose of 20 mg. ***Children 6 to 12 years***—Do not exceed total daily dose of 25 mg. IM: 0.132 mg/kg (not to exceed 10 mg/dose).
- **Anxiety:** ***Adults and children >12 years***—PO: 5 mg 3 to 4 times/day, not to exceed 20 mg/d or longer than 12 weeks. Sustained-release caps may be given as 15 mg once daily or 10 mg twice daily.
- **Nausea and vomiting:** ***Adults***—PO: 5 to 10 mg 3 or 4 times/day. SR caps: 15 mg once daily or 10 mg twice daily. Rectal: 25 mg twice daily. IM: 5 to 10 mg. May repeat every 3 or 4 hours, not to exceed 40 mg/d. ***Children 20 to 29 lb***—PO/Rectal: 2.5 mg 1 or 2 times/day, not to exceed 7.5 mg/d. ***Children 30 to 39 lb***—PO/Rectal: 2.5 mg 2 or 3 times/day, not to exceed 10 mg/d. ***Children 40 to 85 lb***—PO/Rectal: 2.5 mg 3 times/day or 5 mg 2 times/day, not to exceed 15 mg/d. ***Children > 20 lb or 2 years of age***—IM: 0.132 mg/kg. Usually only 1 dose is required.
- **Relief of migraine headache:** ***Adults***—IV: 10 mg.

Thioridazine (Mellaril)

- **Psychotic disorders:** ***Adults***—PO: 50 to 100 mg 3 times/day initially. May be gradually increased to a maximum of 800 mg/d to control symptoms. Gradually reduce to the minimum maintenance dose between 200 and 800 mg/d in 2 to 4 divided doses.
- **Psychoneurotic manifestations:** ***Adults***—PO: Initial dose: 25 mg 3 times/day. Adjust dose from 10 mg 2 to 4 times/day for milder cases to 50 mg 3 or 4 times/day for more severe cases. Total daily dosage range: 20 to 200 mg.
- **Pediatric behavioral disorders:** ***Children ages 2 to 12***—PO: Initial dose: 0.5 mg/kg/d in divided doses. May be gradually increased to a maintenance dose of up to 3 mg/kg/d.

Trifluoperazine (Stelazine)

- **Schizophrenia:** ***Adults***— PO: 2 to 5 mg 2 times/day. Usual optimum dosage range: 15 to 20 mg/d, although a few may require 40 mg/d or more. IM: 1 to 2 mg every 4 to 6 hours, not to exceed 10 mg/24 hours. ***Children 6 to 12 years***—PO: Initial dose: 1 mg once or twice daily. May increase dose gradually to a maximum of 15 mg/d. IM: Not recommended for children, but if required to control severe symptoms, may administer 1 mg once or twice daily.

- **Nonpsychotic anxiety:** ***Adults***— PO: 1 to 2 mg 2 times/day. Do not administer more than 6 mg/d or for longer than 12 weeks.

■ CHEMICAL CLASS: BENZISOXAZOLE

Example

Generic (Trade) Name	Pregnancy Category/ Half-life	Indications	Available Forms (mg)
Risperidone (Risperdal)	C/~20	Schizophrenia	Tabs: 0.25, 0.5, 1, 2, 3, 4 Oral Solution: 1/mL

Action

- Exerts antagonistic effects on dopamine type 2 (D_2), serotonin type 2 ($5HT_2$), α_1- and α_2-adrenergic, and H_1 histaminergic receptors

Contraindications and Precautions

Contraindicated in:

- Known hypersensitivity
- Comatose or severely depressed patients
- Clients with cardiac disease
- Lactation

Use cautiously in:

- Clients with hepatic or renal impairment
- Clients with history of seizures
- Clients exposed to temperature extremes
- Clients with history of suicide attempts
- Pregnancy (safety not established)

Adverse Reactions and Side Effects

- Anxiety
- Agitation
- Insomnia
- Sedation
- Extrapyramidal symptoms
- Dizziness
- Headache
- Constipation
- Nausea
- Rhinitis
- Rash
- Tachycardia

Interactions

- Increased effects of risperidone with **clozapine.**
- Decreased effects of **levodopa** and **other dopamine agonists.**
- Decreased effectiveness of risperidone with **carbamazepine.**
- Additive CNS depression with **CNS depressants,** such as **alcohol, antihistamines, sedative/hypnotics,** and **opioid analgesics.**

Route and Dosage

- **Schizophrenia:** ***Adults***—PO: Initial dose: 1 mg twice daily. May increase by 1 mg twice daily on 2nd and 3rd day to 3 mg twice daily on day 3. Further increments may be made at weekly intervals by 1 mg twice daily (usual range, 4 to 6 mg/d, not to exceed 16 mg/d). Optimum dosage range: 4 to 8 mg/d. ***Elderly and debilitated patients***—PO: Initial dose: 0.5 mg twice daily. May increase by 0.5 mg twice daily, up to 1.5 mg twice daily, then increase at weekly intervals if necessary.

CHEMICAL CLASS: BUTYROPHENONE

Example

Generic (Trade) Name	Pregnancy Category/ Half-life	Indications	Available Forms (mg)
Haloperidol (Haldol)	C/21–24 h (oral, IM lactate); 3 wk (IM decanoate)	Psychotic disorders Tourette's disorder Pediatric behavior problems and hyperactivity *Unlabeled uses:* Intractable hiccups Infantile autism Control in acute psychiatric situations	Tabs: 0.5, 1, 2, 5, 10, 20 Concentrate: 2/mL Injection: 5/mL (lactate) Injection: 50/mL; 100/mL (decanoate)

Action

- Blocks postsynaptic dopamine receptors in the hypothalamus, limbic system, and reticular formation.
- Demonstrates varying affinity for cholinergic, α_1-adrenergic, and histaminic receptors.

Contraindications and Precautions

Contraindicated in:

- Hypersensitivity to the drug
- In comatose or severely CNS-depressed clients

- Clients with blood dyscrasias
- Parkinson's disease
- Glaucoma
- Clients with liver, renal, or cardiac insufficiency

Use cautiously in:

- Severely ill or elderly clients
- Diabetic clients
- Clients with history of seizures
- Clients with respiratory insufficiency
- Prostatic hypertrophy
- Pregnancy and lactation (safety has not been established)

Adverse Reactions and Side Effects

Refer to this section under Phenothiazines.

Interactions

- Additive hypotension with **antihypertensives.**
- Additive anticholinergic effects with other **drugs that have anticholinergic properties.**
- Additive CNS depression with other drugs that cause **CNS depression,** such as **alcohol, antihistamines, opioid analgesics,** and **sedative/hypnotics.**
- Decreased effects of haloperidol with **phenytoin** and **carbamazepine.**
- Increased effects of **tricyclic antidepressants** with haloperidol.
- Decreased effects of **guanethidine** with haloperidol.
- Increased risk of EPS with **fluoxetine.**
- Potential for neurotoxicity with **lithium.**
- Decreased plasma levels of haloperidol with **rifampin.**
- Severe hypotension and tachycardia with **epinephrine.**
- Risk of psychosis with **methyldopa.**

Route and Dosage

- **Psychotic disorders:** ***Adults***—PO: Initial dose: 0.05 to 5 mg 2 to 3 times daily. Patients with severe symptoms may require up to 100 mg/d. ***Elderly or debilitated patients***—PO: 0.5 to 2 mg 2 or 3 times/day. ***Children 3 to 12 years***—PO: 25 to 50 μg/kg/d. May increase in 0.5-mg increments every 5 to 7 days up to 0.15 mg/kg/d given in 2 or 3 divided doses.
- **For control of severe symptoms:** ***Adults***—IM: 2 to 5 mg every 1 to 8 hours.
- **For chronic psychosis requiring prolonged antipsychotic therapy:** ***Adults*—IM decanoate**: 10 to 15 times the previous daily oral dose, not to exceed 100 mg initially. Repeat every 4 weeks, or adjust interval to patient response.
- **Tourette's disorder:** ***Adults***—PO: Initial dose: 0.5 to 1.5 mg 3 times/day. Increase dose gradually as determined by patient

response. Up to about 10 mg/d may be required. ***Children 3 to 12 years***—PO: 0.05 to 0.075 mg/kg/d.

- **Behavioral disorders/hyperactivity:** ***Children 3 to 12 years***—PO: 0.05 to 0.075 mg/kg/d.
- **Intractable hiccups:** ***Adults***—PO: 1.5 mg 3 times/day. ***Adults***—IM/IV: 3 to 15 mg in divided doses.
- **Infantile autism:** ***Children 3 to 12 years***—PO: 0.5 to 4 mg/d.
- **Control in acute psychiatric situations:** IM/IV: 2 to 30 mg, approximately every 60 minutes, at a rate of 5 mg/min.

■ CHEMICAL CLASS: DIBENZOXAZEPINE

Example

Generic (Trade) Name	Pregnancy Category/ Half-life	Indications	Available Forms (mg)
Loxapine (Loxitane)	Initial: 5 h Terminal: 19 h	Schizophrenia	Caps: 5, 10, 25, 50

Action

- Not fully understood
- Thought to act primarily in the reticular formation
- Reduces firing threshold of CNS neurons

Contraindications and Precautions

Contraindicated in:

- Hypersensitivity
- Comatose or severe drug-induced depressed states
- Clients with blood dyscrasias
- Parkinson's disease
- Hepatic, renal, or cardiac insufficiency
- Severe hypotension or hypertension
- Children younger than 16 years; pregnancy and lactation (safety has not been established)

Use cautiously in:

- Patients with history of seizures
- Respiratory insufficiency
- Prostatic hypertrophy
- Elderly or debilitated patients
- Glaucoma

Adverse Reactions and Side Effects

Refer to this section under Phenothiazines.

Interactions

- Increased CNS depression with other drugs that produce CNS depression, such as **alcohol, anxiolytics, antidepressants,** and **sedative/hypnotics.**
- Concomitant use with **lorazepam** may result in respiratory depression, stupor, and/or hypotension.

Route and Dosage

- **Schizophrenia:** ***Adults***— PO: Initial dose: 10 mg 2 times/day. May increase dose fairly rapidly over 7 to 10 days, depending on severity of condition. Optimal maintenance dose: 20 to 60 mg/d (range: 20 to 250 mg/d). Maintain dose at lowest level compatible with control of symptoms.

CHEMICAL CLASS: DIBENZODIAZEPINE

Example

Generic (Trade) Name	Pregnancy Category/ Half-life	Indications	Available Forms (mg)
Clozapine (Clozaril)	B/4–66 h	Refractory schizophrenia	Tabs: 25, 100

Action

- Exerts an antagonistic effect on dopamine receptors, with a particularly high affinity for the D_4 receptor.
- It appears to be more active at limbic that at striatal dopamine receptors.
- Also acts as an antagonist at adrenergic, cholinergic, histaminergic, and serotonergic receptors.

Contraindications and Precautions

Contraindicated in:

- Hypersensitivity
- Myeloproliferative disorders
- History of clozapine-induced agranulocytosis or severe granulocytopenia
- Concomitant use with other drugs that have the potential to suppress bone marrow function
- Severe CNS depression or comatose states
- Uncontrolled epilepsy
- Lactation
- Children (safety has not been established)

Use cautiously in:

- Patients with hepatic, renal, or cardiac insufficiency
- Diabetes mellitus

- Prostatic enlargement
- Narrow-angle glaucoma
- Pregnancy

Adverse Reactions and Side Effects

- Drowsiness, dizziness
- Agranulocytosis
- Seizures (appear to be dose-related)
- Salivation
- Sedation
- Tachycardia
- Constipation
- Fever
- Weight gain
- Orthostatic hypotension
- Neuroleptic malignant syndrome
- Hyperglycemia

Interactions

- Increased effects of **risperidone** with Clozaril.
- Additive anticholinergic effects with other **agents having anticholinergic properties.**
- Additive CNS depression with **alcohol, antidepressants, antihistamines, opioid analgesics,** and **sedative/hypnotics.**
- Increased risk of agranulocytosis with **agents that suppress bone marrow function.**
- Additive hypotensive effects with **antihypertensive agents.**
- Decreased effects of clozaril with **phenytoin, nicotine,** and **rifampin.**
- Increased plasma levels of Clozaril with **cimetidine, caffeine, erythromycin,** and **selective serotonin reuptake inhibitors** (particularly **fluvoxamine**).

Route and Dosage

- **Schizophrenia:** ***Adults***—PO: Initial dose: 12.5 mg once or twice daily. May increase dose by 25 to 50 mg/d over 2 weeks to a target dose of 300 to 450 mg/d. If required, make additional increases in increments of 100 mg not more than once or twice weekly to a maximum dose of 900 mg/d in 3 divided doses. Titrate dose slowly to observe for possible seizures and agranulocytosis. Ordinarily only a 1-week supply of medication is dispensed at a time, and clients are required to present for weekly white blood cell (WBC) counts to monitor for adverse effect of agranulocytosis.

CHEMICAL CLASS: DIBENZOTHIAZEPINE

Example

Generic (Trade) Name	Pregnancy Category/ Half-life	Indications	Available Forms (mg)
Quetiapine (Seroquel)	C/6 h	Schizophrenia	Tabs: 25, 100, 200, 300

Action

- Antipsychotic activity is thought to be mediated through a combination of dopamine type 2 (D_2) and serotonin type 2 ($5HT_2$) antagonism. Other effects may be due to antagonism of histamine H_1 receptors and adrenergic α_1 receptors.

Contraindications and Precautions

Contraindicated in:
- Hypersensitivity
- Lactation
- Children (safety has not been established)

Use cautiously in:
- Clients with hepatic or cardiovascular disease
- Clients with history of seizures
- Comatose or other CNS-depressed clients
- Clients at risk for aspiration pneumonia
- Pregnancy
- Elderly and debilitated clients

Adverse Reactions and Side Effects

- Somnolence
- Dizziness
- Headache
- Constipation
- Dry mouth
- Dyspepsia
- Weight gain
- Orthostatic hypotension
- Neuroleptic malignant syndrome
- Extrapyramidal symptoms
- Tardive dyskinesia
- Cataracts
- Lowered seizure threshold

Interactions

- Additive hypotension with **antihypertensive drugs.**
- Additive CNS depression with **alcohol, antihistamines, opioid analgesics,** and **sedative/hypnotics.**
- May antagonize the effects of **levodopa** and **dopamine agonists.**
- Decreased clearance of **lorazepam** with quetiapine.
- Increased clearance of quetiapine with **thioridazine, phenytoin, carbamazepine, barbiturates, rifampin,** and **glucocorticoids.**
- Decreased clearance of quetiapine with **cimetidine, ketoconazole, itraconazole, fluconazole,** and **erythromycin.**

Route and Dosage

- **Schizophrenia:** ***Adults***—PO: Initial dose: 25 mg 2 times/day. May increase in increments of 25 to 50 mg 2 or 3 times/day on days 2 and 3 to a target dose range of 300 to 400 mg/d (in 2 or 3 divided doses) by day 4. Maximum daily dose: 800 mg.

■ CHEMICAL CLASS: DIHYDROCARBOSTYRIL

Example

Generic (Trade) Name	Pregnancy Category/ Half-life	Indications	Available Forms (mg)
Aripiprazole (Abilify)	C/75 h (aripiprazole); 94 h (metabolite)	Schizophrenia	Tabs: 10, 15, 20, 30

Action

- The efficacy of aripiprazole is thought to occur through a combination of partial agonist activity at D_2 and 5-HT_{1A} receptors and antagonist activity at 5-HT_{2A} receptors.
- Also exhibits antagonist activity at adrenergic α_1 receptors.

Contraindications and Precautions

Contraindicated in:

- Hypersensitivity
- Lactation

Use cautiously in:

- Alzheimer's disease
- History of seizures
- Hepatic or renal impairment
- Known cardiovascular or cerebrovascular disease
- Conditions that cause hypotension (dehydration, hypovolemia, treatment with antihypertensive medication)

- Pregnancy (weigh benefits of the drug against potential risk to fetus)
- Children and adolescents (safety and effectiveness have not been established)

Adverse Reactions and Side Effects

- Headache
- Nausea and vomiting
- Constipation
- Anxiety, restlessness
- Insomnia
- Lightheadedness
- Somnolence
- Weight gain, weight loss
- Blurred vision
- Increased salivation
- Extrapyramidal symptoms

Interactions

- Decreased plasma levels of aripiprazole with **carbamazepine** and **other CYP3A4 inducers.**
- Increased plasma levels and potential for aripiprazole toxicity with **CYP2D6 inhibitors**, such as **quinidine, fluoxetine,** and **paroxetine.**
- Decreased metabolism and increased effects of aripiprazole with **ketoconazole** or **other CYP3A4 inhibitors.**
- Additive hypotensive effects with **antihypertensive drugs.**
- Additive CNS effects with **alcohol.**

Route and Dosage

- **Schizophrenia:** ***Adults***—PO: Initial and target dose: 10 or 15 mg/d as a single dose. Doses up to 30 mg/d have been used but were not more effective than 10 or 15 mg/d. Dose increases should not be made before 2 weeks. Maximum daily dose: 30 mg.

■ CHEMICAL CLASS: DIHYDROINDOLONE

Example

Generic (Trade) Name	Pregnancy Category/ Half-life	Indications	Available Forms (mg)
Molindone (Moban)	C/10–20 h	Psychotic disorders	Tabs: 5, 10, 25, 50, 100 Concentrate: 20/mL

Action

The exact mechanism of action is not fully understood. It is thought that molindone exerts its effect on the ascending reticular activating system.

Contraindications and Precautions

Contraindicated in:

- Hypersensitivity
- Comatose or severely CNS-depressed patients
- Children younger than 12 years (safety has not been established)
- Lactation
- Sensitivity to sulfites (contained in some preparations)

Use cautiously in:

- Patients with history of seizures
- Respiratory, renal, hepatic, thyroid, or cardiovascular disorders
- Elderly or debilitated patients
- Pregnancy

Adverse Reactions and Side Effects

Refer to this section under Phenothiazines.

Interactions

- Additive CNS effects with **CNS depressants.**
- Additive anticholinergic effects with drugs that have anticholinergic properties.
- Decreased absorption of **phenytoin** and **tetracyclines** with molindone.

Route and Dosage

- **Psychotic disorders:** ***Adults***—PO: Initial dose: 50 to 75 mg/d. May increase to 100 mg in 3 or 4 days, up to 225 mg/d if required.
- **Maintenance therapy:** ***Adults***—*Mild symptoms:* PO: 5 to 15 mg 3 or 4 times/day.
- **Moderate symptoms:** PO: 10 to 25 mg 3 or 4 times/day.
- **Severe symptoms:** PO: Up to 225 mg/d may be required.

■ CHEMICAL CLASS: THIENOBENZODIAZEPINE

Example

Generic (Trade) Name	Pregnancy Category/ Half-life	Indications	Available Forms (mg)
Olanzapine (Zyprexa)	C/21–54 h	Schizophrenia Bipolar mania	Tabs: 2.5, 5, 7.5, 10, 15, 20

Action

- Efficacy in schizophrenia is mediated through a combination of dopamine and $5HT_2$ antagonism.
- Also shows antagonism for muscarinic, histaminic, and adrenergic receptors.
- The mechanism of action of olanzapine in the treatment of bipolar mania is unknown.

Contraindications and Precautions

Contraindicated in:

- Hypersensitivity
- Children (safety has not been established)
- Lactation

Use cautiously in:

- Patients with hepatic or cardiovascular disease
- Patients with history of seizures
- Comatose or other CNS-depressed patients
- Patients at risk for aspiration pneumonia
- Prostatic hypertrophy
- Narrow-angle glaucoma
- History of paralytic ileus
- Pregnancy
- Elderly and debilitated patients
- Conditions that may contribute to elevation in core body temperature

Adverse Reactions and Side Effects

- Asthenia
- Somnolence
- Headache
- Fever
- Dizziness
- Dry mouth
- Constipation
- Weight gain
- Orthostatic hypotension
- Tachycardia
- Extrapyramidal symptoms (high-dose–dependent)

Interactions

- Antagonizes the effects of **levodopa** and **dopamine agonists.**
- Additive CNS depression with **alcohol** and other **CNS depressants.**
- Possible additive hypotensive effects with **antihypertensive agents.**

- Decreased olanzapine effects with **carbamazepine, omeprazole,** and **rifampin.**
- Decreased clearance of olanzapine with **fluvoxamine.**
- Concomitant use with **alcohol** or **diazepam** potentiates orthostatic hypotension.

Route and Dosage

- **Schizophrenia:** ***Adults***—PO: Initial dose: 5 to 10 mg/d. May increase at weekly intervals by 5 mg/d (not to exceed 20 mg/d).
- **Bipolar mania:** ***Adults***—PO: Initial dose: 10 to 15 mg/d. May increase every 24 hours by 5 mg/d (not to exceed 20 mg/d).

■ CHEMICAL CLASS: THIOXANTHENE

Example

Generic (Trade) Name	Pregnancy Category/ Half-life	Indications	Available Forms (mg)
Thiothixene (Navane)	C/34 h	Psychotic disorders	Caps: 1, 2, 5, 10, 20 Concentrate: 5/mL Injection: 2/mL; 5/mL

Action

- Blocks postsynaptic dopamine receptors in the hypothalamus, limbic system, and reticular formation.
- Demonstrates varying affinity for cholinergic, α_1-adrenergic, and histaminic receptors.

Contraindications and Precautions

Contraindicated in:

- Hypersensitivity
- Comatose or severely CNS-depressed patients
- Bone marrow depression or blood dyscrasias
- Parkinson's disease
- Severe hypotension or hypertension
- Children younger than 12 years
- Pregnancy and lactation (safety has not been established)

Use cautiously in:

- Patients with history of seizures
- Respiratory, renal, hepatic, thyroid, and cardiovascular disorders
- Elderly or debilitated patients
- Patients exposed to extreme environmental heat
- Patients taking atropine or atropine-like drugs

Adverse Reactions and Side Effects

Refer to this section under Phenothiazines.

Interactions

- Additive CNS depression with **alcohol** and other **CNS depressants.**
- Additive anticholinergic effects with other drugs that have anticholinergic properties.
- Possible additive hypotension with **antihypertensive agents.**

Route and Dosage

- **Psychotic Disorders:** ***Adults***—PO: *Mild conditions:* Initial dose: 2 mg 3 times/day. May increase to 15 mg. *Severe conditions:* Initial dose: 5 mg 2 times/day. Optimal dose is 20 to 30 mg/d. May increase gradually, not to exceed 60 mg/d.
- *In cases in which rapid control is required or oral administration is not indicated:* ***Adults***—IM: Initial dose: 4 mg 2 to 4 times/day. Adjust dose according to patient's response. Maximum daily dose: 30 mg. Switch to oral form as soon as possible.

■ CHEMICAL CLASS: BENZOTHIAZOLYLPIPERAZINE

Example

Generic (Trade) Name	Pregnancy Category/ Half-life	Indications	Available Forms (mg)
Ziprasidone (Geodon)	C/7 h	Schizophrenia	Caps: 20, 40, 60, 80 Injection: 20/mL

Action

- Efficacy in schizophrenia is mediated through a combination of dopamine type 2 (D_2) and serotonin type 2 ($5HT_2$) antagonism.
- May also exhibit antagonism of histamine H_1 receptors and α_1-adrenergic receptors.

Contraindications and Precautions

Contraindicated in:

- Hypersensitivity
- History of QT prolongation or cardiac arrhythmias
- Recent myocardial infarction
- Uncompensated heart failure
- Concurrent use with other drugs that prolong the QT interval
- Hypokalemia or hypomagnesemia
- Lactation

Use cautiously in:

- Concurrent diuretic therapy or diarrhea (may increase the risk of hypotension, hypokalemia, or hypomagnesemia)

- Hepatic or renal insufficiency
- History of cardiovascular or cerebrovascular disease
- History of seizures
- Hypotension, concurrent antihypertensive therapy, dehydration, or hypovolemia (may increase the risk of orthostatic hypotension)
- Patients with Alzheimer's disease or advanced age or others who may be at risk for aspiration pneumonia
- Pregnancy and children (safety has not been established)

Adverse Reactions and Side Effects

- Somnolence
- Headache
- Nausea
- Dyspepsia
- Constipation
- Dizziness
- Diarrhea
- Restlessness
- Extrapyramidal symptoms
- Prolonged QT interval
- Orthostatic hypotension
- Rash

Interactions

- Additive effects with drugs that prolong QT interval. Do not administer with **dofetilide, sotalol, quinidine, other class Ia and III antiarrhythmics, mesoridazine, thioridazine, chlorpromazine, droperidol, pimozide, sparfloxacin, gatifloxacin, moxifloxacin, halofantrine, mefloquine, pentamidine, arsenic trioxide, levomethadyl acetate, dolasetron mesylate, probucol, or tacrolimus.**
- Additive CNS effects with **alcohol** or other **CNS depressants.**
- Additive hypotensive effects with **antihypertensive agents.**
- May antagonize the effects of **levodopa** and **dopamine agonists.**
- Decreased blood levels of ziprasidone with **carbamazepine.**
- Increased blood levels of ziprasidone with **ketoconazole.**

Route and Dosage

- **Schizophrenia:** ***Adults***—PO: Initial dose: 20 mg 2 times/day. May increase dose by intervals of at least 2 days up to a dose of 80 mg 2 times/day.

■ NURSING DIAGNOSES RELATED TO ALL ANTIPSYCHOTIC AGENTS

- Risk for other-directed violence related to panic anxiety and mistrust of others.

- Risk for injury related to medication side effects of sedation, photosensitivity, reduction of seizure threshold, agranulocytosis, extrapyramidal symptoms, tardive dyskinesia, neuroleptic malignant syndrome, and/or QT prolongation.
- Risk for activity intolerance related to medication side effects of sedation, blurred vision, and/or weakness.
- Noncompliance with medication regimen related to suspiciousness and mistrust of others.

■ NURSING IMPLICATIONS FOR ANTIPSYCHOTIC AGENTS

The plan of care should include monitoring for the following side effects from antipsychotic medications. Nursing implications related to each side effect are designated by an asterisk (*).

1. Anticholinergic Effects
   a. Dry mouth
      *Provide client with sugarless candy or gum, ice, and frequent sips of water.
      *Ensure that client practices strict oral hygiene.
   b. Blurred vision
      *Explain that this symptom will most likely subside after a few weeks.
      *Advise client not to drive a car until vision clears.
      *Clear small items from pathway to prevent falls.
   c. Constipation
      *Order foods high in fiber; encourage increase in physical activity and fluid intake if not contraindicated.
   d. Urinary retention
      *Instruct client to report any difficulty urinating; monitor intake and output.
2. Nausea; Gastrointestinal (GI) Upset
   *Tablets or capsules may be administered with food to minimize GI upset.
   *Concentrates may be diluted and administered with fruit juice or other liquid; they should be mixed immediately before administration.
3. Skin Rash
   *Report appearance of any rash on skin to physician.
   *Avoid spilling any of the liquid concentrate on skin; contact dermatitis can occur.
4. Sedation
   *Discuss with physician possibility of administering drug at bedtime.
   *Discuss with physician possible decrease in dose or order for less sedating drug.
   *Instruct client not to drive or operate dangerous equipment while experiencing sedation.

5. Orthostatic Hypotension
   *Instruct client to rise slowly from a lying or sitting position; monitor blood pressure (lying and standing) each shift; document and report significant changes.
6. Photosensitivity
   *Ensure that client wears protective sunscreens, clothing, and sunglasses while spending time outdoors.
7. Hormonal Effects
   a. Decreased libido, retrograde ejaculation, gynecomastia (men)
      *Provide explanation of the effects and reassurance of reversibility. If necessary, discuss with physician possibility of ordering alternate medication.
   b. Amenorrhea (women)
      *Offer reassurance of reversibility; instruct client to continue use of contraception because amenorrhea does not indicate cessation of ovulation.
   c. Weight gain
      *Weigh client every other day; order calorie-controlled diet; provide opportunity for physical exercise; provide diet and exercise instruction.
8. Reduction of Seizure Threshold
   *Closely observe client with history of seizures.
   *NOTE: This is particularly important with clients taking clozapine (Clozaril). Reportedly, seizures affect 1 to 5 percent of individuals who take this drug, depending on the dose.
9. Agranulocytosis
   *Potentially very serious side effect, but relatively rare with most of the antipsychotic drugs. It usually occurs within the first 3 months of treatment. Observe for symptoms of sore throat, fever, and malaise. A complete blood count should be monitored if these symptoms appear.
   *EXCEPTION: With clozapine (Clozaril), agranulocytosis occurs in 1.2 percent of all clients taking the drug (Schatzberg, Cole, & DeBattista, 2003). It is a potentially fatal blood disorder in which the client's WBC count can drop to extremely low levels. Individuals receiving clozapine therapy are required to have blood levels drawn weekly for the first 6 months of therapy, followed by biweekly monitoring for patients with acceptable WBC counts. If the WBC count falls below 3000 mm^3 or the granulocyte count falls below 1500 mm^3, clozapine therapy is discontinued. The disorder is reversible if discovered in the early stages. However, this additional required technology of weekly blood tests has made this drug cost-prohibitive for some people.
10. Salivation (with clozapine)
   *A significant number of clients receiving clozapine (Clozaril) therapy experience extreme salivation. Offer support to

client, as this may be an embarrassing situation. It may even be a safety issue (e.g., risk of aspiration) if the problem is very severe.

11. Extrapyramidal Symptoms
    *Observe for symptoms and report; administer antiparkinsonian drugs as ordered.
    a. Pseudoparkinsonism (tremor, shuffling gait, drooling, rigidity).
       *Symptoms may appear 1 to 5 days following initiation of antipsychotic medication; occurs most often in women, the elderly, and dehydrated clients.
    b. Akinesia (muscular weakness).
       *Same as pseudoparkinsonism.
    c. Akathisia (continuous restlessness and fidgeting).
       *This occurs most frequently in women; symptoms may occur 50 to 60 days following initiation of therapy.
    d. Dystonia (involuntary muscular movements [spasms] of face, arms, legs, and neck).
       *This occurs most often in men and in clients younger than 25 years.
    e. Oculogyric crisis (uncontrolled rolling back of the eyes).
       *This may appear as part of the syndrome described as dystonia. It may be mistaken for seizure activity. Dystonia and oculogyric crisis should be treated as emergency situations. The physician should be contacted, and intravenous benztropine mesylate (Cogentin) is commonly administered. Stay with client, and offer reassurance and support during this frightening time.
12. Tardive Dyskinesia (bizarre facial and tongue movements, stiff neck, and difficulty swallowing).
    a. All clients receiving long-term (months or years) antipsychotic therapy are at risk.
       *Symptoms are potentially irreversible.
       *Drug should be withdrawn at first sign, which is usually vermiform movements of the tongue; prompt action may prevent irreversibility.
13. Neuroleptic Malignant Syndrome (NMS)
    a. NMS is a rare but potentially fatal complication of treatment with neuroleptic drugs. Routine assessments should include temperature and observation for parkinsonian symptoms. Onset can occur within hours or even years after drug initiation, and progression is rapid over the following 24 to 72 hours.
       *Symptoms include severe parkinsonian muscle rigidity, hyperpyrexia up to 107° F, tachycardia, tachypnea, fluctuations in blood pressure, diaphoresis, and rapid deterioration of mental status to stupor and coma.

*Discontinue neuroleptic medication immediately.
*Monitor vital signs, degree of muscle rigidity, intake and output, level of consciousness.
*The physician may order bromocriptine (Parlodel) or dantrolene (Dantrium) to counteract the effects of NMS.

14. ECG Changes
    a. ECG changes, including prolongation of the QT interval, are possible with most of the antipsychotics. This is particularly true with ziprasidone (Geodon). Caution is advised in prescribing this medication to individuals with history of arrhythmias. Conditions that produce hypokalemia and/or hypomagnesemia, such as diuretic therapy or diarrhea, should be taken into consideration when prescribing. Routine ECG should be taken before initiation of therapy and periodically during therapy.
    *Monitor vital signs every shift.
    *Observe for symptoms of dizziness, palpitations, syncope, or weakness.

■ CLIENT/FAMILY EDUCATION RELATED TO ALL ANTIPSYCHOTICS

- Use caution when driving or operating dangerous machinery. Drowsiness and dizziness can occur.
- Do not stop taking the drug abruptly after long-term use. To do so might produce withdrawal symptoms, such as nausea, vomiting, gastritis, headache, tachycardia, insomnia, or tremulousness.
- Use sunscreens, and wear protective clothing when spending time outdoors. Skin is more susceptible to sunburn, which can occur as quickly as 30 minutes.
- Report weekly (if receiving clozapine therapy) to have blood levels drawn and to obtain a weekly supply of the drug.
- Report occurrence of any of the following symptoms to the physician immediately: sore throat, fever, malaise, unusual bleeding, easy bruising, persistent nausea and vomiting, severe headache, rapid heart rate, fainting, difficulty urinating, muscle twitching, tremors, darkly colored urine, pale stools, yellow skin or eyes, muscular incoordination, and skin rash.
- Rise slowly from a sitting or lying position to prevent a sudden drop in blood pressure.
- If experiencing a problem with dry mouth, take frequent sips of water, chew sugarless gum, or suck on hard candy. Good oral care (frequent brushing, flossing) is very important.
- Consult the physician regarding smoking while taking this medication. Smoking increases the metabolism of some antipsychotics, possibly requiring adjustment in dosage to achieve therapeutic effect.

- Dress warmly in cold weather, and avoid extended exposure to very high or low temperatures. Body temperature is harder to maintain with this medication.
- Do not drink alcohol while on antipsychotic therapy. These drugs potentiate each other's effects.
- Do not consume other medications (including over-the-counter products) without physician's approval. Many medications contain substances that interact with antipsychotics in a way that may be harmful.
- Be aware of possible risks of taking antipsychotic medication during pregnancy. Safe use during pregnancy and lactation has not been established. Antipsychotics are thought to readily cross the placental barrier; if so, a fetus could experience adverse effects of the drug. Client should inform the physician immediately if pregnancy occurs, is suspected, or is planned.
- Be aware of side effects of antipsychotic drugs. Refer to written materials furnished by health-care providers for safe self-administration.
- Continue to take medication, even if feeling well and as though it is not needed. Symptoms may return if medication is discontinued.
- Carry card or other identification at all times describing medications being taken.

INTERNET REFERENCES

- http://www.rxlist.com
- http://www.nimh.nih.gov/publicat/medicate.cfm
- http://www.fadavis.com/townsend

CHAPTER 28

Antiparkinsonian Agents

CHEMICAL CLASS: ANTICHOLINERGICS

Examples

Generic (Trade) Name	Pregnancy Category/ Half-life	Indications	Available Forms (mg)
Benztropine (Cogentin)	C/Unknown	Parkinsonism Drug-induced extrapyramidal symptoms	Tabs: 0.5, 1, 2 Injection: 1/mL
Biperiden (Akineton)	C/18.4–24.3 h	Parkinsonism Drug-induced extrapyramidal symptoms	Tabs: 2
Procyclidine (Kemadrin)	C/11.5–12.5 h	Parkinsonism Drug-induced extrapyramidal symptoms	Tabs: 5
Trihexyphenidyl (Artane)	C/5.6–10.2 h	Parkinsonism Drug-induced extrapyramidal symptoms	Tabs: 2, 5 Elixir: 2/5 mL
Diphenhydramine (Benadryl)	B/4–15 h	Parkinsonism Drug-induced extrapyramidal symptoms Motion sickness Allergy reactions Nighttime sleep aid Cough suppressant	Tabs/Caps: 25, 50 Elixir/Syrup: 12.5/5 mL Injection: 50/mL

Action

- Block acetylcholine receptors to diminish excess cholinergic effects. May also inhibit the reuptake and storage of dopamine at central dopamine receptors, thereby prolonging the action of dopamine.

- Diphenhydramine also blocks histamine release by competing with histamine for H_1 receptor sites. Decreased allergic response and somnolence are affected by diminished histamine activity.

Contraindications and Precautions

Contraindicated in:

- Hypersensitivity
- Narrow-angle glaucoma
- Pyloric or duodenal obstruction
- Peptic ulcers
- Prostatic hypertrophy
- Megaesophagus
- Megacolon
- Myasthenia gravis
- Lactation
- Children (*except* diphenhydramine)

Use cautiously in:

- Tachycardia
- Cardiac arrhythmias
- Hypertension
- Hypotension
- Tendency to urinary retention
- Clients exposed to high environmental temperatures
- Pregnancy

Adverse Reactions and Side Effects

- Dry mouth
- Blurred vision
- Constipation
- Paralytic ileus
- Urinary retention
- Tachycardia
- Agitation, nervousness
- Decreased sweating
- Elevated temperature
- Nausea/vomiting
- Sedation
- Dizziness
- Exacerbation of psychoses
- Orthostatic hypotension

Interactions

- **Diphenhydramine:** Additive sedative effects with central nervous system (**CNS**) **depressants.**
- Additive anticholinergic effects with other drugs that have anticholinergic properties.

- Anticholinergic drugs counteract the cholinergic effects of **bethanechol.**
- Possible increased **digoxin** levels with anticholinergics.
- Concomitant use of anticholinergics with **haloperidol** may result in worsening of psychotic symptoms, decreased haloperidol serum levels, and development of tardive dyskinesia.
- Possible decreased efficacy of **phenothiazines** and increased incidence of anticholinergic side effects with concomitant use.

Route and Dosage

Benztropine (Cogentin)

- **Parkinsonism:** ***Adults***—PO: 1 to 2 mg/d in 1 to 2 divided doses (range 0.5 to 6 mg/d).
- **Drug-induced extrapyramidal symptoms:** ***Adults***—PO: 1 to 4 mg given once or twice daily.
- **Acute dystonic reactions:** ***Adults***—IM, IV: 1 to 2 mg, then 1 to 2 mg PO twice daily.

Biperiden (Akineton)

- **Parkinsonism:** ***Adults***—PO: 2 mg 3 or 4 times/day, not to exceed 16 mg/24 h.
- **Drug-induced extrapyramidal symptoms:** ***Adults***—PO: 2 mg 1 to 3 times/day.

Procyclidine (Kemadrin)

- **Parkinsonism:** ***Adults***—PO: Initial dose: 2.5 mg 3 times/day after meals. May increase slowly to 5 mg 3 times/day and, if necessary, at bedtime.
- **Drug-induced extrapyramidal symptoms:** ***Adults***—PO: Initial dose: 2.5 mg 3 times/day. Increase in daily increments of 2.5 mg to maintenance dose of 10 to 20 mg daily.

Trihexyphenidyl (Artane)

- **Parkinsonism:** ***Adults***—PO: Initial dose: 1 to 2 mg the 1st day; increase by 2 mg increments at 3- to 5-day intervals up to a daily dose of 6 to 10 mg in 3 divided doses taken at mealtimes.
- **Drug-induced extrapyramidal symptoms:** ***Adults***—PO: Initial dose: 1 mg. Repeat dose every few hours until symptoms are controlled. Maintenance or prophylactic use: 5 to 15 mg/d.

Diphenhydramine (Benadryl)

- **Parkinsonism and drug-induced extrapyramidal symptoms/Motion sickness/Allergy reactions:** ***Adults***—PO: 25 to 50 mg 3 or 4 times/day. IM/IV: 10 to 50 mg. Maximum daily dosage: 400 mg. ***Children >10 kg***—PO: 12.5 to 25 mg 3 or 4 times/day or 5 mg/kg/d, not to exceed 300 mg/d. IM/IV: 5 mg/kg/d divided into 4 doses, not to exceed 300 mg/d.
- **Nighttime sleep aid:** ***Adults and children ≥12 years***—50 mg at bedtime.

- **Cough suppressant (syrup only):** ***Adults***—PO: 25 mg every 4 hours, not to exceed 100 mg in 24 hours. ***Children 6 to 12 years***—PO: 12.5 mg every 4 hours, not to exceed 50 mg in 24 hours. ***Children 2 to 6 years***—PO: 6.25 mg every 4 hours, not to exceed 25 mg in 24 hours.

■ CHEMICAL CLASS: DOPAMINERGIC AGONISTS

Examples

Generic (Trade) Name	Pregnancy Category/ Half-life	Indications	Available Forms (mg)
Amantadine (Symmetrel)	C/10–25 h	Parkinsonism Drug induced extrapyramidal symptoms Prophylaxis and treatment of influenza A viral infection	Caps: 100 Syrup: 50/5mL
Bromocriptine (Parlodel)	B/6–8 h	Parkinsonism Hyperprolactinemia-associated dysfunctions Acromegaly Neuroleptic malignant syndrome	Tabs: 2.5 Caps: 5

Action

Increase the content of dopamine in the brain directly by stimulating dopamine receptors, by releasing intact dopamine stores, or by blocking neuronal dopamine reuptake.

Contraindications and Precautions

Contraindicated in:

Amantadine:

- Hypersensitivity to the drug
- Safe use in pregnancy, lactation, and in children younger than 1 year has not been established.
- Angle-closure glaucoma

Bromocriptine:

- Hypersensitivity to this drug, other ergot alkaloids, or sulfites (contained in some preparations)
- Clients with severe peripheral vascular disease
- Pregnancy and lactation; children younger than 15 years (safety has not been established)

Use cautiously in:

- Hepatic or renal impairment
- Uncontrolled psychiatric disturbances

- History of congestive heart failure, myocardial infarction, or ventricular arrhythmia
- Elderly or debilitated clients
- Orthostatic hypotension

Amantadine:

- Clients with a history of seizures
- Concurrent use of CNS stimulants

Bromocriptine:

- Clients with acromegaly

Adverse Reactions and Side Effects

Refer to this section under Anticholinergics.

Interactions

- Additive anticholinergic effects with other drugs that have anticholinergic properties.
- Increased CNS stimulation with **CNS stimulants.**
- Increased plasma levels of amantadine with **trimethoprim-sulfamethoxazole, quinine,** or **quinidine.**
- Increased levels of bromocriptine with **erythromycin.**
- Concurrent use with **phenothiazines, haloperidol, methyldopa, reserpine,** and **tricyclic antidepressants** reduces bromocriptine's ability to decrease prolactin levels.
- Additive CNS effects with **alcohol.**

Route and Dosage

Amantadine (Symmetrel)

- **Parkinsonism:** ***Adults***—PO: 100 mg 1 to 2 times/day (up to 400 mg/d).
- **Drug-induced extrapyramidal symptoms:** ***Adults***—PO: 100 mg 2 times/day (up to 300 mg/d in divided doses).
- **Influenza A viral infection:** ***Adults and children >12 years***—PO: 200 mg/d as a single dose or 100 mg 2 times/day (not >100 mg/d in geriatric clients). ***Children 9 to12 years***—PO: 100 mg twice daily. ***Children 1 to 9 years***—PO: 4.4 to 8.8 mg/kg/d given once daily or divided twice daily, not to exceed 150 mg/d.

Bromocriptine (Parlodel)

- **Parkinsonism:** ***Adults***— PO: Initial dose: 1.25 mg 2 times/day with meals. May increase dose every 2 to 4 weeks by 2.5 mg/d with meals. Usual range is 10 to 40 mg/d.
- **Hyperprolactinemia-associated dysfunctions:** ***Adults***—PO: Initial dose: 0.5 to 2.5 mg/d with meals. May increase by 2.5 mg every 3 to 7 days. Usual therapeutic dosage range: 2.5 to 15 mg/d.
- **Acromegaly:** ***Adults***—PO: Initial dose: 1.25 to 2.5 mg for 3 days (with food) at bedtime. May increase by 1.25 to 2.5 mg/d every

3 to 7 days. Usual therapeutic dosage range: 20 to 30 mg/d. Maximum dosage: 100 mg/d.

- **Neuroleptic malignant syndrome: *Adults*—**PO: 2.5 to 5 mg 3 times/day.

NURSING DIAGNOSES RELATED TO ANTIPARKINSONIAN AGENTS

1. Risk for injury related to symptoms of Parkinson's disease or drug-induced EPS.
2. Hyperthermia related to anticholinergic effect of decreased sweating.
3. Activity intolerance related to side effects of drowsiness, dizziness, ataxia, weakness, or confusion.
4. Deficient knowledge related to medication regimen.

NURSING IMPLICATIONS FOR ANTIPARKINSONIAN AGENTS

The plan of care should include monitoring for the following side effects from antiparkinsonian medications. Nursing implications related to each side effect are designated by an asterisk (*).

1. Anticholinergic Effects. These side effects are identical to those produced by antipsychotic drugs. Taking both medications compounds these effects. For this reason, the physician may elect to prescribe an antiparkinsonian agent only at the onset of EPS rather than as routine adjunctive therapy.
   a. Dry mouth
      *Offer sugarless candy or gum, ice, frequent sips of water.
      *Ensure that client practices strict oral hygiene.
   b. Blurred vision
      *Explain that symptom will most likely subside after a few weeks.
      *Offer to assist with tasks requiring visual acuity.
   c. Constipation
      *Order foods high in fiber; encourage increase in physical activity and fluid intake, if not contraindicated.
   d. Paralytic ileus
      *A rare but potentially very serious side effect of anticholinergic drugs. Monitor for abdominal distention, absent bowel sounds, nausea, vomiting, and epigastric pain.
      *Report any of these symptoms to physician immediately.
   e. Urinary retention
      *Instruct client to report any difficulty urinating; monitor intake and output.
   f. Tachycardia, decreased sweating, elevated temperature
      *Assess vital signs each shift; document and report significant changes to physician.

*Ensure that client remains in cool environment, because the body is unable to cool itself naturally with this medication.

2. Nausea, Gastrointestinal (GI) Upset
   *May administer tablets or capsules with food to minimize GI upset.
3. Sedation, Drowsiness, Dizziness
   *Discuss with physician possibility of administering drug at bedtime.
   *Discuss with physician possible decrease in dosage or ordering less sedating drug.
   *Instruct client not to drive or use dangerous equipment while experiencing sedation or dizziness.
4. Exacerbation of Psychoses
   *Assess for signs of loss of contact with reality.
   *Intervene during a hallucination; talk about real people and real events; reorient client to reality.
   *Stay with client during period of agitation and delirium; remain calm, and reassure client of his or her safety.
   *Discuss with physician possible decrease in dosage or change in medication.
5. Orthostatic Hypotension
   *Instruct client to rise slowly from a lying or sitting position; monitor blood pressure (lying and standing) each shift; document and report significant changes.

■ CLIENT/FAMILY EDUCATION RELATED TO ALL ANTIPARKINSONIAN AGENTS

- Take the medication with food if GI upset occurs.
- Use caution when driving or operating dangerous machinery. Drowsiness and dizziness can occur.
- Do not stop taking the drug abruptly. To do so might produce unpleasant withdrawal symptoms.
- Report occurrence of any of the following symptoms to the physician immediately: pain or tenderness in area in front of ear; extreme dryness of mouth; difficulty urinating; abdominal pain; constipation; fast, pounding heart beat; rash; visual disturbances; mental changes.
- Rise slowly from a sitting or lying position to prevent a sudden drop in blood pressure.
- Stay inside in air-conditioned room when weather is very hot. Perspiration is decreased with antiparkinsonian agents, and the body cannot cool itself as well. There is greater susceptibility to heat stroke. Inform physician if air-conditioned housing is not available.
- Take frequent sips of water, chew sugarless gum, or suck on hard candy if dry mouth is a problem. Good oral care (frequent brushing, flossing) is very important.

- Do not drink alcohol while on antiparkinsonian therapy.
- Do not consume other medications (including over-the-counter products) without physician's approval. Many medications contain substances that interact with antiparkinsonian agents in a way that may be harmful.
- Be aware of possible risks due to taking antiparkinsonian agents during pregnancy. Safe use during pregnancy and lactation has not been fully established. It is thought that antiparkinsonian agents readily cross the placental barrier; if so, fetus could experience adverse effects of the drug. Inform physician immediately if pregnancy occurs, is suspected, or is planned.
- Be aware of side effects of antiparkinsonian agents. Refer to written materials furnished by health-care providers for safe self-administration.
- Continue to take medication, even if feeling well and as though it is not needed. Symptoms may return if medication is discontinued.
- Carry card or other identification at all times describing medications being taken.

INTERNET REFERENCES

- http://www.rxlist.com/
- http://www.nimh.nih.gov/publicat/medicate.cfm
- http://www.fadavis.com/townsend

CHAPTER 29

Sedative-Hypnotics

CHEMICAL CLASS: BENZODIAZEPINES

Examples

Generic (Trade) Name	Controlled/ Pregnancy Category	Half-life	Indications	Available Forms (mg)
Estazolam (ProSom)	CIV/X	8–28 h	Insomnia	Tabs: 1, 2
Flurazepam (Dalmane)	CIV/NR	2–3 (active metabolite, 47–100) h	Insomnia	Caps: 15, 30
Quazepam (Doral)	CIV/X	41 (active metabolite, 47–100) h	Insomnia	Tabs: 7.5, 15
Temazepam (Restoril)	CIV/X	9–15 h	Insomnia	Caps: 7.5, 15, 30
Triazolam (Halcion)	CIV/X	1.5–5.5 h	Insomnia	Tabs: 0.125, 0.25

Action

- Potentiate gamma aminobutyric acid (GABA) neuronal inhibition.
- The sedative effects involve GABA receptors in the limbic, neocortical, and mesencephalic reticular systems.

Contraindications and Precautions

Contraindicated in:

- Hypersensitivity to these or other benzodiazepines
- Pregnancy and lactation
- **Quazepam:** established or suspected sleep apnea
- **Triazolam:** concurrent use with ketoconazole, itraconazole, or nefazodone, medications that impair the metabolism of triazolam by cytochrome P450 3A (CYP3A)
- **Flurazepam:** Children younger than 15 years

- **Estazolam, quazepam, temazepam, triazolam:** Children younger than 18 years

Use cautiously in:

- Elderly and debilitated patients
- Hepatic or renal dysfunction
- Patients with history of drug abuse and dependence
- Depressed or suicidal patients
- Respiratory depression and sleep apnea

Adverse Reactions and Side Effects

- Drowsiness
- Headache
- Confusion
- Lethargy
- Tolerance
- Physical and psychological dependence
- Potentiates the effects of other central nervous system (CNS) depressants
- May aggravate symptoms in depressed persons
- Palpitations; tachycardia; hypotension
- Paradoxical excitement
- Dry mouth
- Nausea and vomiting
- Blood dyscrasias

Interactions

- Additive CNS depression with **alcohol** and **other CNS depressants.**
- Decreased clearance and increased effects of benzodiazepines with **cimetidine, oral contraceptives, disulfiram,** and **isoniazid.**
- More rapid onset or more prolonged benzodiazepine effect with **probenecid.**
- Increased clearance and decreased half-life of benzodiazepines with **rifampin.**
- Increased benzodiazepine clearance with **cigarette smoking.**
- Antagonism of benzodiazepines with **theophylline.**
- Increased bioavailability of triazolam with **macrolides.**
- Benzodiazepines may increase serum levels of **digoxin** and **phenytoin** and increase risk of toxicity.

Route and Dosage

Estazolam (ProSom)

- **Insomnia:** ***Adults*—PO:** 1 to 2 mg at bedtime. ***Healthy elderly patients*—PO:** 1 mg at bedtime. Increase with caution. ***Debilitated or small elderly patients*—PO:** 0.5 mg at bedtime.

Flurazepam (Dalmane)

- **Insomnia**: ***Adults***—PO: 15 to 30 mg at bedtime. ***Elderly or debilitated patients***—PO: 15 mg at bedtime.

Quazepam (Doral)

- **Insomnia: *Adults***—PO: 7.5 to 15 mg at bedtime.

Temazepam (Restoril)

- **Insomnia:** *Adults*—PO: 15 to 30 mg at bedtime. ***Elderly or debilitated patients***—PO: 15 mg at bedtime.

Triazolam (Halcion)

- **Insomnia: *Adults***—PO: 0.125 to 0.5 mg at bedtime. ***Elderly or debilitated patients***—PO: 0.125 to 0.25 mg at bedtime.

■ CHEMICAL CLASS: BARBITURATES

Examples

Generic (Trade) Name	Controlled/ Pregnancy Category	Half-life	Indications	Available Forms (mg)
Amobarbital (Amytal)	CII/D	16–40 h	Sedation Insomnia	Injection: powder, 250/vial, 500/vial
Butabarbital (Butisol)	CIII/D	66–140 h	Sedation Insomnia	Tabs: 15, 30, 50, 100 Elixir: 30/5 mL
Mephobarbital (Mebaral)	CIV/D	11–67 h	Sedation Epilepsy	Tabs: 32, 50, 100
Pentobarbital (Nembutal)	CII/D	15–50 h	Sedation Insomnia	Caps: 30, 100 Injection: 50/mL
Phenobarbital (Luminal)	CIV/D	53–118 h	Sedation Insomnia Epilepsy	Tabs: 15, 16, 30, 60, 90, 100 Caps: 16 Elixir: 15/5 mL; 20/5 mL Injection (mg/mL): 30, 60, 65, 130
Secobarbital (Seconal)	CII/D	15–40 h	Sedation Insomnia	Caps: 100

Action

- Depress the sensory cortex, decrease motor activity, and alter cerebellar function.
- All levels of CNS depression can occur, from mild sedation to hypnosis to coma to death.
- Can induce anesthesia in sufficiently high therapeutic doses.

Contraindications and Precautions

Contraindicated in:

- Hypersensitivity to barbiturates
- Severe hepatic, renal, cardiac, or respiratory disease
- Individuals with history of drug abuse or dependence
- Porphyria
- Intra-arterial or subcutaneous administration

Use cautiously in:

- Elderly and debilitated patients
- Patients with hepatic, renal, cardiac, or respiratory impairment
- Depressed or suicidal patients
- Children
- Pregnancy and lactation

Adverse Reactions and Side Effects

- Bradycardia
- Hypotension
- Somnolence
- Agitation
- Confusion
- Nausea, vomiting
- Constipation
- Skin rashes
- Respiratory depression
- Physical and psychological dependence

Interactions

- Additive CNS depression with **alcohol** and **other CNS depressants.**
- Possible decreased effects from the following drugs with barbiturates: **chloramphenicol, anticoagulants, beta blockers, carbamazepine, clonazepam, oral contraceptives, corticosteroids, digitoxin, doxorubicin, doxycycline, felodipine, fenoprofen, griseofulvin, metronidazole, phenylbutazone, quinidine, theophylline,** and **verapamil.**
- Possible decreased effects of barbiturates with **chloramphenicol** and **rifampin.**
- Possible increased effects of barbiturates with **monoamine oxidase inhibitors** and **valproic acid.**
- Concomitant use with **methoxyflurane** may enhance renal toxicity.

Route and Dosage

Amobarbital (Amytal)

- **Sedation:** ***Adults***—IM: 30 to 50 mg 2 or 3 times/day.
- **Insomnia:** ***Adults***—IM: 65 to 200 mg.
- NOTE: Do not inject a volume >5 mL at any one site regardless of drug concentration. Tissue damage can occur.

Butabarbital (Butisol)

- **Daytime Sedation:** ***Adults***—PO: 15 to 30 mg 3 or 4 times/day.
- **Insomnia:** ***Adults***—PO: 50 to 100 mg at bedtime.
- **Preoperative sedation:** ***Adults***—PO: 50 to 100 mg 60 to 90 minutes before surgery. ***Children***—PO: 2 to 6 mg/kg; maximum 100 mg.

Mephobarbital (Mebaral)

- **Sedation:** ***Adults***—PO: 32 to 100 mg 3 or 4 times/day. Optimum dose: 50 mg 3 or 4 times/day. ***Children***—PO: 16 to 32 mg 3 or 4 times/day.
- **Epilepsy:** ***Adults***—PO: 400 to 600 mg daily. ***Children <5 years***—PO: 16 to 32 mg 3 or 4 times/day. ***Children >5 years***—PO: 32 to 64 mg 3 or 4 times/day.

Pentobarbital (Nembutal)

- **Sedation:** ***Adults***—PO: 20 mg 3 or 4 times/day. ***Children***—PO: 2 to 6 mg/kg/d, depending on age, weight, and amount of sedation desired. Maximum dose: 100 mg.
- **Insomnia:** ***Adults***—PO: 100 mg at bedtime. ***Children***—PO: Base dose on age and weight. ***Adults***—IM: Usual dose: 150 to 200 mg. ***Children***—IM: 2 to 6 mg/kg as a single IM injection, not to exceed 100 mg. NOTE: Inject deeply into large muscle mass. Do not exceed a volume of 5 mL at any one site because of possible tissue irritation.

Phenobarbital (Luminal)

- **Sedation:** ***Adults***—PO: 30 to 120 mg/d in 2 to 3 divided doses not to exceed 400 mg in 24 hours. IM or IV: 30 to 120 mg/d in 2 to 3 divided doses. ***Children***—PO: 8 to 32 mg.
- **Preoperative sedation:** ***Adults***—IM only: 100 to 200 mg 60 to 90 minutes before surgery ***Children***—IM or IV: 1 to 3 mg/kg.
- **Insomnia:** ***Adults***—PO: 100 to 200 mg at bedtime. ***Children***—PO: Determined by age and weight.
- **Epilepsy:** ***Adults***—PO: 60 to 100 mg/d. ***Children***—PO: 3 to 6 mg/kg/d.

Secobarbital (Seconal)

- **Preoperative sedation:** ***Adults***—PO: 200 to 300 mg 1 to 2 hours before surgery.
- ***Children***—PO: 2 to 6 mg/kg, not to exceed 100 mg.
- **Insomnia:** ***Adults***—PO: 100 mg at bedtime.

CHEMICAL CLASS: MISCELLANEOUS

Examples

Generic (Trade) Name	Controlled/ Pregnancy Category	Half-life	Indications	Available Forms (mg)
Chloral hydrate (Noctec)	CIV/C	7–10 h	Sedation Insomnia	Caps: 500 Syrup: 250/5 mL; 500/5 mL Suppositories: 324, 648
Zaleplon (Sonata)	CIV/C	1 h	Insomnia	Caps: 5, 10
Zolpidem (Ambien)	CIV/B	2–3 h	Insomnia	Tabs: 5, 10

Action

Zolpidem and Zaleplon

Bind to GABA receptors in the CNS. Appear to be selective for the ω_1-receptor subtype.

Chloral Hydrate

- Action unknown. Produces a calming effect through depression of the CNS.
- Has generally been replaced by safer and more effective agents.

Contraindications and Precautions

Contraindicated in:

- Hypersensitivity
- In combination with other CNS depressants
- Pregnancy and lactation

Zolpidem, zaleplon:

- Children

Chloral hydrate

- Severe hepatic, renal, or cardiac impairment
- Esophagitis, gastritis, or peptic ulcer disease (oral form)

Use cautiously in:

- Elderly or debilitated patients
- Depressed or suicidal patients
- Patients with history of drug abuse or dependence
- Patients with hepatic, renal, or respiratory dysfunction

Adverse Reactions and Side Effects

- Headache
- Drowsiness

- Dizziness
- Amnesia
- Nausea
- Myalgia
- Paradoxical excitement
- Physical and/or psychological dependence

Chloral hydrate:

- Skin rash

Interactions

- Peak concentration levels are decreased and time-to-peak concentration is prolonged when zolpidem is taken with food and when zaleplon is taken following a high-fat meal.
- Additive CNS depression with **alcohol and other CNS depressants.**
- Reduced effectiveness of **hydantoins** with chloral hydrate.
- Increased effects of **oral anticoagulants** with chloral hydrate.
- Decreased effects of zaleplon with drugs that induce the CYP3A4 enzyme system, including **rifampin, phenytoin, carbamazepine,** and **phenobarbital.**
- **Cimetidine** decreases metabolism and increases effects of zaleplon.
- IV **furosemide** administered following a dose of chloral hydrate may result in sweating, hot flashes, tachycardia, hypertension, weakness, and nausea.

Route and Dosage

Chloral Hydrate

- **Sedation:** ***Adults***—PO: 250 mg 3 times/day after meals. Maximum daily dose: 2 g. ***Children***—PO: 25 mg/kg/d, not to exceed 500 mg per single dose. May be given in divided doses.
- **Insomnia:** ***Adults***—PO: 500 mg to 1 g 15 to 30 minutes before bedtime. ***Children***—PO: 50 mg/kg/d, up to 1 g per single dose. May be given in divided doses.

Zaleplon (Sonata)

- **Insomnia**: ***Adults***—PO: 10 mg (range 5 to 20 mg) at bedtime. ***Elderly and debilitated patients***—PO: 5 mg at bedtime, not to exceed 10 mg.

Zolpidem (Ambien)

- **Insomnia:** ***Adults***—PO: 10 mg at bedtime. ***Elderly and debilitated patients***—PO: Initial dose: 5 mg, not to exceed 10 mg.

■ NURSING DIAGNOSES RELATED TO ALL SEDATIVE-HYPNOTICS

1. Risk for injury related to abrupt withdrawal from long-term use or decreased mental alertness caused by residual sedation.
2. Disturbed sleep pattern related to situational crises, physical condition, or severe level of anxiety.
3. Risk for activity intolerance related to side effects of lethargy, drowsiness, and dizziness.
4. Risk for acute confusion related to action of the medication on the CNS.

■ NURSING IMPLICATIONS FOR SEDATIVE-HYPNOTICS

The nursing care plan should include monitoring for the following side effects from sedative-hypnotics. Nursing implications related to each side effect are designated by an asterisk (*):

1. Drowsiness, Confusion, Lethargy (most common side effects)
   *Instruct client not to drive or operate dangerous machinery while taking the medication.
2. Tolerance, Physical and Psychological Dependence
   *Instruct client to take the medication exactly as directed. Do not take more than the amount prescribed because of the habit-forming potential. Recommended for short-term use only. Abrupt withdrawal after long-term use may result in serious, even life-threatening, symptoms.
3. Potentiates the Effects of Other CNS Depressants
   *Instruct client not to drink alcohol or take other medications that depress the CNS while taking this medication.
4. May Aggravate Symptoms in Depressed Persons
   *Assess mood daily.
   *Take necessary precautions for potential suicide.
5. Orthostatic Hypotension; Palpitations; Tachycardia
   *Monitor lying and standing blood pressure and pulse every shift.
   *Instruct client to arise slowly from a lying or sitting position.
   *Monitor pulse rate and rhythm, and report any significant change to the physician.
6. Paradoxical Excitement
   *Withhold drug, and notify the physician.
7. Dry Mouth
   *Have client take frequent sips of water or ice chips, suck on hard candy, or chew sugarless gum.
8. Nausea and Vomiting
   *Have client take drug with food or milk.

9. Blood Dyscrasias
   *Symptoms of sore throat, fever, malaise, easy bruising, or unusual bleeding should be reported to the physician immediately.

CLIENT/FAMILY EDUCATION RELATED TO ALL SEDATIVE-HYPNOTICS

- Do not drive or operate dangerous machinery. Drowsiness and dizziness can occur.
- Do not stop taking the drug abruptly after prolonged use. Can produce serious withdrawal symptoms, such as depression, insomnia, anxiety, abdominal and muscle cramps, tremors, vomiting, sweating, convulsions, and delirium.
- Do not consume other CNS depressants (including alcohol).
- Do not take nonprescription medication without approval from physician.
- Rise slowly from the sitting or lying position to prevent a sudden drop in blood pressure.
- Report to physician immediately symptoms of sore throat, fever, malaise, easy bruising, unusual bleeding, or motor restlessness.
- Be aware of risks of taking these drugs during pregnancy. (Congenital malformations have been associated with use during the first trimester.) If pregnancy is suspected or planned, notify the physician of the desirability to discontinue the drug.
- Be aware of possible side effects. Refer to written materials furnished by health-care providers regarding the correct method of self-administration.
- Carry card or piece of paper at all times describing medications being taken.

INTERNET REFERENCES

- http://www.rxlist.com/
- http://www.drugguide.com/
- http://www.nimh.nih.gov/publicat/medicate.cfm
- http://www.fadavis.com/townsend

CHAPTER 30

Central Nervous System Stimulants

NOTE: *The FDA recently approved the medication atomoxetine (Strattera) as an agent for attention deficit hyperactivity disorder (ADHD). Because of atomoxetine's chemical classification, it is covered in Chapter 25: Antidepressants.*

CHEMICAL CLASS: AMPHETAMINES

Examples

Generic (Trade) Name	Controlled/ Pregnancy Category	Half-life	Indications	Available Forms (mg)
Amphetamine/ dextroamphetamine mixtures (Adderall; Adderall XR)	C-II/C	9–13 h	Narcolepsy ADHD in children	Tabs: 5, 7.5, 10, 12.5, 15, 20, 30 Caps (XR): 5, 10, 15, 20, 25, 30
Dextroamphetamine sulfate (Dexedrine; Dextrostat)	C-II/C	~12 h	Narcolepsy ADHD in children	Tabs: 5, 10 Caps (SR): 5, 10, 15
Methamphetamine (Desoxyn)	C-II/C	4–5 h	ADHD in children Exogenous obesity	Tabs: 5

Action

- Central nervous system (CNS) stimulation is mediated by release of norepinephrine from central noradrenergic

neurons in cerebral cortex, reticular activating system, and brain stem.
- At higher doses, dopamine may be released in the mesolimbic system.
- Action in the treatment of ADHD is unclear.

Contraindications and Precautions

Contraindicated in:

- Advanced arteriosclerosis
- Symptomatic cardiovascular disease
- Moderate to severe hypertension
- Hyperthyroidism
- Hypersensitivity or idiosyncrasy to the sympathomimetic amines
- Glaucoma
- Agitated states
- History of drug abuse
- During or within 14 days following administration of monoamine oxidase (MAO) inhibitors (hypertensive crisis may occur)
- Children younger than 3 years
- Pregnancy and lactation

Use cautiously in:

- Patients with mild hypertension
- Children with psychoses (may exacerbate symptoms)
- Tourette's disorder (may exaggerate tics)
- Anorexia
- Insomnia
- Elderly, debilitated, or asthenic patients
- Patients with suicidal or homicidal tendencies

Adverse Reactions and Side Effects

- Overstimulation
- Restlessness
- Dizziness
- Insomnia
- Headache
- Palpitations
- Tachycardia
- Elevation of blood pressure
- Anorexia
- Weight loss
- Dry mouth
- Tolerance
- Physical and psychological dependence
- Suppression of growth in children (with long-term use)

Interactions

- Increased sensitivity to amphetamines with **furazolidone.**
- Use of amphetamines with **MAO inhibitors** can result in hypertensive crisis.
- Increased effects of amphetamines and risk of serotonin syndrome with **selective serotonin reuptake inhibitors (SSRIs).**
- Prolonged effects of amphetamines with **urinary alkalinizers.**
- Hastened elimination of amphetamines with **urinary acidifiers.**
- Amphetamines may reverse the hypotensive effects of **guanethidine.**
- **Phenothiazines** may antagonize the CNS stimulant action of amphetamines.
- Patients with diabetes mellitus who take amphetamines may require **insulin** adjustment.

Route and Dosage

AMPHETAMINE/DEXTROAMPHETAMINE MIXTURES (Adderall; Adderall XR)

- **Narcolepsy:** (Adults ≥ 12 years) **PO:** Initial dose: 10 mg/day; may increase in increments of 10 mg/day at weekly intervals up to a maximum of 60 mg/day. Give first dose on awakening and 1 or 2 additional doses at intervals of 4 to 6 hours. (Children 6 to 12 years of age): Narcolepsy is rare in children younger than 12 years. When it does occur, initial dose is 5 mg/day. May increase in increments of 5 mg/day in weekly intervals up to a maximum of 60 mg/day.
- **ADHD in children:** (not recommended for children < 3 years of age) (Children 3 to 6 years) **PO:** Initial dose: 2.5 mg/day. May increase in increments of 2.5 mg/day at weekly intervals. (Children ≥ 6 years): Initial dose: 5 mg 1 or 2 times daily. May increase in increments of 5 mg/day at weekly intervals.
- **Extended-release caps:** (Children ≥ 6 years): **PO:** Initial dose: 10 mg once daily in the morning. May increase daily dosage in increments of 10 mg at weekly intervals. Maximum dosage: 30 mg/day.

DEXTROAMPHETAMINE SULFATE (Dexedrine; Dextrostat)

- **Narcolepsy:** (Adults ≥ 12 years) **PO:** Initial dose: 10 mg/day; may increase in increments of 10 mg/day at weekly intervals up to a maximum of 60 mg/day. Give first dose on awakening and 1 or 2 additional doses at intervals of 4 to 6 hours. (Children 6 to 12 years of age): Narcolepsy is rare in children younger than 12 years. When it does occur, initial dose is 5 mg/day. May increase in increments of 5 mg/day in weekly intervals up to a maximum of 60 mg/day.
- **ADHD in children:** (not recommended for children < 3 years of age) (Children 3 to 6 years) **PO:** Initial dose: 2.5 mg/day. May

increase in increments of 2.5 mg/day at weekly intervals. (Children ≥ 6 years): Initial dose: 5 mg 1 or 2 times daily. May increase in increments of 5 mg/day at weekly intervals.

- **Sustained-release caps** may be used for once-a-day dosage. Give first dose on awakening and 1 or 2 additional doses at intervals of 4 to 6 hours.

METHAMPHETAMINE (Desoxyn)

- **ADHD in children:** 5 mg once or twice daily. May increase in increments of 5 mg at weekly intervals. Usual effective dose is 20 to 25 mg/day.
- **Exogenous obesity:** 5 mg 30 minutes before each meal.

■ CHEMICAL CLASS: ANOREXIANTS

Examples

Generic (Trade) Name	Controlled/ Pregnancy Category	Half-life	Indications	Available Forms (mg)
Benzphetamine (Didrex)	C-III/X	7–33 h	Obesity	Tabs: 50
Diethylpropion (Tenuate)	C-IV/B	1–3.5 h	Obesity	Tabs: 25 Tabs (CR): 75
Phendimetrazine (Bontril; Bontril PDM)	C-III/C	1.9–9.8 h	Obesity	Tabs: 35 Caps (SR): 105
Phentermine (Adipex-P, Ionamin)	C-IV/C	19–24 h	Obesity	Tabs: 37.5 Caps: 15, 30, 37.5
Sibutramine (Meridia)	C-IV/C	1.1 h	Obesity	Caps: 5, 10, 15

Action

- The exact mechanism of action is unclear.
- It is thought that appetite suppression is produced by a direct stimulant effect on the satiety center in the hypothalamic and limbic regions.

Diethylpropion, phentermine, benzphetamine, phendimetrazine:

- Act by modulating central norepinephrine and dopamine receptors through the promotion of catecholamine release.

Sibutramine:

- Inhibits the reuptake of norepinephrine, serotonin, and dopamine.

Contraindications and Precautions

Contraindicated in:

- Advanced arteriosclerosis
- History of cardio- or cerebrovascular disease
- Moderate to severe hypertension
- Hyperthyroidism
- Known hypersensitivity or idiosyncrasy to sympathomimetic amines
- Glaucoma
- Agitated states
- History of drug abuse
- During or within 14 days following administration of MAO inhibitors
- Coadministration with other CNS stimulants
- Pregnancy and lactation
- Children younger than 12 years

Sibutramine:

- Anorexia nervosa
- Severe renal impairment
- Children younger than 16 years
- Concomitantly with other SSRIs (may cause serotonin syndrome)

Use cautiously in:

- Mild hypertension
- Diabetes mellitus
- Elderly or debilitated patients
- Patients with a history of seizures

Adverse Reactions and Side Effects

- Overstimulation
- Restlessness
- Dizziness
- Insomnia
- Headache
- Palpitations
- Tachycardia
- Elevation of blood pressure
- Dry mouth
- Tolerance
- Physical and psychological dependence

Interactions

Benzphetamine; diethylpropion; phendimetrazine; phentermine:

- Possible hypertensive crisis and intracranial hemorrhage with **MAO inhibitors** or **furazolidone.**
- Possible increased CNS effects and risk of serotonin syndrome with **SSRIs.**
- Decreased hypotensive effect of **guanethidine** with anorexiants.
- Possible increased effects of **tricyclic antidepressants** with anorexiants.

Sibutramine:

- Concomitant use with **other centrally acting anorexiants, MAO inhibitors, SSRIs, naratriptan, frovatriptan, rizatriptan, zolmitriptan, sumatriptan, dihydroergotamine, methysergide, dextromethorphan, meperidine, pentazocine, fentanyl, lithium,** or **tryptophan** may result in potentially fatal serotonin syndrome. Allow 2 weeks between use of MAO inhibitors and sibutramine.
- Decreased metabolism and increased blood levels and effects of sibutramine with **ketoconazole, cimetidine,** and **erythromycin.**
- Concomitant use with cough, cold, and allergy medications that contain **ephedrine** or **pseudoephedrine** may cause hypertension.

Route and Dosage

Benzphetamine (Didrex)

- **Obesity:** ***Adults***—PO: Initial dose: 25 to 50 mg once daily, mid-morning or mid-afternoon. Increase dosage according to client response. Dosage range: 25 to 50 mg 1 to 3 times daily.

Diethylpropion (Tenuate)

- **Obesity:** ***Adults***—PO: *Immediate-release tablets:* 25 mg 3 times/day 1 hour before meals.
- *Controlled-release tablets:* 75 mg once daily in mid-morning.

Phendimetrazine (Bontril)

- **Obesity:** ***Adults***—PO: *Immediate-release tablets:* 35 mg 2 or 3 times/day 1 hour before meals. *Sustained-release tablets:* 105 mg once daily in the morning 30 to 60 minutes before the morning meal.

Phentermine (Ionamin; Adipex-P)

- **Obesity:** ***Adults***—PO: 15 to 37.5 mg once daily before breakfast or 10 to 14 hours before bedtime.

Sibutramine (Meridia)

- **Obesity:** ***Adults***—PO: 10 mg once daily in the morning; may be increased to 15 mg/d after 4 weeks. Clients who do not tolerate an initial dose of 10 mg/d may be started on 5 mg/d. Maximum daily dose: 15 mg.

CHEMICAL CLASS: MISCELLANEOUS

Examples

Generic (Trade) Name	Controlled/ Pregnancy Category	Half-life	Indications	Available Forms (mg)
Dexmethylphenidate (Focalin)	C-II/C	2.2 h	ADHD	Tabs: 2.5, 5, 10
Methylphenidate (Ritalin; Metadate ER; Metadate CD; Concerta; Ritalin-SR; Ritalin-LA)	C-II/C	3–3.5 h	ADHD Narcolepsy	Immediate release tabs: 5, 10, 20 Metadate ER: Tabs: 10, 20 Metadate CD: Caps: 20 Concerta: Tabs: 18, 27, 36, 54 Ritalin-SR: Tabs: 20 Ritalin-LA: Caps: 20, 30, 40
Modafinil (Provigil)	C-IV/C	15 h	Narcolepsy	Tabs: 100, 200
Pemoline (Cylert)	C-IV/B	12 h	ADHD	Tabs: 18.75, 37.5, 75 Tabs (chewable): 37.5

Actions

- Dexmethylphenidate blocks the reuptake of norepinephrine and dopamine into the presynaptic neuron and increases the release of these amines into the extraneuronal space.
- Methylphenidate activates the brain stem arousal system and cortex to produce its stimulant effect.
- Modafinil binds to the dopamine reuptake site and causes an increase in extracellular dopamine.
- The exact mechanism of action of pemoline is unknown, but it is thought to act through dopaminergic mechanisms.
- Action in the treatment of ADHD is unknown.

Contraindications and Precautions

Contraindicated in:

- Hypersensitivity
- Pregnancy, lactation, and children younger than 6 years (safety has not been established)

Dexmethylphenidate; methylphenidate:

- Clients with marked anxiety, tension, or agitation
- History of glaucoma
- Motor tics or family history or diagnosis of Tourette's syndrome

- During or within 14 days of treatment of MAO inhibitors (hypertensive crisis can occur)

Pemoline:

- Hepatic insufficiency (NOTE: Pemoline has been associated with life-threatening hepatic failure and should not ordinarily be considered as first-line therapy for ADHD.)

Use cautiously in:

- Patients with history of seizure disorder and/or EEG abnormalities
- Hypertension
- History of drug or alcohol dependence
- Emotionally unstable patient
- Renal or hepatic insufficiency

Adverse Reactions and Side Effects

- Headache
- Nausea
- Rhinitis
- Fever
- Anorexia
- Insomnia
- Tachycardia
- Nervousness
- Abdominal pain
- Growth suppression in children (with long-term use)

Interactions

- **Modafinil** absorption is delayed by **methylphenidate.**
- Increased levels of **tricyclic antidepressants, phenytoin,** and **warfarin.**
- Reduced effectiveness of **oral contraceptives** with modafinil.
- Decreased effectiveness of **antihypertensive agents** with methylphenidate and dexmethylphenidate.
- Increased serum levels of **anticonvulsants, tricyclic antidepressants,** and **SSRIs** with methylphenidate and dexmethylphenidate.
- Increased levels of **warfarin** with dexmethylphenidate.
- Decreased effectiveness of **anticonvulsants** with pemoline.

Route and Dosage

Dexmethylphenidate (Focalin)

- **ADHD:** ***Adults and children ≥6 years***—Administer doses 2 times/day at least 4 hours apart. ***Clients new to the medication:*** Starting dose: 2.5 mg 2 times/day. May increase dosage in 2.5- to 5-mg increments at weekly intervals to a maximum of 20 mg/d (10 mg 2 times/ day).
- **Clients currently taking methylphenidate:** Starting dose: Half of the dose of methylphenidate being taken. Maximum recommended dose of dexmethylphenidate: 20 mg/d (10 mg 2 times/day).

Methylphenidate (Ritalin; Ritalin-SR; Metadate ER; Concerta)

- **ADHD: Ritalin immediate release:** ***Adults***—PO: Range 10 to 60 mg/d in divided doses 2 or 3 times/day preferably 30 to 45 minutes before meals. Average dose is 20 to 30 mg/d. To prevent interruption of sleep, take last dose of the day before 6 p.m. ***Children ≥6 years***—PO: Individualize dose. May start with low dose of 5 mg 2 times/day before breakfast and lunch. May increase dosage in 5- to 10-mg increments at weekly intervals. Maximum daily dose: 60 mg. **Ritalin-SR and Metadate ER:** ***All patients***—PO: May be used in place of the immediate-release tablets when the 8-hour dose corresponds to the titrated 8-hour dose of the immediate-release tablets. **Ritalin-LA and Metadate CD:** ***All patients***—PO: Initial dose: 20 mg once daily in the morning. May increase dosage in 10- to 20-mg increments at weekly intervals to a maximum of 60 mg taken once daily in the morning. Capsules may be swallowed whole with liquid or opened and contents sprinkled on soft food (e.g., applesauce). Ensure that entire contents of capsule are consumed when taken in this manner. **Concerta:** ***All patients***—PO: Should be taken once daily in the morning. Must be swallowed whole and not chewed, divided, or crushed. ***Clients new to methylphenidate***—18 mg once daily in the morning. May adjust dose at weekly intervals to maximum of 54 mg/d taken once daily in the morning. ***Clients currently using methylphenidate***—Should use following conversion table:

Previous methylphenidate dose	***Recommended Concerta dose***
5 mg 2 or 3 times/day or 20 mg (SR)	18 mg every morning
10 mg 2 or 3 times/day or 40 mg (SR)	36 mg every morning
15 mg 2 or 3 times/day or 60 mg (SR)	54 mg every morning

- **Narcolepsy:** ***Adults***—PO: **Ritalin, Ritalin-SR, and Metadate ER** indicated for this use. Dose as provided for ADHD for these three medications.

Modafinil (Provigil)

- **Narcolepsy:** ***Adults***—PO: 200 mg/d taken as a single dose in the morning.

Pemoline (Cylert)

- **ADHD:** ***Adults and children ≥6 years***—Initial dose: 37.5 mg/d as a single dose in the morning. May increase in 18.75-mg increments at weekly intervals until desired response is achieved. Usual effective dose range: 56.25 to 75 mg/d. Maximum recommended daily dose: 112.5 mg.

NURSING DIAGNOSES RELATED TO CNS STIMULANTS

1. Risk for injury related to overstimulation and hyperactivity.
2. Risk for suicide related to abrupt withdrawal after extended use.
3. Imbalanced nutrition, less than body requirements, related to side effects of anorexia and weight loss.
4. Imbalanced nutrition, more than body requirements, related to excess intake in relation to metabolic needs.
5. Disturbed sleep pattern related to overstimulation resulting from use of the medication.

NURSING IMPLICATIONS FOR CNS STIMULANTS

The plan of care should include monitoring for the following side effects from CNS stimulants. Nursing implications related to each side effect are designated by an asterisk (*).

1. Overstimulation, Restlessness, Insomnia
   * Assess mental status for changes in mood, level of activity, extent of stimulation, and aggressiveness.
   *Ensure that client is protected from injury.
   *Keep stimuli low and environment as quiet as possible to discourage overstimulation.
   *To prevent insomnia, administer the last dose at least 6 hours before bedtime.
   *Administer sustained-release forms in the morning.
2. Palpitations, Tachycardia
   *Monitor and record vital signs at regular intervals (2 or 3 times/day) throughout therapy. Report significant changes to the physician immediately.
3. Anorexia, Weight Loss
   *If the medication is being taken by children with behavior disorders (and not as an anorexiant): to reduce anorexia, administer the medication immediately after meals. The client should be weighed regularly (at least weekly) during hospitalization and at home while receiving therapy with CNS stimulants because of the potential for anorexia and weight loss as well as temporary interruption of growth and development.
4. Tolerance, Physical and Psychological Dependence
   *Tolerance develops rapidly. If anorexigenic effects begin to diminish, client should notify the physician immediately. Client should be on reduced-calorie diet and program of regular exercise in addition to the medication.
   *In children with behavior disorders, a drug "holiday" should be attempted periodically under direction of the physician to determine the effectiveness of the medication and the need for continuation.

*The drug should not be withdrawn abruptly. To do so could initiate the following syndrome of symptoms: nausea, vomiting, abdominal cramping, headache, fatigue, weakness, mental depression, suicidal ideation, increased dreaming, and psychotic behavior.

CLIENT/FAMILY EDUCATION RELATED TO ALL CNS STIMULANTS

- Use caution in driving or operating dangerous machinery. Dizziness and blurred vision can occur.
- Do not stop taking the drug abruptly. To do so could produce serious withdrawal symptoms.
- Avoid taking medication late in the day to prevent insomnia. Take no later than 6 hours before bedtime.
- Do not take other medications (including over-the-counter drugs) without physician's approval. Many medications contain substances that, in combination with CNS stimulants, can be harmful.
- Diabetic clients should monitor blood sugar two or three times a day or as instructed by the physician. Be aware of need for possible alteration in insulin requirements due to changes in food intake, weight, and activity.
- Avoid consumption of large amounts of caffeinated products (coffee, tea, colas, chocolate), as they may enhance the stimulant effect of these medications.
- Follow a reduced-calorie diet provided by the dietitian as well as a program of regular exercise. Do not exceed the recommended dose if the appetite suppressant effect diminishes. Contact the physician.
- Notify physician if symptoms of restlessness, insomnia, anorexia, or dry mouth become severe or if rapid, pounding heartbeat becomes evident.
- Be aware of possible risks of taking CNS stimulants during pregnancy. Safe use during pregnancy and lactation has not been established. Inform the physician immediately if pregnancy is suspected or planned.
- Be aware of potential side effects of CNS stimulants. Refer to written materials furnished by health-care providers for safe self-administration.
- Carry a card or other identification at all times describing medications being taken.

INTERNET REFERENCES

- http://www.rxlist.com
- http://www.drugguide.com
- http://www.nimh.nih.gov/publicat/medicate.cfm
- http://www.fadavis.com/townsend

Bibliography

Accent on today's woman: Sugar blues. The Sunday Oklahoman, August 2, 1998.

Aguilera, DC: Crisis Intervention: Theory and Methodology, ed 8. St. Louis: CV Mosby, 1998.

American Academy of Child and Adolescent Psychiatry: Children of alcoholics, 1999. Retrieved February 19, 2002, from http://www.aacap.org/publications/factsfam/Alcoholic.htm

American Medical Association: Strategies for the treatment and prevention of sexual assault, 1999. Available at http://www.ama-assn.org/ public/releases/assault/sa-guide.htm

American Nurses Association: Nursing: A Social Policy Statement. American Nurses Association, Kansas City, MO, 1980.

American Nurses Association: Standards of Clinical Nursing Practice, ed. 2. Kansas City, MO: American Nurses Association, 1998.

American Psychiatric Association: Diagnostic and Statistical Manual of Mental Disorders, ed 4., Text Revision. Washington, DC: American Psychiatric Association, 2000.

Avants, SK, Margolin, A, Holford, TR, et al: (2000). A randomized controlled trial of auricular acupuncture for cocaine dependence. Arch Intern Med 160:2305–2312, 2000.

Bagley, C, and Mallick, K: Spiraling up and spiraling down: Implications of a long-term study of temperament and conduct disorder for social work with children. Child Fam Social Work 5:291–301, 2000.

Bartlett, JG, and Finkbeiner, AK: The Guide to Living with HIV Infection, ed 3. Baltimore: Johns Hopkins University Press, 1996.

Bateman, AL: Understanding the process of grieving and loss: A critical social thinking perspective. J Am Psychiatr Nurse Assoc 5:139–147, 1999.

Beck, A, et al: Cognitive Theory of Depression. New York: Guilford Press, 1979.

Becker, JV, and Kavoussi, RJ: Sexual and gender identity disorders. In Hales, RE, Yudofsky, SC, and Talbott, JA (eds.): Textbook of Psychiatry, ed 2. Washington, DC: American Psychiatric Press, 1994.

Bennett, G, and Woolf, DS: Substance Abuse: Pharmacologic, Developmental, and Clinical Perspectives, ed 2. New York: John Wiley & Sons, 1991.

Bernier, SL: Mental health issues and nursing in corrections. In McFarland GK, and Thomas, MD (eds.): Psychiatric Mental Health Nursing: Application of the Nursing Process. Philadelphia: JB Lippincott, 1991.

Black, DW, and Andreasen, NC: Schizophrenia, schizophreniform disorder, and delusional (paranoid) disorders. In Hales, RE, and Yudofsky, SC (eds.): Essentials of Clinical Psychiatry. Washington, DC: American Psychiatric Press, 1999.

Black, DW, and Andreasen, NC: Schizophrenia, schizophreniform disorder, and delusional (paranoid) disorder. In Hales, RE, Yudofsky, SC, and Talbott, JA (eds.): Textbook of Psychiatry, ed 2. Washington, DC: American Psychiatric Press, 1994.

Blumenthal, M (ed.): The complete German Commission E monographs: Therapeutic Guide to Herbal Medicines. Austin, TX: American Botanical Garden, 1998.

Bowlby, J: Processes of mourning. Int J Psychoanal, 42:22 1961.

Burgess, AW: Intra-familial sexual abuse. In Campbell, J, and Humphreys, J (eds.): Nursing Care of Victims of Family Violence. Reston, VA: Reston Publishing, 1984.

Burgess, AW: Psychiatric Nursing in the Hospital and the Community, ed 5. Norwalk, CT: Appleton & Lange, 1990.

Cadoret, R: Antisocial personality. In Winokur, G, and Clayton, PJ (eds.): The Medical Basis of Psychiatry. Philadelphia: WB Saunders, 1994.

Case, J: Special focus: Psychiatric services. Hosp Home Health 10:61–68, 1993.

Cath, SH., and Sadavoy, J: Psychosocial aspects. In Sadavoy, J, Lazarus LW, and Jarvik LF (eds.): Comprehensive Review of Geriatric Psychiatry. Washington, DC: American Psychiatric Press, 1991.

Celano, MP: Activities and games for group psychotherapy with sexually abused children. Int J Group Psychother 40:419–428, 1990.

Chess, S, Thomas, A, and Birch, H: The origins of personality. Sci Am 223:102, 1970.

Cloninger, CR: Somatoform and dissociative disorders. In Winokur, G, and Clayton, PJ (eds.): The Medical Basis of Psychiatry, ed 2. Philadelphia: W.B. Saunders, 1994.

Clunn, P: Child Psychiatric Nursing. St. Louis: Mosby–Year Book, 1991.

Complementary and Alternative Medicine: Complementary and Alternative Medicine Newsletter, v 2. Silver Spring, MD: Office of Alternative Medicine Clearinghouse, 1998.

Coniglione, T: Our doctors must begin looking at the total person. InBalance. Oklahoma City, OK: The Balanced Healing Medical Center, 1998.

Credit, LP, Hartunian, SG, and Nowak, MJ: Your Guide To Complementary Medicine. Garden City Park, NY: Avery Publishing Group, 1998.

Deglin, JH, and Vallerand, AH: Davis's Drug Guide for Nurses, ed 8. Philadelphia: FA Davis, 2003.

Doenges, M, and Moorhouse, M: Nurse's Pocket Guide: Diagnoses, Interventions, and Rationales, ed 7. Philadelphia: FA Davis, 2000.

Doenges, M, Townsend, M, and Moorhouse, M: Psychiatric Care Plans: Guidelines for Client Care, ed 3. Philadelphia: FA Davis, 1998.

Dopheide, JA: ADHD Part 1: Current status, diagnosis, etiology/pathophysiology. From the American Pharmaceutical Association 148th Annual Meeting, 2001. Retrieved October 11, 2001, from http://www.medscape.com/Medscape/CNO/2001/AphA/AphA-01.html

Dopheide, JA and Theesen, KA: Disorders of childhood. In Dipiro, JT, Talbert, RL, and Yee, GC (eds.): Pharmacotherapy: A Pathophysiological Approach, ed 4. New York: McGraw-Hill, 1999.

Duffey, JM, and Miller, MP: Toward resolving the issue: In-home psychiatric nursing. J Am Psychiatr Nurse Assoc 2:104–106, 1996.

Eckert, ED, and Mitchell, JE: Anorexia nervosa and bulimia nervosa. In Winokur, G, and Clayton, PJ (eds.): The Medical Basis of Psychiatry, ed 2. Philadelphia: WB Saunders, 1994.

Eisendrath, SJ: Psychiatric disorders. In Tierney, LM, McPhee, SJ, and Papadakis, MA (eds.): Current Medical Diagnosis and Treatment, ed 35. Norwalk, CT: Appleton & Lange, 1996.

Engel, G: Grief and grieving. Am J Nurs 64:93, 1964.
Erikson, EH: Childhood and Society. New York: WW Norton, 1963.
Finkelman, AW: Psychiatric Home Care. Gaithersburg, MD: Aspen Publications, 1997.
Frackiewicz, EJ, and Shiovitz, TM: Evaluation and management of premenstrual syndrome. J Am Pharm Assoc 41:437–447, 2001.
Freud, S: The neuropsychoses of defense (1894). In Strachey, J (ed): Standard Edition of the Complete Psychological Works of Sigmund Freud, vol 3. London: Hogarth Press, 1962.
Friedmann, E, and Thomas, SA: Pet ownership, social support, and one-year survival after acute myocardial infarction in the cardiac arrhythmia suppression trial. Am J Cardiol 76: 1213, 1995.
Goodwin, FK, and Jamison, KR: Manic-depressive illness. New York: Oxford University Press, 1990.
Gordon, M: Nursing Diagnosis: Process and Application, ed 2. New York: McGraw-Hill, 1987.
Guinness, AE (ed.): Family Guide to Natural Medicine. Pleasantville, NY: The Reader's Digest Association, 1993.
Haddad, PM: Antidepressant discontinuation syndromes: Clinical relevance, prevention, and management. Drug Safety, 24:183–197, 2001.
Halmi, KA: Eating disorders: Anorexia nervosa, bulimia nervosa, and obesity. In Hales, RE, Yudofsky, SC, and Talbott, JA (eds.): Textbook of Psychiatry, ed 2. Washington, DC: American Psychiatric Press, 1994.
Halstead, HL: Spirituality in older adults. In Stanley, M, and Beare, PG (eds.): Gerontological Nursing: A Health Promotion/Protection Approach, ed 2. Philadelphia: FA Davis, 1999.
Hellwig, K: Psychiatric home care nursing: Managing patients in the community setting. J Psychosocial Nurs 31:21–24, 1993.
Hermes, WJ: Substance Abuse. New York: Chelsea House Publishers, 1993.
Hollandsworth, JG: The Physiology of Psychological Disorders. New York: Plenum Press, 1990.
Hufft, A, and Peternelj-Taylor, C: Forensic nursing: An emerging specialty. In Catalano, JT (ed.): Contemporary Professional Nursing Update. Philadelphia: FA Davis, 1999.
Hunter, JK: Making a difference for homeless patients. RN, December 1992.
Institute for Natural Resources: Alternative Medicine: An Objective View, ed 2. Berkeley, CA: Institute for Natural Resources, 1998.
International Association of Forensic Nurses and American Nurses Association: Scope and Standards of Forensic Nursing Practice. Washington, DC: American Nurses Publishing, 1997.
Johnson, C, and Dorman, B: What is autism? Autism Society of America. Available at http://www.autism-society.org/autism.html
Julien, RM: A primer of drug action: A concise nontechnical guide to the actions, uses, and side effects of psychoactive drugs, ed 9. San Francisco: W.H. Freeman, 2001.
Kansas Child Abuse Prevention Council: A Guide About Child Abuse and Neglect. Wichita, KS: National Committee for Prevention of Child Abuse and Parents Anonymous, Inc, 1992.
Kaplan, HI, and Sadock, B.J: Synopsis of Psychiatry: Behavioral Sciences/Clinical Psychiatry, ed 8. Baltimore: Williams & Wilkins, 1998.
Kaplan, HI, Sadock, BJ, and Grebb, JA: Kaplan and Sadock's Synopsis of Psychiatry, ed 7. Baltimore: Williams & Wilkins, 1994.

Kelsoe, JR: Molecular genetics of mood disorders. J California Alliance Mentally Ill 2:20–22, 1991.

Koegel, P, Burnam, MA, and Baumohl, J: The causes of homelessness. In Baumohl, J (ed.): Homelessness in America. Phoenix, AZ: Oryx Press, 1996.

Kübler-Ross, E: On Death and Dying. New York: Macmillan, 1969.

Kuhn, MA: Pharmacotherapeutics: A Nursing Process Approach, ed 4. Philadelphia: FA Davis, 1998.

Ladd, GW: Peer relationships and social competence during early and middle childhood. Ann Rev Psych 50:333–359, 1999.

Ledray, LE, and Arndt, S: Examining the sexual assault victim: A new model for nursing care. J Psychosoc Nurs 32:7–12, 1994.

Lego, S: Book review: "Live from death row." J Am Psychiatr Nurses Assoc, 1:171–174, 1995.

Leiblum, SR: Sexual problems and dysfunction: Epidemiology, classification, and risk factors. J Gender-Specific Med 2:41–45, 1999.

Lutz, CA, and Przytulski, KR: Nutrition and Diet Therapy, ed. 3. Philadelphia: FA Davis, 2001.

Lynch, VA: Clinical forensic nursing: A new perspective in the management of crime victims from trauma to trial. Critical Care Nurs Clin North Am 7:489–507, 1995.

Mahler, M, et al: Psychological Birth of the Human Infant: Symbiosis and Individuation. Basic Books, New York, 1975.

MoneyWorld. Hocus pocus comes of age. November, 1997, p 17.

Murray, RB, and Zentner, JP: Health Assessment and Promotion Strategies Through the Life Span, ed 6. Stamford, CT: Appleton & Lange, 1997.

National Association for Home Care: How to choose a home care provider. Available at http://www.nahc.org/Consumer/wihc.html

National Association for Home Care: Basic statistics about home care. Retrieved May 28, 2002, from http://www.nahc.org/Consumer/hcstats.html

National Clearinghouse on Child Abuse and Neglect: What is child maltreatment? Retrieved May 4, 2002, from http://www.calib.com/nccanch/pubs/facttsheets/childmal.cfm

National Coalition for the Homeless: How many people experience homelessness? Available at http://nch.ari.net/numbers.html

National Institutes of Health: NIH consensus report on acupuncture 15:1997.

National Institutes of Mental Health: Autism. NIH Publication No. 97. Retrieved February 1, 2002, from http://www.nimh.nih.gov/publicat/autism.cfm#aut10

North American Nursing Diagnosis Association: Nursing Diagnoses: Definitions and Classification, 2003–2004. Philadelphia: NANDA, 2003.

Nowak, TJ, and Handford, AG: Essentials of Pathophysiology. Dubuque, IA: Wm. C. Brown, 1994.

Peplau, HE: Interpersonal techniques: The crux of psychiatric nursing. Am J Nurs 62:50–54, 1962.

Peplau, HE: Interpersonal Relations in Nursing. New York: Springer, 1991.

Periyakoil, VJ: Is it grief or depression? End-of-Life Physician Education Resource Center. Retrieved October 27, 2002, from www.eperc.mcw.edu/educate/flash/fastfact/226.htm

Peschel, E, and Peschel, R: Neurobiological disorders. J California Alliance Mentally Ill 2:4, 1991.

Phillips, NA: Female sexual dysfunction: Evaluation and treatment. Am Fam Physician 62:127–136, 141–142, 2000.

Phillips, KA, Yen, S, and Gunderson, JG: Personality disorders. In Hales, RE, and Yudofsky, SC (eds.): Textbook of Clinical Psychiatry, ed 4. Washington, DC: American Psychiatric Publishing, 2003.

Piaget, J, and Inhelder, B: The Psychology of the Child. New York: Basic Books, 1969.

Popper, CW, and Steingard, RJ: Disorders usually first diagnosed in infancy, childhood, or adolescence. In Hales, RE, Yudofsky, SC, and Talbott, JA (eds.): The American Psychiatric Press Textbook of Psychiatry, ed 2. Washington, DC: The American Psychiatric Press, 1994.

Rice, ME, Harris, GT, and Quinsey, VL: Treatment for forensic patients. In Sales, BD, and Shah, SA (eds.): Mental Health and Law: Research, Policy and Services. Durham, NC: Carolina Academic Press, 1996.

Rosner, TA, and Pollice, SA: Tourette's syndrome. J Psychosocial Nurs 29:4–9, 1991.

Sackeim, HA, and Mukherjee, S: Schizophrenia. In Kass, FI, Oldham, JM, and Pardes, H (eds.): The Columbia University College of Physicians and Surgeons Complete Home Guide to Mental Health. New York: Henry Holt, 1992.

Scanlon, VC, and Sanders, T: Essentials of Anatomy and Physiology, ed. 2. Philadelphia: FA Davis, 1995.

Schatzberg, AF, Cole, JO, and Debattista, C: Manual of clinical psychopharmacology, ed 4. Washington, DC: American Psychiatric Publishing, 2003.

Scheibel, A: Schizophrenia: Cells in disarray. J California Alliance Mentally Ill, 2:9–10, 1991.

Schmitt, K: Development, administration, and scoring of the NCLEX-RN. In Beare, PG (ed.): Davis's NCLEX-RN Review, ed 2. Philadelphia: FA Davis, 1996.

Schoenen, J, Jacquy, J., and Lenaerts, M: Effectiveness of high-dose riboflavin in migraine prophylaxis: A randomized controlled trial. Neurology 50:466–469, 1998.

Seligman, M: Depression and learned helplessness. In Friedman, R, and Katz, M (eds.): The Psychology of Depression: Contemporary Theory and Research. Washington, DC: V.H. Winston & Sons, 1974.

Selye, H: The Stress of Life. New York: McGraw-Hill, 1956.

Silver, JM, and Yudofsky, S: Violence and aggression. In Kass, FI, Oldham, JM, and Pardes, H (eds.): The Columbia University College of Physicians and Surgeons Complete Home Guide to Mental Health. New York: Henry Holt, 1992.

Smith, LS: Sexual Assault: The Nurse's Role. AD Nurse 2:24–28, 1987a

Smith, LS: Battered women: The nurse's role. AD Nurse 2:21–24, 1987b.

Sobel, DS, and Ornstein, R: The healthy mind, healthy body handbook. Los Altos, CA: DRx, 1996.

Sullivan, HS: The Interpersonal Theory of Psychiatry. New York: WW Norton, 1953.

Sullivan, HS: Clinical Studies in Psychiatry. New York: WW Norton, 1956.

Sullivan, HS: Schizophrenia as a Human Process. New York: WW Norton, 1962.

Tardiff, K: Violence. In Hales, RE, Yudofsky, SC, and Talbott, JA (eds.): Textbook of Psychiatry, ed 2. Washington, DC: American Psychiatric Press, 1994.

Townsend, MC: Drug Guide for Psychiatric Nursing, ed 2. Philadelphia: FA Davis, 1995.

Townsend, MC: Essentials of Psychiatric/Mental Health Nursing, ed 2. Philadelphia: FA Davis, 2002.
Townsend, MC: Psychiatric Mental Health Nursing: Concepts of Care, ed 4. Philadelphia: FA Davis, 2003.
US Conference of Mayors: A status report on hunger and homelessness in America's cities: 2001. Washington, DC: US Conference of Mayors, 2001.
US Conference of Mayors: A status report on hunger and homelessness in America's cities: 1998. Washington, DC: US Conference of Mayors, 1998.
US Department of Agriculture and US Department of Health and Human Services: Nutrition and your health: Dietary guidelines for Americans, ed 4. Washington, DC: USDA and USDHHS, 1995.
VandeVusse, L, and Simandl, G: Sexuality patterns, altered. In Gettrust, KV and Brabec, PD (eds.): Nursing Diagnosis in Clinical Practice: Guides for Care Planning. New York: Delmar, Albany, 1992.
Wallsten, SM: Geriatric mental health: A portrait of homelessness. J Psychosoc Nurs 30:20–24, 1992.
Wark, D: Prison violence: Homicide, assault, and rape. Retrieved April 6, 1999, from http://oak.cats.ohiou.edu/~dw101094/esp/soc4661.html/
Waziri, R: The amnestic syndrome. In Winokur, G, and Clayton, PJ (eds): The Medical Basis of Psychiatry, ed 2. Philadelphia: WB Saunders, 1994.
Wheeler, K: Psychiatric clinical pathways in home care. In Dykes, PC (ed.): Psychiatric Clinical Pathways: An Interdisciplinary Approach. Gaithersburg, MD: Aspen Publishers, 1998.
Whitaker, J: Pet owners are a healthy breed. Health Healing 10:1–8, 2000.
Wise, MG, Gray, KF: Delirium, dementia, and amnestic disorders. In Hales, RE, Yudofsky, SC, and Talbott, JA (eds.): The American Psychiatric Press Textbook of Psychiatry, ed 2. Washington, DC: The American Psychiatric Press, 1994.
Wolfelt, A: Death and Grief: A Guide for the Clergy. New York: Taylor & Francis, 1988.
Worden, JW: Grief Counseling and Grief Therapy: A Handbook for the Mental Health Practitioner, ed 2. New York: Springer, 1991.
Yates, WR: Other psychiatric syndromes: Adjustment disorder, factitious disorder, illicit steroid abuse. In Winokur, G, and Clayton, PJ (eds.): The Medical Basis of Psychiatry. Philadelphia: WB Saunders, 1994.
Yeager, S: New Foods for Healing. Emmaus, PA: Rodale Press, 1998.

APPENDIX A

*Ego Defense Mechanisms**

Defense Mechanisms	Example	Defense Mechanisms	Example
Compensation: Covering up a real or perceived weakness by emphasizing a trait considered more desirable.	A physically handicapped boy is unable to participate in football, so he compensates by becoming a great scholar.	**Rationalization:** Attempting to make excuses or formulate logical reasons to justify unacceptable feelings or behaviors.	John tells the rehabilitation nurse, "I drink because it's the only way I can deal with my bad marriage and my worse job."
Denial: Refusing to acknowledge the existence of a real situation or the feelings associated with it.	A woman who drinks alcohol every day and cannot stop fails to acknowledge that she has a problem.	**Reaction Formation:** Preventing unacceptable or undesirable thoughts or behaviors from being expressed by exaggerating opposite thoughts or types of behaviors.	Jane hates nursing. She attended nursing school to please her parents. During career day, she speaks to prospective students about the excellence of nursing as a career.
Displacement: The transfer of feelings from one target to another that is considered less threatening or neutral.	A client is angry at his physician, does not express it, but becomes verbally abusive with the nurse.	**Regression:** Retreating in response to stress to an earlier level of development and the comfort measures associated with that level of functioning.	When 2-year-old Jay is hospitalized for tonsillitis he will drink only from a bottle, even though his mother states he has been drinking from a cup for 6 months.

*From Townsend, 2003, p. 20, with permission.

Defense Mechanisms	Example	Defense Mechanisms	Example
Identification: An attempt to increase self-worth by acquiring certain attributes and characteristics of an admired individual.	A teenager who required lengthy rehabilitation after an accident decides to become a physical therapist as a result of his experiences.	**Repression:** The involuntary blocking of unpleasant feelings and experiences from one's awareness.	An accident victim can remember nothing about her accident.
Intellectualization: An attempt to avoid expressing actual emotions associated with a stressful situation by using the intellectual processes of logic, reasoning, and analysis.	Susan's husband has a job transfer to a city far away from her parents. She hides anxiety by explaining to her parents the advantages associated with the move.	**Sublimation:** Rechanneling of drives or impulses that are personally or socially unacceptable into activities that are constructive.	A mother whose son was killed by a drunk driver channels her anger and energy into being the president of the local chapter of Mothers Against Drunk Drivers.
Introjection: Integrating the beliefs and values of another individual into one's own ego structure.	Children integrate their parents' value system into the process of conscience formation. A child says to a friend, "Don't cheat. It's wrong."	**Suppression:** The voluntary blocking of unpleasant feelings and experiences from one's awareness.	Scarlett O'Hara says, "I don't want to think about that now. I'll think about that tomorrow."
Isolation: Separating a thought or memory from the feeling tone, or emotion associated with it.	A young woman describes being attacked and raped, without showing any emotion.	**Undoing:** Symbolically negating or canceling out an experience that one finds intolerable.	Joe is nervous about his new job and yelled at his wife. On his way home he stops and buys her some flowers.

Defense Mechanisms	Example	Defense Mechanisms	Example
Projection Attributing feelings or impulses unacceptable to one's self to another person	Sue feels a strong sexual attraction to her track coach and tells her friend, "He's coming on to me!"		

APPENDIX B

*Levels of Anxiety**

Level	Perceptual Field	Ability to Learn	Physical Characteristics	Emotional/ Behavioral Characteristics
Mild	Heightened perception (e.g., noises may seem louder; details within the environment are clearer) Increased awareness Increased alertness	Learning is enhanced	Restlessness Irritability	May remain superficial with others. Rarely experienced as distressful. Motivation is increased.
Moderate	Reduction in perceptual field Reduced alertness to environmental events (e.g., someone talking may not be heard; part of the room may not be noticed)	Learning still occurs, but not at optimal ability Decreased attention span Decreased ability to concentrate	Increased restlessness Increased heart and respiration rate Increased perspiration Gastric discomfort Increased muscular tension Increase in speech rate, volume, and pitch	A feeling of discontent. May lead to some amount of impairment in interpersonal relationships as individual begins to focus on self and the need to relieve personal discomfort.

*From Townsend, 2003, p. 19, with permission.

Level	Perceptual Field	Ability to Learn	Physical Character istics	Emotional/ Behavioral Characteristics
Severe	Greatly diminished Only extraneous details are perceived, or fixation on a single detail may occur May not take notice of an event even when attention is directed by another	Extremely limited attention span Unable to concentrate or problem-solve Effective learning cannot occur	Headaches Dizziness Nausea Trembling Insomnia Palpitations Tachycardia Hyperventilation Urinary frequency Diarrhea	Feelings of dread, loathing, horror. Total focus on self and intense desire to relieve the anxiety.
Panic	Unable to focus on even one detail within the environment Misperceptions of the environment common (e.g., a perceived detail may be elaborated and out of proportion)	Learning cannot occur Unable to concentrate Unable to comprehend even simple directions	Dilated pupils Labored breathing Severe trembling Sleeplessness Palpitations Diaphoresis and pallor Muscular incoordination Immobility or purposeless hyperactivity Incoherence or inability to verbalize	Sense of impending doom. Terror. Bizarre behavior, including shouting, screaming, running about wildly, clinging to anyone or anything from which a sense of safety and security is derived. Hallucinations; delusions. Extreme withdrawal into self.

APPENDIX C

*Medication Assessment Tool**

Date ____________ Client's Name ______________________ Age ______

Marital Status ____________ Children ____________________ Occupation ____________

Presenting Symptoms (subjective/objective) ______________________________

Diagnosis (***DSM-IV-TR***) ______________________________

Current Vital Signs: Blood Pressure: Sitting _____/___; Standing ____/___; Pulse________ ; Respirations ______

CURRENT/PAST USE OF PRESCRIPTION DRUGS (Indicate C or P beside name of drug whether current or past use):

Name	Dosage	How Long Used	Why Prescribed	By Whom	Side Effects/Results

CURRENT/PAST USE OF OVER-THE-COUNTER DRUGS (Indicate C or P beside name of drug whether current or past use):

Name	Dosage	How Long Used	Why Prescribed	By Whom	Side Effects/Results
______	______	______	______	______	______
______	______	______	______	______	______
______	______	______	______	______	______

CURRENT/PAST USE OF STREET DRUGS, ALCOHOL, NICOTINE, AND/OR CAFFEINE:

Name	Amount Used	How Often Used	When Last Used	Effects Produced
______	______	______	______	______
______	______	______	______	______
______	______	______	______	______

Any allergies to food or drugs? ______________________________

Any special diet considerations? ______________________________

Do you have (or have you ever had) any of the following? If yes, provide explanation on the back of this sheet.

	Yes	No		Yes	No		Yes	No
1. Difficulty swallowing	____	____	7. Seizures	____	____	14. Fainting spells	____	____
2. Delayed wound healing	____	____	8. Headaches	____	____	15. Swollen ankles/legs/ hands	____	____
3. Constipation problems	____	____	9. Dizziness	____	____			
4. Urination problems	____	____	10. High blood pressure	____	____	16. Asthma	____	____
5. Recent change in elimination patterns	____	____	11. Palpitations	____	____	17. Varicose veins	____	____
			12. Chest pain			18. Numbness/tingling (location?)	____	____
6. Weakness or tremors	____	____	13. Blood clots/pain in legs	____	____			

	Yes	No		Yes	No		Yes	No
19. Ulcers	____	____	24. Lumps in your breasts	____	____	29. Diabetes	____	____
20. Nausea/vomiting	____	____	25. Blurred or double vision	____	____	30. Hepatitis (or other liver disease)	____	____
21. Problems with diarrhea	____	____	26. Ringing in the ears	____	____			
22. Shortness of breath	____	____	27. Insomnia	____	____	31. Kidney disease	____	____
23. Sexual dysfunction	____	____	28. Skin Rashes	____	____	32. Glaucoma	____	____

Are you pregnant or breast feeding?______________ Date of last menses__________ Type of contraception used__________

Describe any restrictions/limitations that might interfere with your use of medication for your current problem.____________

Prescription orders:

Patient teaching related to medications prescribed:

Lab work ordered:

____
Nurse's Signature

____
Client's Signature

*Adapted from Townsend, 2003, p. 292, with permission.

APPENDIX D

*Cultural Assessment Tool**

Client's name______________________________
Ethnic origin______________________________
Address______________________________
Birth date______________________________
Name of significant other____________________
Relationship______________________________
Primary language spoken____________________
Second language spoken____________________
How does client usually communicate with people who speak a different language?____________________
Is an interpreter required?____________ Available?______
Highest level of education achieved________________
Occupation______________________________
Presenting problem________________________
Has this problem ever occurred before?______________
If so, in what manner was it handled previously?________________________
What is client's usual manner of coping with stress?________________________
Who is(are) the client's main support system(s)?________________________
Describe the family living arrangements________________________
Who is the major decision maker in the family?________________________
Describe client's/family members' roles within the family________________________
____
Describe religious beliefs and practices________________________
Are there any religious requirements or restrictions that place limitations on the client's care ?____________________

*From Townsend, 2003, p. 95, with permission.

If so, describe________________________________
Who in the family takes responsibility for health concerns?________________________________
Describe any special health beliefs and practices________________________________
From whom does family usually seek medical assistance in time of need?________________________________
Describe client's usual emotional/behavioral response to:

- Anxiety________________________________
- Anger________________________________
- Loss/change/failure__________________________
- Pain________________________________
- Fear________________________________

Describe any topics that are particularly sensitive or that the client is unwilling to discuss (because of cultural taboos)________________
Describe any activities in which the client is unwilling to participate (because of cultural customs or taboos) ________________
What are the client's personal feelings regarding touch?________________________________
What are the client's personal feelings regarding eye contact?________________________________
What is the client's personal orientation to time? (past, present, future)________________________________
Describe any particular illnesses to which the client may be bioculturally susceptible (e.g., hypertension and sickle cell anemia in African Americans) ________________________
Describe any nutritional deficiencies to which the client may be bioculturally susceptible (e.g., lactose intolerance in Native and Asian Americans) ________________________
Describe client's favorite foods________________________________
Are there any foods the client requests or refuses because of cultural beliefs related to this illness? (e.g., "hot" and "cold" foods for Hispanic and Asian Americans). If so, please describe____________

____

Describe client's perception of the problem and expectations of health care________________________________

APPENDIX E

The DSM-IV-TR Multiaxial Evaluation System

The American Psychiatric Association endorses case evaluation on a multiaxial system in order "to facilitate comprehensive and systematic evaluation with attention to the various mental disorders and general medical conditions, psychosocial and environmental problems, and level of functioning that might be overlooked if the focus were on assessing a single presenting problem." Each individual is evaluated on five axes. They are defined by the *DSM-IV-TR* in the following manner:

Axis I—Clinical Disorders and Other Conditions That May Be a Focus of Clinical Attention

These include all mental disorders (except personality disorders and mental retardation).

Axis II—Personality Disorders and Mental Retardation

These disorders usually begin in childhood or adolescence and persist in a stable form into adult life.

Axis III—General Medical Conditions

These include any current general medical condition that is potentially relevant to the understanding or management of the individual's mental disorder.

Axis IV—Psychosocial and Environmental Problems

These are problems that may affect the diagnosis, treatment, and prognosis of mental disorders named on axes I and II. Examples include: problems with primary support group, problems related to the social environment, educational problems, occupational problems, housing problems, economic problems, problems with access to health-care services, and problems related to interaction with the legal system.

Axis V—Global Assessment of Functioning

This allows the clinician to rate the individual's overall functioning on the Global Assessment of Functioning (GAF) Scale. This scale represents in global terms a single measure of the individual's psychological, social, and occupational functioning. A copy of the GAF Scale appears in Appendix F.

APPENDIX F

Global Assessment of Functioning (GAF) Scale

Consider psychological, social, and occupational functioning on a hypothetical continuum of mental health-illness. Do not include impairment in functioning due to physical (or environmental) limitations.

Code (**Note:** Use intermediate codes when appropriate, e.g., 45, 68, 72)

100–91: Superior functioning in a wide range of activities, life's problems never seem to get out of hand, is sought out by others because of his or her many positive qualities. No symptoms.

90–81: Absent or minimal symptoms (e.g., mild anxiety before an exam), **good functioning in all areas, interested and involved in a wide range of activities, socially effective, generally satisfied with life, no more than everyday problems or concerns** (e.g., an occasional argument with family members).

80–71: If symptoms are present, they are transient and expectable reactions to psychosocial stressors (e.g., difficulty concentrating after family argument); **no more than slight impairment in social, occupational, or school functioning** (e.g., temporarily falling behind in schoolwork).

70–61: Some mild symptoms (e.g., depressed mood and mild insomnia) **OR some difficulty in social, occupational, or school functioning** (e.g., occasional truancy, or theft within the household), **but generally functioning pretty well, has some meaningful interpersonal relationships.**

60–51: Moderate symptoms (e.g., flat affect and circumstantial speech, occasional panic attacks) **OR moderate difficulty in social, occupational, or school functioning** (e.g., few friends, conflicts with peers or co-workers).

50–41: Serious symptoms (e.g., suicidal ideation, severe obsessional rituals, frequent shoplifting) **OR any serious impairment in**

social, occupational, or school functioning (e.g., no friends, unable to keep a job).

40–31: Some impairment in reality testing or communication (e.g., speech is at times illogical, obscure, or irrelevant) **OR major impairment in several areas, such as work or school, family relations, judgment, thinking, or mood** (e.g., depressed man avoids friends, neglects family, and is unable to work; child frequently beats up younger children, is defiant at home, and is failing at school).

30–21: Behavior is considerably influenced by delusions or hallucinations OR serious impairment in communication or judgment (e.g., sometimes incoherent, acts grossly inappropriately, suicidal preoccupation) **OR inability to function in almost all areas** (e.g., stays in bed all day; no job, home, or friends).

20–11: Some degree of hurting self or others (e.g., suicide attempts without clear expectation of death; frequently violent; manic excitement) **OR occasionally fails to maintain minimal personal hygiene** (e.g., smears feces) **OR gross impairment in communication** (e.g., largely incoherent or mute).

10–1: Persistent danger of severely hurting self or others (e.g., recurrent violence) **OR persistent inability to maintain minimal personal hygiene OR serious suicidal act with clear expectation of death.**

0: Inadequate information.

SOURCE: From the *Diagnostic and Statistical Manual of Mental Disorders, 4th Edition, Text Revision, 2000.* Used with permission from the American Psychiatric Association.

APPENDIX G

DSM-IV-TR Classification: Axes I and II Categories and Codes

Disorders Usually First Diagnosed in Infancy, Childhood, or Adolescence

Mental Retardation

Note: These are coded on Axis II.

317 Mild Mental Retardation
318.0 Moderate Mental Retardation
318.1 Severe Mental Retardation
318.2 Profound Mental Retardation
319 Mental Retardation, Severity Unspecified

Learning Disorders

315.00 Reading Disorder
315.1 Mathematics Disorder
315.2 Disorder of Written Expression
315.9 Learning Disorder Not Otherwise Specified (NOS)

Motor Skills Disorder

315.4 Developmental Coordination Disorder

Communication Disorders

315.31 Expressive Language Disorder
315.32 Mixed Receptive-Expressive Language Disorder
315.39 Phonological Disorder
307.0 Stuttering
307.9 Communication Disorder NOS

Pervasive Developmental Disorders

299.00 Autistic Disorder
299.80 Rett's Disorder
299.10 Childhood Disintegrative Disorder
299.80 Asperger's Disorder
299.80 Pervasive Developmental Disorder NOS

Attention-Deficit and Disruptive Behavior Disorders

314.xx Attention-Deficit/Hyperactivity Disorder
.01 Combined Type
.00 Predominantly Inattentive Type
.01 Predominantly Hyperactive-Impulsive Type
314.9 Attention-Deficit/Hyperactivity Disorder NOS
312.xx Conduct Disorder
.81 Childhood-Onset Type
.82 Adolescent-Onset Type
.89 Unspecified Onset
313.81 Oppositional Defiant Disorder
312.9 Disruptive Behavior Disorder NOS

Feeding and Eating Disorders of Infancy or Early Childhood

307.52 Pica
307.53 Rumination Disorder
307.59 Feeding Disorder of Infancy or Early Childhood

Tic Disorders

307.23 Tourette's Disorder
307.22 Chronic Motor or Vocal Tic Disorder
307.21 Transient Tic Disorder
307.20 Tic Disorder NOS

Elimination Disorders

_____ Encopresis
787.6 With Constipation and Overflow Incontinence
307.7 Without Constipation and Overflow Incontinence
307.6 Enuresis (Not Due to a General Medical Condition)

Other Disorders of Infancy, Childhood, or Adolescence

309.21 Separation Anxiety Disorder
313.23 Selective Mutism
313.89 Reactive Attachment Disorder of Infancy or Early Childhood
307.3 Stereotypic Movement Disorder
313.9 Disorder of Infancy, Childhood, or Adolescence NOS

Delirium, Dementia, and Amnestic and Other Cognitive Disorders

Delirium

293.0 Delirium Due to *(indicate the General Medical Condition)*
_____ Substance Intoxication Delirium *(refer to Substance-Related Disorders for substance-specific codes)*

_____ Substance Withdrawal Delirium *(refer to Substance-Related Disorders for substance-specific codes)*
_____ Delirium Due to Multiple Etiologies *(code each of the specific etiologies)*
780.09 Delirium NOS

Dementia

294.xx Dementia of the Alzheimer's Type, With Early Onset
.10 Without Behavioral Disturbance
.11 With Behavioral Disturbance
294.xx Dementia of the Alzheimer's Type, With Late Onset
.10 Without Behavioral Disturbance
.11 With Behavioral Disturbance
290.xx Vascular Dementia
.40 Uncomplicated
.41 With Delirium
.42 With Delusions
.43 With Depressed Mood
294.1x Dementia Due to HIV Disease
294.1x Dementia Due to Head Trauma
294.1x Dementia Due to Parkinson's Disease
294.1x Dementia Due to Huntington's Disease
294.1x Dementia Due to Pick's Disease
294.1x Dementia Due to Creutzfeldt-Jakob Disease
294.1x Dementia Due to *(indicate the General Medical Condition not listed above)*
_____ Substance-Induced Persisting Dementia *(refer to Substance-Related Disorders for substance-specific codes)*
_____ Dementia Due to Multiple Etiologies *(code each of the specific etiologies)*
294.8 Dementia NOS

Amnestic Disorders

294.0 Amnestic Disorder Due to *(indicate the General Medical Condition)*
_____ Substance-Induced Persisting Amnestic Disorder *(refer to Substance-Related Disorders for substance-specific codes)*
294.8 Amnestic Disorder NOS

Other Cognitive Disorders

294.9 Cognitive Disorder NOS

Mental Disorders Due to a General Medical Condition Not Elsewhere Classified

293.89 Catatonic Disorder Due to *(indicate the General Medical Condition)*

310.1 Personality Change Due to *(indicate the General Medical Condition)*
293.9 Mental Disorder NOS Due to *(indicate the General Medical Condition)*

Substance-Related Disorders

Alcohol-Related Disorders

Alcohol Use Disorders

303.90 Alcohol Dependence
305.00 Alcohol Abuse

Alcohol-Induced Disorders

303.00 Alcohol Intoxication
291.81 Alcohol Withdrawal
291.0 Alcohol Intoxication Delirium
291.0 Alcohol Withdrawal Delirium
291.2 Alcohol-Induced Persisting Dementia
291.1 Alcohol-Induced Persisting Amnestic Disorder
291.x Alcohol-Induced Psychotic Disorder
.5 With Delusions
.3 With Hallucinations
291.89 Alcohol-Induced Mood Disorder
291.89 Alcohol-Induced Anxiety Disorder
291.89 Alcohol-Induced Sexual Dysfunction
291.89 Alcohol-Induced Sleep Disorder
291.9 Alcohol-Related Disorder NOS

Amphetamine (or Amphetamine-Like)-Related Disorders

Amphetamine Use Disorders

304.40 Amphetamine Dependence
305.70 Amphetamine Abuse

Amphetamine-Induced Disorders

292.89 Amphetamine Intoxication
292.0 Amphetamine Withdrawal
292.81 Amphetamine Intoxication Delirium
292.xx Amphetamine-Induced Psychotic Disorder
.11 With Delusions
.12 With Hallucinations
292.84 Amphetamine-Induced Mood Disorder
292.89 Amphetamine-Induced Anxiety Disorder
292.89 Amphetamine-Induced Sexual Dysfunction
292.89 Amphetamine-Induced Sleep Disorder
292.9 Amphetamine-Related Disorder NOS

Caffeine-Related Disorders

Caffeine-Induced Disorders

305.90 Caffeine Intoxication
292.89 Caffeine-Induced Anxiety Disorder
292.89 Caffeine-Induced Sleep Disorder
292.9 Caffeine-Related Disorder NOS

Cannabis-Related Disorders

Cannabis Use Disorders

304.30 Cannabis Dependence
305.20 Cannabis Abuse

Cannabis-Induced Disorders

292.89 Cannabis Intoxication
292.81 Cannabis Intoxication Delirium
292.xx Cannabis-Induced Psychotic Disorder
.11 With Delusions
.12 With Hallucinations
292.89 Cannabis-Induced Anxiety Disorder
292.9 Cannabis-Related Disorder NOS

Cocaine-Related Disorders

Cocaine Use Disorders

304.20 Cocaine Dependence
305.60 Cocaine Abuse

Cocaine-Induced Disorders

292.89 Cocaine Intoxication
292.0 Cocaine Withdrawal
292.81 Cocaine Intoxication Delirium
292.xx Cocaine-Induced Psychotic Disorder
.11 With Delusions
.12 With Hallucinations
292.84 Cocaine-Induced Mood Disorder
292.89 Cocaine-Induced Anxiety Disorder
292.89 Cocaine-Induced Sexual Dysfunction
292.89 Cocaine-Induced Sleep Disorder
292.9 Cocaine-Related Disorder NOS

Hallucinogen-Related Disorders

Hallucinogen Use Disorders

304.50 Hallucinogen Dependence
305.30 Hallucinogen Abuse

Hallucinogen-Induced Disorders

292.89 Hallucinogen Intoxication
292.89 Hallucinogen Persisting Perception Disorder (Flashbacks)
292.81 Hallucinogen Intoxication Delirium
292.xx Hallucinogen-Induced Psychotic Disorder
.11 With Delusions
.12 With Hallucinations
292.84 Hallucinogen-Induced Mood Disorder
292.89 Hallucinogen-Induced Anxiety Disorder
292.9 Hallucinogen-Related Disorder NOS

Inhalant-Related Disorders

Inhalant Use Disorders

304.60 Inhalant Dependence
305.90 Inhalant Abuse

Inhalant-Induced Disorders
292.89 Inhalant Intoxication
292.81 Inhalant Intoxication Delirium
292.82 Inhalant-Induced Persisting Dementia
292.xx Inhalant-Induced Psychotic Disorder
.11 With Delusions
.12 With Hallucinations
292.84 Inhalant-Induced Mood Disorder
292.89 Inhalant-Induced Anxiety Disorder
292.9 Inhalant-Related Disorder NOS

Nicotine-Related Disorders
Nicotine Use Disorders
305.1 Nicotine Dependence
Nicotine-Induced Disorders
292.0 Nicotine Withdrawal
292.9 Nicotine-Related Disorder NOS

Opioid-Related Disorders
Opioid Use Disorders
304.00 Opioid Dependence
305.50 Opioid Abuse
Opioid-Induced Disorders
292.89 Opioid Intoxication
292.0 Opioid Withdrawal
292.81 Opioid Intoxication Delirium
292.xx Opioid-Induced Psychotic Disorder
.11 With Delusions
.12 With Hallucinations
292.84 Opioid-Induced Mood Disorder
292.89 Opioid-Induced Sexual Dysfunction
292.89 Opioid-Induced Sleep Disorder
292.9 Opioid-Related Disorder NOS

Phencyclidine (or Phencyclidine-Like)–Related Disorders
Phencyclidine Use Disorders
304.60 Phencyclidine Dependence
305.90 Phencyclidine Abuse
Phencyclidine-Induced Disorders
292.89 Phencyclidine Intoxication
292.81 Phencyclidine Intoxication Delirium
292.xx Phencyclidine-Induced Psychotic Disorder
.11 With Delusions
.12 With Hallucinations
292.84 Phencyclidine-Induced Mood Disorder
292.89 Phencyclidine-Induced Anxiety Disorder
292.9 Phencyclidine-Related Disorder NOS

Sedative-, Hypnotic-, or Anxiolytic-Related Disorders
Sedative, Hypnotic, or Anxiolytic Use Disorders
304.10 Sedative, Hypnotic, or Anxiolytic Dependence

305.40 Sedative, Hypnotic, or Anxiolytic Abuse

Sedative-, Hypnotic-, or Anxiolytic-Induced Disorders

292.89 Sedative, Hypnotic, or Anxiolytic Intoxication
292.0 Sedative, Hypnotic, or Anxiolytic Withdrawal
292.81 Sedative, Hypnotic, or Anxiolytic Intoxication Delirium
292.81 Sedative, Hypnotic, or Anxiolytic Withdrawal Delirium
292.82 Sedative-, Hypnotic-, or Anxiolytic-Induced Persisting Dementia
292.83 Sedative-, Hypnotic-, or Anxiolytic-Induced Persisting Amnestic Disorder
292.xx Sedative-, Hypnotic-, or Anxiolytic-Induced Psychotic Disorder
.11 With Delusions
.12 With Hallucinations
292.84 Sedative-, Hypnotic-, or Anxiolytic-Induced Mood Disorder
292.89 Sedative-, Hypnotic-, or Anxiolytic-Induced Anxiety Disorder
292.89 Sedative-, Hypnotic-, or Anxiolytic-Induced Sexual Dysfunction
292.89 Sedative-, Hypnotic-, or Anxiolytic-Induced Sleep Disorder
292.9 Sedative-, Hypnotic-, or Anxiolytic-Related Disorder NOS

Polysubstance-Related Disorder

304.80 Polysubstance Dependence

Other (or Unknown) Substance-Related Disorders

Other (or Unknown) Substance Use Disorders

304.90 Other (or Unknown) Substance Dependence
305.90 Other (or Unknown) Substance Abuse

Other (or Unknown) Substance-Induced Disorders

292.89 Other (or Unknown) Substance Intoxication
292.0 Other (or Unknown) Substance Withdrawal
292.81 Other (or Unknown) Substance-Induced Delirium
292.82 Other (or Unknown) Substance-Induced Persisting Dementia
292.83 Other (or Unknown) Substance-Induced Persisting Amnestic Disorder
292.xx Other (or Unknown) Substance-Induced Psychotic Disorder
.11 With Delusions
.12 With Hallucinations
292.84 Other (or Unknown) Substance-Induced Mood Disorder

292.89 Other (or Unknown) Substance-Induced Anxiety Disorder
292.89 Other (or Unknown) Substance-Induced Sexual Dysfunction
292.89 Other (or Unknown) Substance-Induced Sleep Disorder
292.9 Other (or Unknown) Substance-Related Disorder NOS

Schizophrenia and Other Psychotic Disorders

295.xx Schizophrenia
.30 Paranoid type
.10 Disorganized type
.20 Catatonic type
.90 Undifferentiated type
.60 Residual type
295.40 Schizophreniform Disorder
295.70 Schizoaffective Disorder
297.1 Delusional Disorder
298.8 Brief Psychotic Disorder
297.3 Shared Psychotic Disorder
293.xx Psychotic Disorder Due to *(indicate the General Medical Condition)*
.81 With Delusions
.82 With Hallucinations
_____ Substance-Induced Psychotic Disorder *(refer to Substance-Related Disorders for substance-specific codes)*
298.9 Psychotic Disorder NOS

Mood Disorders

(Code current state of Major Depressive Disorder or Bipolar I Disorder in fifth digit: 0 = unspecified; 1 = mild; 2 = moderate; 3 = severe, without psychotic features; 4 = severe, with psychotic features; 5 = in partial remission; 6 = in full remission.)

Depressive Disorders

296.xx Major Depressive Disorder
.2x Single episode
.3x Recurrent
300.4 Dysthymic Disorder
311 Depressive Disorder NOS

Bipolar Disorders

296.xx Bipolar I Disorder
.0x Single Manic Episode
.40 Most Recent Episode Hypomanic
.4x Most Recent Episode Manic
.6x Most Recent Episode Mixed
.5x Most Recent Episode Depressed
.7 Most Recent Episode Unspecified

296.89 Bipolar II Disorder *(specify current or most recent episode: Hypomanic or Depressed)*
301.13 Cyclothymic Disorder
296.80 Bipolar Disorder NOS
293.83 Mood Disorder Due to *(indicate the General Medical Condition)*
_____ Substance-Induced Mood Disorder *(refer to Substance-Related Disorders for substance-specific codes)*
296.90 Mood Disorder NOS

Anxiety Disorders

300.01 Panic Disorder Without Agoraphobia
300.21 Panic Disorder With Agoraphobia
300.22 Agoraphobia Without History of Panic Disorder
300.29 Specific Phobia
300.23 Social Phobia
300.3 Obsessive-Compulsive Disorder
309.81 Posttraumatic Stress Disorder
308.3 Acute Stress Disorder
300.02 Generalized Anxiety Disorder
293.89 Anxiety Disorder Due to *(indicate the General Medical Condition)*
_____ Substance-Induced Anxiety Disorder *(refer to Substance-Related Disorders for substance-specific codes)*
300.00 Anxiety Disorder NOS

Somatoform Disorders

300.81 Somatization Disorder
300.82 Undifferentiated Somatoform Disorder
300.11 Conversion Disorder
307.xx Pain Disorder
    .80 Associated with Psychological Factors
    .89 Associated with Both Psychological Factors and a General Medical Condition
300.7 Hypochondriasis
300.7 Body Dysmorphic Disorder
300.82 Somatoform Disorder NOS

Factitious Disorders

300.xx Factitious Disorder
    .16 With Predominantly Psychological Signs and Symptoms
    .19 With Predominantly Physical Signs and Symptoms
    .19 With Combined Psychological and Physical Signs and Symptoms
300.19 Factitious Disorder NOS

Dissociative Disorders

300.12 Dissociative Amnesia
300.13 Dissociative Fugue
300.14 Dissociative Identity Disorder
300.6 Depersonalization Disorder
300.15 Dissociative Disorder NOS

Sexual and Gender Identity Disorders

Sexual Dysfunctions

Sexual Desire Disorders

302.71 Hypoactive Sexual Desire Disorder
302.79 Sexual Aversion Disorder

Sexual Arousal Disorders

302.72 Female Sexual Arousal Disorder
302.72 Male Erectile Disorder

Orgasmic Disorders

302.73 Female Orgasmic Disorder
302.74 Male Orgasmic Disorder
302.75 Premature Ejaculation

Sexual Pain Disorders

302.76 Dyspareunia (Not Due to a General Medical Condition)
306.51 Vaginismus (Not Due to a General Medical Condition)

Sexual Dysfunction Due to a General Medical Condition

625.8 Female Hypoactive Sexual Desire Disorder Due to *(indicate the General Medical Condition)*
608.89 Male Hypoactive Sexual Desire Disorder Due to *(indicate the General Medical Condition)*
607.84 Male Erectile Disorder Due to *(indicate the General Medical Condition)*
625.0 Female Dyspareunia Due to *(indicate the General Medical Condition)*
608.89 Male Dyspareunia Due to *(indicate the General Medical Condition)*
625.8 Other Female Sexual Dysfunction Due to *(indicate the General Medical Condition)*
608.89 Other Male Sexual Dysfunction Due to *(Indicate the General Medical Condition)*
_____ Substance-Induced Sexual Dysfunction *(refer to Substance-Related Disorders for substance-specific codes)*
302.70 Sexual Dysfunction NOS

Paraphilias

302.4 Exhibitionism
302.81 Fetishism
302.89 Frotteurism
302.2 Pedophilia

302.83 Sexual Masochism
302.84 Sexual Sadism
302.3 Transvestic Fetishism
302.82 Voyeurism
302.9 Paraphilia NOS

Gender Identity Disorders

302.xx Gender Identity Disorder
.6 In Children
.85 In Adolescents or Adults
302.6 Gender Identity Disorder NOS
302.9 Sexual Disorder NOS

Eating Disorders

307.1 Anorexia Nervosa
307.51 Bulimia Nervosa
307.50 Eating Disorder NOS

Sleep Disorders

Primary Sleep Disorders

Dyssomnias

307.42 Primary Insomnia
307.44 Primary Hypersomnia
347 Narcolepsy
780.59 Breathing-Related Sleep Disorder
307.45 Circadian Rhythm Sleep Disorder
307.47 Dyssomnia NOS

Parasomnias

307.47 Nightmare Disorder
307.46 Sleep Terror Disorder
307.46 Sleepwalking Disorder
307.47 Parasomnia NOS

Sleep Disorders Related to Another Mental Disorder

307.42 Insomnia Related to *(indicate the Axis I or Axis II Disorder)*
307.44 Hypersomnia Related to (*indicate the Axis I or Axis II Disorder)*

Other Sleep Disorders

780.xx Sleep Disorder Due to *(indicate the General Medical Condition)*
.52 Insomnia type
.54 Hypersomnia type
.59 Parasomnia type
.59 Mixed type
_____ Substance-Induced Sleep Disorder *(refer to Substance-Related Disorders for substance-specific codes)*

Impulse Control Disorders not Elsewhere Classified

312.34 Intermittent Explosive Disorder
312.32 Kleptomania

312.33 Pyromania
312.31 Pathological Gambling
312.39 Trichotillomania
312.30 Impulse Control Disorder NOS

Adjustment Disorders

309.xx Adjustment Disorder
.0 With Depressed Mood
.24 With Anxiety
.28 With Mixed Anxiety and Depressed Mood
.3 With Disturbance of Conduct
.4 With Mixed Disturbance of Emotions and Conduct
.9 Unspecified

Personality Disorders

Note: These are coded on Axis II.

301.0 Paranoid Personality Disorder
301.20 Schizoid Personality Disorder
301.22 Schizotypal Personality Disorder
301.7 Antisocial Personality Disorder
301.83 Borderline Personality Disorder
301.50 Histrionic Personality Disorder
301.81 Narcissistic Personality Disorder
301.82 Avoidant Personality Disorder
301.6 Dependent Personality Disorder
301.4 Obsessive-Compulsive Personality Disorder
301.9 Personality Disorder NOS

Other Conditions that may be a Focus of Clinical Attention

Psychological Factors Affecting Medical Condition

316 *Choose name based on nature of factors:*
Mental Disorder Affecting Medical Condition
Psychological Symptoms Affecting Medical Condition
Personality Traits or Coping Style Affecting Medical Condition
Maladaptive Health Behaviors Affecting Medical Condition
Stress-Related Physiological Response Affecting Medical Condition
Other or Unspecified Psychological Factors Affecting Medical Condition

Medication-Induced Movement Disorders

332.1 Neuroleptic-Induced Parkinsonism
333.92 Neuroleptic Malignant Syndrome
333.7 Neuroleptic-Induced Acute Dystonia
333.99 Neuroleptic-Induced Acute Akathisia
333.82 Neuroleptic-Induced Tardive Dyskinesia
333.1 Medication-Induced Postural Tremor
333.90 Medication-Induced Movement Disorder NOS

Other Medication-Induced Disorder

995.2 Adverse Effects of Medication NOS

Relational Problems

V61.9 Relational Problem Related to a Mental Disorder or General Medical Condition
V61.20 Parent-Child Relational Problem
V61.10 Partner Relational Problem
V61.8 Sibling Relational Problem
V62.81 Relational Problem NOS

Problems Related to Abuse or Neglect

V61.21 Physical Abuse of Child
V61.21 Sexual Abuse of Child
V61.21 Neglect of Child
_____ Physical Abuse of Adult
V61.12 (if by partner)
V62.83 (if by person other than partner)
_____ Sexual Abuse of Adult
V61.12 (if by partner)
V62.83 (if by person other than partner)

Additional Conditions that may be a Focus of Clinical Attention

V15.81 Noncompliance with Treatment
V65.2 Malingering
V71.01 Adult Antisocial Behavior
V71.02 Childhood or Adolescent Antisocial Behavior
V62.89 Borderline Intellectual Functioning (coded on Axis II)
780.9 Age-Related Cognitive Decline
V62.82 Bereavement
V62.3 Academic Problem
V62.2 Occupational Problem
313.82 Identity Problem
V62.89 Religious or Spiritual Problem
V62.4 Acculturation Problem
V62.89 Phase of Life Problem

Additional Codes

300.9 Unspecified Mental Disorder (nonpsychotic)
V71.09 No Diagnosis or Condition on Axis I
799.9 Diagnosis or Condition Deferred on Axis I
V71.09 No Diagnosis on Axis II
799.9 Diagnosis Deferred on Axis II

SOURCE: From the *Diagnostic and Statistical Manual of Mental Disorders, 4th Edition, Text Revision, 2000.* Used with permission from the American Psychiatric Association.

APPENDIX H

*Mental Status Assessment**

Gathering the correct information about the client's mental status is essential to the development of an appropriate plan of care. The mental status examination is a description of all the areas of the client's mental functioning. The following are the components that are considered critical in the assessment of a client's mental status.

Identifying Data

1. Name
2. Gender
3. Age
4. Race/culture
5. Occupational/financial status
6. Educational level
7. Significant other
8. Living arrangements
9. Religious preference
10. Allergies
11. Special diet considerations
12. Chief complaint
13. Medical diagnosis

General Description

Appearance

1. Grooming and dress
2. Hygiene
3. Posture
4. Height and weight
5. Level of eye contact
6. Hair color and texture
7. Evidence of scars, tattoos, or other distinguishing skin marks
8. Evaluation of client's appearance compared with chronological age

*From Townsend, 2003, pp. 874–875, with permission.

Motor Activity

1. Tremors
2. Tics or other stereotypical movements
3. Mannerisms and gestures
4. Hyperactivity
5. Restlessness or agitation
6. Aggressiveness
7. Rigidity
8. Gait patterns
9. Echopraxia
10. Psychomotor retardation
11. Freedom of movement (range of motion)

Speech Patterns

1. Slowness or rapidity of speech
2. Pressure of speech
3. Intonation
4. Volume
5. Stuttering or other speech impairments
6. Aphasia

General Attitude

1. Cooperative/uncooperative
2. Friendly/hostile/defensive
3. Uninterested/apathetic
4. Attentive/interested
5. Guarded/suspicious

Emotions

Mood

1. Sad
2. Depressed
3. Despairing
4. Irritable
5. Anxious
6. Elated
7. Euphoric
8. Fearful
9. Guilty
10. Labile

Affect

1. Congruence with mood
2. Constricted or blunted (diminished amount/range and intensity of emotional expression)
3. Flat (absence of emotional expression)
4. Appropriate or inappropriate (defines congruence of affect with the situation or with the client's behavior)

Thought Processes

Form of Thought

1. Flight of ideas

2. Associative looseness
3. Circumstantiality
4. Tangentiality
5. Neologisms
6. Concrete thinking
7. Clang associations
8. Word salad
9. Perseveration
10. Echolalia
11. Mutism
12. Poverty of speech (restriction in the amount of speech)
13. Ability to concentrate
14. Attention span

Content of Thought

1. Delusions
   a. Persecutory
   b. Grandiose
   c. Reference
   d. Control or influence
   e. Somatic
   f. Nihilistic
2. Suicidal or homicidal ideas
3. Obsessions
4. Paranoia/suspiciousness
5. Magical thinking
6. Religiosity
7. Phobias
8. Poverty of content (vague, meaningless responses)

Perceptual Disturbances

1. Hallucinations
   a. Auditory
   b. Visual
   c. Tactile
   d. Olfactory
   e. Gustatory
2. Illusions
3. Depersonalization (altered perception of the self)
4. Derealization (altered perception of the environment)

Sensorium and Cognitive Ability

1. Level of alertness/consciousness
2. Orientation
   a. Time
   b. Place
   c. Person
   d. Circumstances

3. Memory
   a. Recent
   b. Remote
   c. Use of confabulation
4. Capacity for abstract thought

Impulse Control

1. Ability to control impulses related to the following:
   a. Aggression
   b. Hostility
   c. Fear
   d. Guilt
   e. Affection
   f. Sexual feelings

Judgment and Insight

1. Ability to solve problems
2. Ability to make decisions
3. Knowledge about self
   a. Awareness of limitations
   b. Awareness of consequences of actions
   c. Awareness of illness
4. Adaptive/maladaptive use of coping strategies and ego defense mechanisms

APPENDIX I

*Assigning Nursing Diagnoses to Client Behaviors**

Following is a list of client behaviors and the NANDA nursing diagnoses that correspond to the behaviors and that may be used in planning care for the client exhibiting the specific behavioral symptoms.

Behaviors	**NANDA Nursing Diagnoses**
Aggression; hostility	Risk for injury; Risk for other-directed violence
Anorexia or refusal to eat	Imbalanced nutrition: Less than body requirements
Anxious behavior	Anxiety (Specify level)
Confusion; memory loss	Confusion, acute/chronic; Disturbed thought processes
Delusions	Disturbed thought processes
Denial of problems	Ineffective denial
Depressed mood or anger turned inward	Dysfunctional grieving
Detoxification; withdrawal from substances	Risk for injury
Difficulty making important life decision	Decisional conflict (specify)
Difficulty with interpersonal relationships	Impaired social interaction
Disruption in capability to perform usual responsibilities	Ineffective role performance
Dissociative behaviors (depersonalization; derealization)	Disturbed sensory perception (kinesthetic)

*From Townsend, 2003, pp. 886–887, with permission.

Behaviors	NANDA Nursing Diagnoses
Expresses feelings of disgust about body or body part	Disturbed body image
Expresses lack of control over personal situation	Powerlessness
Flashbacks, nightmares, obsession with traumatic experience	Post-trauma syndrome
Hallucinations	Disturbed sensory perception (auditory; visual)
Highly critical of self or others	Low self-esteem (chronic; situational)
HIV-positive; altered immunity	Ineffective protection
Inability to meet basic needs	Self-care deficit (feeding; bathing/hygiene; dressing/grooming; toileting)
Insomnia or hypersomnia	Disturbed sleep pattern
Loose associations or flight of ideas	Impaired verbal communication
Manic hyperactivity	Risk for injury
Manipulative behavior	Ineffective coping
Multiple personalities; gender identity disturbance	Disturbed personal identity
Orgasm, problems with; lack of sexual desire	Sexual dysfunction
Overeating, compulsive	Risk for imbalanced nutrition: More than body requirements
Phobias	Fear
Physical symptoms as coping behavior	Ineffective coping
Projection of blame; rationalization of failures; denial of personal responsibility	Defensive coping
Ritualistic behaviors	Anxiety (severe); ineffective coping
Seductive remarks; inappropriate sexual behaviors	Impaired social interaction
Self-mutilative behaviors	Self-mutilation; Risk for self-mutilation
Sexual behaviors (difficulty, limitations, or changes in; reported dissatisfaction)	Ineffective sexuality patterns

Behaviors	NANDA Nursing Diagnoses
Stress from caring for chronically ill person	Caregiver role strain
Stress from locating to new environment	Relocation stress syndrome
Substance use as a coping behavior	Ineffective coping
Substance use (denies use is a problem)	Ineffective denial
Suicidal	Risk for suicide; Risk for self-directed violence
Suspiciousness	Disturbed thought processes; ineffective coping
Vomiting, excessive, self-induced	Risk for deficient fluid volume
Withdrawn behavior	Social isolation

Index

Page numbers followed by "f" indicate figures; those followed by "t" indicate tabular material.

Drug Index

Page numbers followed by "t" indicate tabular material. Trade names appear in bold.

Index of Nursing Diagnoses